OTHER TITLES (

CODING AND REIN

Codelink® CPT & ICD-9-CM Code Linkage Series
Collections Made Easy!
CPT & HCPCS Coding Made Easy!
E/M Coding Made Easy!
4-in-1 Master Coder Series
HCPCS Coders Choice®, Color Coded, Thumb Indexed
Health Insurance Carrier Directory
ICD-9-CM, Coders Choice®, Thumb Indexed
ICD-9-CM, TimeSaver®, Ring Binder, Tab Indexed
ICD-9-CM Coding For Physicians' Offices
ICD-9-CM Coding Made Easy!
Medicare Rules and Regulations
Physicians Fees
Reimbursement Manual for the Medical Office
Working with Insurance and Managed Care Plans

PRACTICE MANAGEMENT

365 Ways to Manage the Business Private Practice
Capitation: Tools, Trends, Traps & Techniques
Computerizing Your Medical Office
Designing and Building Your Professional Office
Doctor Business
Encyclopedia of Practice and Financial Management
Getting Paid for What You Do
Health Information Management
The Managed Care Handbook
Managing Medical Office Personnel
Marketing Strategies for Physicians
McGraw-Hill Pocket Guide to Managed Care
Medical Marketing Handbook
Medical Office Policy Manual
Medical Practice Forms
Medical Practice Handbook
Medical Staff Privileges
Negotiating Managed Care Contracts
Patient Satisfaction
Patients Build Your Practice
Physician's Office Laboratory
Professional and Practice Development
Promoting Your Medical Practice
Surviving a Competitive Health Care Market

**AVAILABLE FROM YOUR LOCAL MEDICAL
BOOK STORE OR CALL 1-800-MED-SHOP**

OTHER TITLES OF INTEREST

FINANCIAL MANAGEMENT

Accounts Receivable Management for the Medical Practice
Achieving Profitability with a Medical Office System
Business Ventures for Physicians
Financial Planning Workbook for Physicians
Financial Valuation of Your Practice
Pension Plan Strategies
Physician Financial Planning in a Changing Environment
Securing Your Assets
Selling or Buying a Medical Practice

RISK MANAGEMENT

Behavioral Types and the Art of Patient Management
Belli: For Your Malpractice Defense
Law, Liability and Ethics for Medical Office Personnel
Malpractice Depositions
Medical Malpractice: A Physician's Guide
Testifying in Court

DICTIONARIES AND OTHER REFERENCE

Health & Medicine on the Internet
Isler's Patient Guide to Medical Terminology
Medical Acronyms, Eponyms and Abbreviations
Medical Phrase Index
Medical Word Building
Medico Mnemonica
Medico-Legal Glossary
Spanish/English Handbook for Medical Professionals

MEDICAL REFERENCE AND CLINICAL

Drugs of Abuse
Gastroenterology: Problems in Primary Care
Hematology: Diagnosis and Treatment of Blood Disorders
Medical Procedures for Referral
Neurology: Problems in Primary Care
Orthopaedics: Problems in Primary Care
Patient Care Emergency Handbook
Patient Care Flowchart Manual
Patient Care Procedures for Your Practice
Pulmonary Medicine: Problems in Primary Care
Urology: Problems in Primary Care

**AVAILABLE FROM YOUR LOCAL MEDICAL
BOOK STORE OR CALL 1-800-MED-SHOP**

H·C·P·C·S

MILLENNIUM EDITION

Health Care
Procedure Coding System

National Level II
Medicare Codes

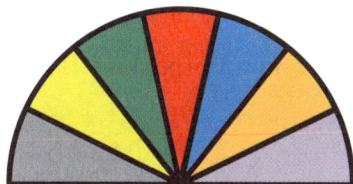

Color Coded

2002

PMIC

ISBN 1-57066-230-4 (Coder's Choice)
ISBN 1-57066-231-2 (Timesaver Binder)
ISBN 1-57066-232-0 (Codes on Disk)

Practice Management Information Corporation (PMIC)
4727 Wilshire Boulevard, Suite 300
Los Angeles, California 90010
1-800-MED-SHOP

http://www.medicalbookstore.com

Printed in China

Additional copies of this book may be purchased from any medical book
store, from PMIC by mail to the above address, by visiting our web site
at http://www.medicalbookstore.com, or by calling 1-800-MED-SHOP.

FOREWORD

The Health Care Procedure Coding System (HCPCS), National Level II, is a listing of codes and descriptive terminology used for reporting the provision of supplies, materials, injections and certain services and procedures to Medicare. HCPCS 2002 is the most recent revision of the HCPCS National Level II codes. The changes that appear in this revision have been prepared by our editorial staff using the November 2001 HCPCS revisions released by the Center for Medicare and Medicaid Services (CMS), formerly known as the Health Care Financing Administration (HCFA), which is overseen by the Department of Health and Human Services (DHHS). HCPCS National Level II codes are now effective January 1st of each year.

Even though HCPCS National Level II codes have been in use since 1983, there is still some confusion among health care professionals regarding when and how to use these codes instead of the more familiar CPT codes. In addition, due to what is known as "carrier discretion," the use, interpretation, and reimbursement policies for HCPCS National Level II codes, which should be uniform nationwide, vary from carrier to carrier. Add to this a third coding system, known as HCPCS Local Level III, and the confusion becomes more understandable. Unfortunately, many health care professionals deal with the confusion by ignoring this coding system, to the serious detriment of their reimbursement.

One of our goals as a publisher is to educate our customers about the business of medicine. One of our most successful methods of accomplishing this goal is to create publications about new or unfamiliar concepts, such as HCPCS, that are similar in format and content to related publications, such as CPT. This provides our customers with an opportunity to learn and implement new concepts of vital importance to their medical practice using formats, conventions and terminology that they already use and understand.

James B. Davis, President

DISCLAIMER

This publication is designed to offer basic information regarding coding and billing of medical services, supplies and procedures using the HCPCS coding system. The information presented is based upon material obtained from the Center for Medicare and Medicaid Services (CMS), formerly known as HCFA, and the experience and interpretations of the editors and publisher. Though all of the information has been carefully researched and checked for accuracy and completeness, the publisher accepts no responsibility or liability with regard to errors, omissions, misuse or misinterpretation.

CONTENTS

INTRODUCTION

HCPCS is an acronym for Health Care Procedure Coding System. This coding system was developed in 1983 by the Health Care Financing Administration (HCFA) for the purpose of standardizing the coding systems used to process Medicare claims. In 2001, HCFA changed its name to the Center for Medicare and Medicaid Services (CMS) to reflect its increased emphasis on improving Medicare and Medicaid beneficiary services and information.

The HCPCS coding system is primarily used to bill Medicare for supplies, materials and injections. It is also used to bill for certain services and procedures which are not defined in CPT. HCPCS codes must be used when billing Medicare carriers, and in some states, Medicaid carriers. Some private insurance carriers also allow or mandate the use of HCPCS codes, mostly those that are processing Medicare claims.

STRUCTURE OF HCPCS

HCPCS is a systematic method for coding supplies, materials, injections and services performed by health care professionals. Each supply, material, injection or service is identified with a five digit alphanumeric code. With the HCPCS coding system, the supplies, materials and injections can be accurately identified and properly reimbursed. There are three levels of codes within the HCPCS coding system.

LEVEL I CPT CODES

The major portion of the HCPCS coding system, referred to as Level I, is CPT. Most of the procedures and services you perform, even for Medicare patients, are billed using CPT codes. However, one of the major deficiencies of CPT is that it has limited code selections to describe supplies, materials and injections.

LEVEL II NATIONAL CODES

HCPCS National Level II codes are alphanumeric codes which start with a letter followed by four numbers. The range of HCPCS National Level II codes is from A0000 through V0000. There are also HCPCS National Level II modifiers. HCPCS National Level II codes are uniform in description throughout the United States. However, due to what is known as "carrier discretion" the processing and reimbursement of HCPCS National Level II codes is not necessarily uniform.

There are over 2,400 HCPCS National Level II codes covering supplies, materials, injections and services. A fundamental understanding of when and how to use HCPCS National Level II or Local Level III codes can have a significant impact on your Medicare reimbursement. The majority of health care professionals use codes from the Medical and Surgical Supplies section and Drugs Administered by Other Than Oral Method, commonly referred to as "A" codes and "J" codes.

LEVEL III LOCAL CODES

HCPCS Local Level III codes are also alphanumeric codes which start with a letter followed by four numbers. The range of HCPCS Local Level III codes is from W0000 to Z0000. Local Level III codes are assigned and maintained by your local Medicare carrier and will vary from carrier to carrier. HCPCS Local Level III codes are often used to describe new services, supplies and materials, or to report procedures and services which have been deleted from CPT, but which the local Medicare carrier still recognizes and reimburses. HCPCS Local Level III codes may be obtained from your local Medicare carrier.

HCPCS CODE OVERLAP

As may be expected, there is some overlap among the three HCPCS code levels. On occasion you may have a coding situation where a specific code exists at all three levels for the same service or material. When faced with this situation, the general rule is that Local Level III codes have the highest priority, followed by National Level II codes, followed by CPT codes. You should consult your local Medicare carrier if you have any questions regarding HCPCS code overlap.

SECTIONS

The main body of HCPCS National Level II codes is divided into 22 sections. The supplies, materials, injections and services are presented in alphanumeric order within each section. The sections of HCPCS National Level II are:

TRANSPORTATION SERVICES	A0000-A0999
MEDICAL AND SURGICAL SUPPLIES	A4000-A4999
MISCELLANEOUS AND EXPERIMENTAL	A9000-A9999
ENTERAL AND PARENTERAL THERAPY	B4000-B9999
TEMPORARY HOSPITAL OUTPATIENT PPS	C0000-C9999
DENTAL PROCEDURES	D0000-D9999
DURABLE MEDICAL EQUIPMENT (DME)	E0000-E9999
PROCEDURES/SERVICES TEMPORARY	G0000-G9999

INSTRUCTIONS FOR USE OF HCPCS NATIONAL LEVEL II

A health care professional using the HCPCS National Level II codes selects the name of the material, supply, injection, service or procedure that most accurately identifies the service performed or supply delivered. Most often, HCPCS National Level II codes will be used instead of, or in addition to, CPT codes for visits, evaluation and management services, or other procedures performed at the same time or during the same visit. All services, procedures, supplies, materials and injections should be properly documented in the medical record.

The listing of a supply, material, injection or service and its code number in a specific section of HCPCS does not usually restrict its use to a specific profession or specialty group. However, there are some HCPCS National Level II codes that are by definition, profession or specialty specific.

FORMAT OF THE TERMINOLOGY

HCPCS National Level II terminology has been developed as stand-alone descriptions of supplies, materials, injections, services and procedures. However, some of the procedures in HCPCS National Level II are not printed in their entirety but refer back to a common portion of the procedure listed in a preceding entry. This is evident when an entry is followed by one or more indentations. For example:

L1610   Hip orthosis (HO), abduction control of hip joints; flexible, (Frejka cover only), prefabricated, includes fitting and adjustment

L1640   static, pelvic band or spreader bar, thigh cuffs, custom fabricated

Note that the common part of code L1610 (the part before the semicolon) should be considered part of code L1640. Therefore the full procedure description represented by code L1640 would read:

L1640   Hip orthosis (HO), abduction control of hip joints; static, pelvic band or spreader bar, thight cuffs, custom fabricated

GUIDELINES

Specific GUIDELINES are presented at the beginning of most of the sections. These GUIDELINES define items that are necessary to appropriately interpret and report the supplies, materials, injections, services and procedures listed in that section.

HCPCS MODIFIERS

A modifier provides the means by which the health care professional can indicate that a service or procedure that has been performed has been altered by some specific circumstance but not changed in its definition or code. HCPCS modifiers may be used to indicate the following:

- A service was supervised by an anesthesiologist

- A service was performed by a specific health care professional, for example, a clinical psychologist, clinical social worker, nurse practitioner, or physician assistant.

- A service was provided as part of a specific government program

- A service was provided to a specific side of the body

- Equipment was purchased or rented

- Single or multiple patients were seen during nursing home visits

It is important to note that HCPCS National Level II modifiers can be combined with CPT codes when reporting services to Medicare.

An example of the use of HCPCS National Level II modifiers is:

E1280-NR Heavy duty wheelchair; detachable arms (desk or full length) elevating leg rests - new when rented

A listing of modifiers pertinent to each section of HCPCS National Level II are located in the GUIDELINES of each section. A complete listing of HCPCS National Level II modifiers is found in APPENDIX A.

In addition to HCPCS National Level II modifiers, local Medicare carriers also created Local Level III modifiers. These modifiers usually begin with W, X, Y or Z and can be obtained from your local Medicare carrier.

UNLISTED PROCEDURE OR SERVICE

A service or procedure may be provided that is not listed in this edition of HCPCS National Level II. When reporting such a service, the appropriate "unlisted procedure" code may be used to indicate the service, identifying it by "special report" as defined below. HCPCS National Level II terminology is inconsistent in defining unlisted procedures. The procedure definition may include the term(s) "unlisted," "not otherwise classified," "unspecified," "unclassified," "other" and "miscellaneous." Prior to using these codes, try to determine if a Local Level III or CPT code is available. When an unlisted procedure code is used, the supply, material, injection, service or procedure must be described. Each of these unlisted procedure codes relates to a specific section of HCPCS National Level II and is presented in the GUIDELINES of that section.

SPECIAL REPORT

A supply, material, injection, service or procedure that is rarely provided, unusual, variable or new may require a special report for reimbursement purposes. Pertinent information should include an adequate definition or description of the nature, extent, and need for the supply, material, injection, service or procedure.

HCPCS CODE CHANGES

Each year numerous codes are added, changed or deleted. A summary of revisions to HCPCS 2002 is found in APPENDIX B. The following symbols, identical to those used in CPT, are used to indicate additions, changes and deletions in HCPCS National Level II.

ADDITIONS TO HCPCS

New HCPCS National Level II codes are identified with a small black circle placed to the left of the code number. An example of a new code in HCPCS 2002 is:

● **A4706**   Bicarbonate concentrate, solution, for hemodialysis, per gallon

CHANGES TO HCPCS

Changes in HCPCS National Level II code definitions are identified with a small black triangle placed to the left of the code number. An example of a changed code in HCPCS 2002 is:

▲ **E1820**   Replacement soft interface material, dynamic adjustable extension/flexion device

DELETIONS FROM HCPCS

Deleted HCPCS National Level II codes are enclosed within parenthesis, along with an italicized reference to replacement codes when available. An example of a code deleted from HCPCS 2002 is:

(L5310)   Code deleted 2002; use L5311

SPECIAL COVERAGE SYMBOLS

NOT VALID FOR MEDICARE

There are codes listed in HCPCS which are not valid for Medicare. These codes are identified by a red bar over the HCPCS code. These codes should not be used to report services to Medicare.

NON-COVERED BY MEDICARE

There are numerous supplies, materials, injections, services and procedures which are not covered by Medicare, either by program definition or by legislative statute. Examples of non-covered services include routine services and appliances, foot care and supportive devices for feet, custodial care, personal comfort items, and cosmetic surgery. These codes are identified by an orange bar over the HCPCS code. These codes should not be used to report services to Medicare; however, in most cases, you may bill the patient directly for non-covered services.

SPECIAL COVERAGE INSTRUCTIONS

Your local Medicare carrier has specific coverage instructions for processing certain HCPCS codes. These codes are identified by a yellow bar over the HCPCS code. While these codes are covered by the Medicare program, the use of these codes does not guarantee payment. If you have a question about a specific code in this category, review your Medicare provider manual or consult with your local Medicare carrier.

CARRIER DISCRETION

Processing and payment for these codes is done at the discretion of each insurance carrier. These codes are identified by a blue bar over the HCPCS code. For codes in this category, you should check with your Medicare carrier for proper billing instructions prior to filing an insurance claim.

DURABLE MEDICAL EQUIPMENT REGIONAL CARRIERS (DMERCS)

All Medicare claims for durable medical equipment (DME), prosthetics, orthotics and supplies go to one of four durable medical equipment regional carriers, or DMERCs.

MEDICARE SUPPLIER NUMBER

Before submitting claims to DMERCs, you must apply for a supplier number. You must use this number when submitting claims to all four carriers. To find out more information, go to the Medicare website at http://www.hcfa.gov/medicare.

REGIONALIZATION OF CLAIM PROCESSING

In accordance with Section 1834(a) of Title XVIII of the Social Security Act, the Center for Medicare and Medicaid Services (formerly HCFA) has contracted with four carriers to process Part B Medicare claims for durable medical equipment, prosthetics, orthotics, and supplies. Listed below are the contracted carriers and the states that they serve. The residence of the beneficiary is what determines which regional carrier processes the claim.

Region A: Connecticut, Delaware, Maine, Massachusetts, New Hampshire, New Jersey, New York, Pennsylvania, Rhode Island, Vermont

HealthNow New York, Inc.
60 E. Main Street
Naticoke, PA 18634
(570) 735-9400
(570) 735-9402 fax

Region B: District of Columbia, Illinois, Indiana, Maryland, Michigan, Minnesota, Ohio, Virginia, West Virginia, Wisconsin

AdminaStar Federal, Inc.
8115 Knue Road
Indianapolis, IN 46250
(317) 841-4400
(877) 299-7900
(317) 841-4691 fax

Region C: Alabama, Arkansas, Colorado, Florida, Georgia, Kentucky, Louisiana, Mississippi, New Mexico, North Carolina, Oklahoma, Puerto Rico, South Carolina, Tennessee, Texas, Virgin Islands

**Blue Cross & Blue Shield of South Carolina/
Palmetto Government Benefits Administrators**
I-20 at Alpine Road
Columbia, SC 29219
(803) 735-1034
(866) 238-9650
(803) 786-4636 fax

Region D: Alaska, Arizona, California, Guam, Hawaii, Idaho, Iowa, Kansas, Missouri, Montana, Nebraska, Nevada, North Dakota, Oregon, South Dakota, Utah, Washington, Wyoming

CIGNA Medicare
2 Vantage Way
Metro Exchange Building
Nashville, TN 37228
(866) 520-4025
(615) 244-6242 fax

CHANGE OF CLAIM JURISDICTION

Prior to October 1, 1993, Medicare carriers processed durable medical equipment (DME), prosthetics, and orthotics claims based on where the transaction for the sale or rental took place. This is called the point of sale. Beginning October 1, 1993 and according to the state by state transfer schedule, regional processing of supplier claims began using beneficiary residence to determine which regional carrier had claim jurisdiction.

ELECTRONIC CLAIM FILING

The Center for Medicare and Medicaid Services (formerly known as HCFA) is strongly encouraging electronic claims submission to DMERCs. Suppliers submitting claims electronic must use the designated National Standard Format which meets all Medicare billing requirements and is accepted by other third-party insurance carriers. The regional carriers will assist you in converting to electronic claims submission. You can contact the Electronic Media Coordinater (EMC) at the DMERCs listed above.

HCPCS 2002 ON DISK

HCPCS 2002 procedure codes and descriptions are also available on disk for IBM PC-compatible computer systems. The HCPCS Short Description disk includes all HCPCS National Level II codes with descriptions of 28 characters or less. The HCPCS disk contains only data files in ASCII format. It does not contain a program or other operating software. For information regarding HCPCS codes on disk, call PMIC at 1-800-MED-SHOP, or visit our web site and virtual bookstore at http://www.medicalbookstore.com.

TRANSPORTATION SERVICES

Guidelines

In addition to the information presented in the INTRODUCTION, several other items unique to this section are defined or identified here:

1. **VEHICLE AND CREW REQUIREMENTS:** The ambulance must be designed and equipped for transporting the sick or injured and include patient care equipment, such as a stretcher, clean linens, first aid supplies, oxygen equipment and other safety and lifesaving equipment required by state or local authorities. The ambulance crew must have two members, one of which has medical training equivalent to the standard and advanced Red Cross training. The vehicle and personnel supplier must provide a statement that describes the first-aid, safety and other patient-care items in the vehicle, the extent of first-aid training of the personnel and the supplier's agreement to notify Medicare of any changes that could affect coverage.

2. **AIR AMBULANCE SERVICE:** Air ambulance services are covered when the point of pick-up is inaccessible by land vehicle; distances or other obstacles are involved in getting the patient to the nearest hospital with appropriate facilities; and, all other conditions of coverage are met.

3. **AMBULANCE SERVICE CLAIMS:** Reimbursement may be made for expenses incurred for ambulance services when specific conditions have been met and the appropriate medical documentation is provided.

4. **MATERIALS SUPPLIED BY AMBULANCE SERVICE:** Reusable devices, such as back boards, neck boards and inflatable leg and arm splints, are considered part of general ambulance services and included in the charge for the trip. A separate reasonable charge may be recognized for non-reusable items and disposable supplies, such as oxygen, gauze and dressings, that are required for patient care during the trip.

5. **UNLISTED SERVICE OR PROCEDURE:** A service or procedure may be provided that is not listed in this edition of HCPCS. When reporting such a service, the appropriate "unlisted procedure" code may be used to indicate the service, identifying it by "special report" as defined below. HCPCS terminology is inconsistent in defining

unlisted procedures. The procedure definition may include the term(s) "unlisted", "not otherwise classified", "unspecified", "unclassified", "other" and "miscellaneous". Prior to using these codes, try to determine if a Local Level III code or CPT code is available. The "unlisted procedures" and accompanying codes for **TRANSPORTATION SERVICES** are as follows:

A0999 Unlisted ambulance service

6. **SPECIAL REPORT:** A service, material or supply that is rarely provided, unusual, variable or new may require a special report in determining medical appropriateness for reimbursement purposes. Pertinent information should include an adequate definition or description of the nature, extent, and need for the service, material or supply.

7. **MODIFIERS:** Listed services may be modified under certain circumstances. When appropriate, the modifying circumstance is identified by adding a modifier to the basic procedure code. CPT and HCPCS National Level II modifiers may be used with CPT and HCPCS National Level II procedure codes. One digit codes are to be used in combination. The first digit should indicate the origin; the second digit should indicate the destination.

The Level II modifiers commonly used with TRANSPORTATION codes are as follows:

-GM Multiple patients on one ambulance trip

-QM Ambulance service provided under arrangement by a provider of services

-QN Ambulance services furnished directly by a provider of services

AMBULANCE SERVICE MODIFIERS

For ambulance service, one-digit modifiers are combined to form a two-digit modifier that identifies the ambulance's place of origin with the first digit, and ambulance's destination with the second digit. They are used in items 12 and 13 on the HCFA Form 1491.

One digit ambulance modifiers:

-D   Diagnostic or therapeutic site other than -P or -H when these are used as origin codes

-E   Residential, domiciliary, custodial facility (other than an 1819 facility)

-H   Hospital

-N   Skilled nursing facility (SNF) (1819 facility)

-P   Physician's office

-R   Residence

-S   Scene of accident or acute event

-X   (Destination code only) Intermediate stop at physician's office on the way to the hospital

8. CPT CODE CROSS-REFERENCE: Unless specified otherwise, there is no equivalent CPT code for listings in this section.

Transportation Services Including Ambulance

A0021   Ambulance service; outside state per mile, transport (Medicaid only)

(A0030)   Code deleted 2001; use A0430

(A0040)   Code deleted 2001; use A0431

(A0050)   Code deleted 2001; use A0429

Ambulance Waiting Time Table

Units	Time (Hrs)	Units	Time (Hrs)
1	1/2 to 1	6	3 to 3 1/2
2	1 to 1 1/2	7	3 1/2 to 4
3	1 1/2 to 2	8	4 to 4 1/2
4	2 to 2 1/2	9	4 1/2 to 5
5	2 to 3	10	5 to 5 1/2

A0080   Non-emergency transportation; per mile—volunteer, with no vested or personal interest

A0090   per mile—volunteer, interested individual, neighbor

A0100   taxi—intra city

A0110   and bus, intra or inter state carrier

A0120   mini-bus, mountain area transports, other non-profit transportation systems

A0130   wheel-chair van

A0140   and air travel (private or commercial) intra or inter state

A0160   per mile—case worker or social worker

A0170   ancillary: parking fees, tolls, other

A0180   ancillary: lodging-recipient

A0190   ancillary: meals-recipient

A0200   ancillary: lodging-escort

A0210   ancillary: meals-escort

A0225 Ambulance service; neonatal transport, base rate, emergency transport, one way

(A0300) Code deleted 2001; use A0428

(A0302) Code deleted 2001; use A0429

(A0304) Code deleted 2001; use A0428

(A0306) Code deleted 2001; use A0426

(A0308) Code deleted 2001; use A0429

(A0310) Code deleted 2001; use A0427

(A0320) Code deleted 2001; use A0428

(A0322) Code deleted 2001; use A0429

(A0324) Code deleted 2001; use A0428

(A0326) Code deleted 2001; use A0426

(A0328) Code deleted 2001; use A0429

(A0330) Code deleted 2001; use A0427

(A0340) Code deleted 2001; use A0428

(A0342) Code deleted 2001; use A0429

(A0344) Code deleted 2001; use A0428

(A0346) Code deleted 2001; use A0426

(A0348) Code deleted 2001; use A0429

(A0350) Code deleted 2001; use A0427

(A0360) Code deleted 2001; use A0428

(A0362) Code deleted 2001; use A0429

(A0364) Code deleted 2001; use A0428

(A0366) Code deleted 2001; use A0426

(A0368) Code deleted 2000

(A0370) Code deleted 2001; use A0427

(A0380) Code deleted 2001; use A0425

A0382 BLS routine disposable supplies

A0384 BLS specialized service disposable supplies, defibrillation (used by ALS ambulances and BLS ambulances in jurisdictions where defibrillation is permitted in BLS ambulances)

(A0390) Code deleted 2001; use A0425

A0392 ALS specialized service disposable supplies; defibrillation (to be used only in jurisdictions where defibrillation cannot be performed in BLS ambulances)

A0394 ALS specialized service disposable supplies; IV drug therapy

A0396 ALS specialized service disposable supplies; esophageal intubation

A0398 ALS routine disposable supplies

A0420 Ambulance waiting time (ALS or BLS), one-half (1/2) hour increments

A0422 Ambulance (ALS or BLS) oxygen and oxygen supplies, life sustaining situation

A0424 Extra ambulance attendant, ALS or BLS (requires medical review)

A0425 Ground mileage, per statue mile

A0426 Ambulance service, advanced life support, non-emergency transport, level 1 (ALS1)

A0427 Ambulance service, advanced life support, emergency transport, level 1 (ALS1-emergency)

A0428 Ambulance service, basic life support, non-emergency transport (BLS)

A0429 Ambulance service, basic life support, emergency transport (BLS-emergency)

A0430 Ambulance service, conventional air services, transport, one way (fixed wing)

A0431 Ambulance service, conventional air services, transport, one way (rotary wing)

A0432 Paramedic intercept (PI), rural area, transport furnished by a volunteer ambulance company which is prohibited by state law from billing third party payers

A0433 Advanced life support, level 2 (ALS2)

A0434 Specialty care transport (SCT)

A0435 Fixed wing air mileage, per statute mile

A0436 Rotary wing air mileage, per statute mile

A0888 Noncovered ambulance mileage, per mile (e.g., for miles traveled beyond closest appropriate facility)

A0999 Unlisted ambulance service

● New code ▲ Revised code ( ) Deleted code

MEDICAL AND SURGICAL SUPPLIES

Guidelines

In addition to the information presented in the INTRODUCTION, several other items unique to this section are defined or identified here:

1. **SUBSECTION INFORMATION:** Some of the listed subheadings or subsections have special needs or instructions unique to that section. Where these are indicated, special "notes" will be presented preceding or following the listings. Those subsections within the MEDICAL AND SURGICAL SUPPLIES section that have "notes" are as follows:

Subsection	Code Numbers
External urinary supplies	A4356-A4359
Tracheostomy supplies	A4622-A4626
Supplies for ESRD	A4650-A4927

2. **UNLISTED SERVICE OR PROCEDURE:** A service or procedure may be provided that is not listed in this edition of HCPCS. When reporting such a service, the appropriate "unlisted procedure" code may be used to indicate the service, identifying it by "special report" as defined below. HCPCS terminology is inconsistent in defining unlisted procedures. The procedure definition may include the term(s) "unlisted", "not otherwise classified", "unspecified", "unclassified", "other" and "miscellaneous". Prior to using these codes, try to determine if a Local Level III code or CPT code is available. The "unlisted procedures" and accompanying codes for MEDICAL AND SURGICAL SUPPLIES are as follows:

A4335   Incontinence supply; miscellaneous
A4421   Ostomy supply; miscellaneous
A4649   Surgical supply; miscellaneous
A4913   Miscellaneous dialysis supplies, not otherwise specified
A6261   Wound filler, gel/paste, per fluid ounce, not elsewhere classified
A6262   Wound filler, dry foam, per gram, not elsewhere classified

3. **SPECIAL REPORT:** A service, material or supply that is rarely provided, unusual, variable or new may require a special report in determining medical appropriateness for reimbursement purposes.

Pertinent information should include an adequate definition or description of the nature, extent, and need for the service, material or supply.

4. **MODIFIERS:** Listed services may be modified under certain circumstances. When appropriate, the modifying circumstance is identified by adding a modifier to the basic procedure code. CPT and HCPCS National Level II modifiers may be used with CPT and HCPCS National Level II procedure codes. Modifiers commonly used with MEDICAL AND SURGICAL SUPPLIES are as follows:

   -CC Procedure code change (use "CC" when the procedure code submitted was changed either for administrative reasons or because an incorrect code was filed)

   -LT Left side (used to identify procedures performed on the left side of the body)

   -RT Right side (used to identify procedures performed on the right side of the body)

5. **CPT CODE CROSS-REFERENCE:** Unless specified otherwise, the equivalent CPT code for all listings in this section is 99070.

6. **DURABLE MEDICAL EQUIPMENT REGIONAL CARRIERS (DMERCS)**: Effective October 1, 1993 claims for supplies must be billed to one of four regional carriers depending upon the residence of the beneficiary. The transition dates for DMERC claims is from November 1, 1993 to March 1, 1994, also depending upon the state you practice in. See the Introduction for a complete discussion of DMERCs.

Medical And Surgical Supplies

A4206   Syringe with needle; sterile 1cc, each

A4207   sterile 2cc, each

A4208   sterile 3cc, each

A4209   sterile 5cc or greater, each

A4210   Needle-free injection device, each

A4211   Supplies for self-administered injections

A4212 Non-coring needle or stylet with or without catheter

A4213 Syringe, sterile, 20cc or greater, each

A4214 Sterile saline or water, 30cc vial

A4215 Needles only, sterile, any size, each

A4220 Refill kit for implantable infusion pump

A4221 Supplies for maintenance of drug infusion catheter, per week (list drug separately)

A4222 Supplies for external drug infusion pump, per cassette or bag (list drug separately)

A4230 Infusion set for external insulin pump, non needle cannula type

A4231 Infusion set for external insulin pump, needle type

A4232 Syringe with needle for external insulin pump, sterile, 3cc

A4244 Alcohol or peroxide, per pint

A4245 Alcohol wipes, per box

A4246 Betadine or phisohex solution, per pint

A4247 Betadine or iodine swabs/wipes, per box

A4250 Urine test or reagent strips or tablets (100 tablets or strips)

A4253 Blood glucose test or reagent strips for home blood glucose monitor, per 50 strips

A4254 Replacement battery, any type, for use with medically necessary home blood glucose monitor owned by patient, each

A4255 Platforms for home blood glucose monitor, 50 per box

A4256 Normal, low and high calibrator solution/chips

● **A4257** Replacement lens shield cartridge for use with laser skin piercing device, each

A4258   Spring-powered device for lancet, each

A4259   Lancets, per box of 100

A4260   Levonorgestrel (contraceptive) implants system, including implants and supplies

A4261   Cervical cap for contraceptive use

A4262   Temporary, absorbable lacrimal duct implant, each

A4263   Permanent, long term, non-dissolvable lacrimal duct implant, each

A4265   Paraffin, per pound

A4270   Disposable endoscope sheath, each

A4280   Adhesive skin support attachment for use with external breast prosthesis, each

A4290   Sacral nerve stimulation test lead, each

VASCULAR CATHETERS

▲A4300   Implantable access catheter, (eg, venous, arterial, epidural subarachnoid, or peritoneal, etc) External access

▲A4301   Implantable access total system; catheter, port/reservoir (eg, venous, arterial, epidural, or subarachnoid, etc) Percutaneous access

INCONTINENCE APPLIANCES AND CARE SUPPLIES

A4305   Disposable drug delivery system, flow rate of 50 ml or greater per hour

A4306   Disposable drug delivery system, flow rate of 5 ml or less per hour

A4310   Insertion tray without drainage bag; and without catheter (accessories only)

A4311   Insertion tray without drainage bag; with indwelling catheter, foley type, two-way latex with coating (teflon, silicone, silicone elastomer or hydrophilic, etc.)

A4312 with indwelling catheter, foley type, two-way, all silicone

A4313 with indwelling catheter, foley type, three-way, for continuous irrigation

A4314 Insertion tray with drainage bag; with indwelling catheter, foley type, two-way latex with coating (teflon, silicone, silicone elastomer or hydrophilic, etc.)

A4315 with indwelling catheter, foley type, two-way, all silicone

A4316 with indwelling catheter, foley type, three-way, for continuous irrigation

A4319 Sterile water irrigation solution, 1000 ml

A4320 Irrigation tray with bulb or piston syringe, any purpose

A4321 Therapeutic agent for urinary catheter irrigation

A4322 Irrigation syringe, bulb or piston, each

A4323 Sterile saline irrigation solution, 1000 ml

A4324 Male external catheter, with adhesive coating, each

A4325 Male external catheter, with adhesive strip, each

A4326 Male external catheter specialty type, (e.g., inflatable, faceplate, etc;) each

A4327 Female external urinary collection device; meatal cup, each

A4328 pouch, each

(A4329) Code deleted 2002.

A4330 Perianal fecal collection pouch with adhesive, each

A4331 Extension drainage tubing, any type, any length, with connector/adaptor, for use with urinary leg bag or urostomy pouch, each

A4332 Lubricant, individual sterile packet, for insertion of urinary catheter, each

URINARY CATHETERS

A4333 Urinary catheter anchoring device, adhesive skin attachment, each

A4334 Urinary catheter anchoring device, leg strap, each

A4335 Incontinence supply; miscellaneous

A4338 Indwelling catheter; foley type, two-way latex with coating (teflon, silicone, silicone elastomer, or hydrophilic, etc.), each

A4340 Indwelling catheter; specialty type, (e.g.; coude, mushroom, wing, etc.), each

A4344 Indwelling catheter, foley type; two-way all silicone, each

A4346 three-way for continuous irrigation, each

A4347 Male external catheter, with or without adhesive, with or without anti-reflux device; per dozen

A4348 Male external catheter with integral collection compartment, extended wear, each, (e.g., 2 per month)

▲ **A4351** Intermittent urinary catheter; straight tip, with or without coating (teflon, silicone, silicone elastomer, or hydrophilic, etc), each

▲ **A4352** Intermittent urinary catheter; coude (curved) tip, with or without coating (teflon, silicone, silicone elastomer, or hydrophilic, etc), each

A4353 Intermittent urinary catheter, with insertion supplies

A4354 Insertion tray with drainage bag, but without catheter

A4355 Irrigation tubing set for continuous bladder irrigation through a three-way indwelling foley catheter, each

EXTERNAL URINARY SUPPLIES

A4356 External urethral clamp or compression device (not to be used for catheter clamp), each

---

A4357 Bedside drainage bag, day or night with or without anti-reflux device, with or without tube, each

▲**A4358** Urinary drainage bag, leg or abdomen, vinyl, with or without tube, with straps, each

A4359 Urinary suspensory without leg bag, each

●**A4360** Adult incontinence garment (e.g., brief, diaper), each

NOTE: See DME section for male or female urinals

OSTOMY SUPPLIES

A4361 Ostomy faceplate, each

A4362 Skin barrier; solid, 4 x 4 or equivalent; each

(A4363) Code deleted 2000; use A4369, A4370, A4371

A4364 Adhesive, liquid or equal, any type, per ounce

A4365 Adhesive remover wipes, any type, per 50

A4367 Ostomy belt, each

A4368 Ostomy filter, any type, each

A4369 Ostomy skin barrier, liquid (spray, brush, etc.), per oz.

A4370 Ostomy skin barrier, paste, per oz.

A4371 Ostomy skin barrier, powder, per oz.

A4372 Ostomy skin barrier, solid 4x4 or equivalent, standard wear, with built-in convexity, each

A4373 Ostomy skin barrier, with flange (solid, flexible or accordion), standard wear, with built-in convexity, any size, each

A4374 Ostomy skin barrier, with flange (solid, flexible or accordion), extended wear, with built-in convexity, any size, each

A4375 Ostomy pouch, drainable, with faceplate attached, plastic, each

| Not valid for Medicare | Non-covered by Medicare | Special coverage instructions | Carrier discretion |

A4376 Ostomy pouch, drainable, with faceplate attached, rubber each

A4377 Ostomy pouch, drainable, for use on faceplate, plastic, each

A4378 Ostomy pouch, drainable, for use on faceplate, rubber, each

A4379 Ostomy pouch, urinary, with faceplate attached, plastic, each

A4380 Ostomy pouch, urinary, with faceplate attached, rubber, each

A4381 Ostomy pouch, urinary, for use on faceplate, plastic, each

A4382 Ostomy pouch, urinary, for use on faceplate, heavy plastic, each

A4383 Ostomy pouch, urinary, for use on faceplate, rubber, each

A4384 Ostomy faceplate equivalent, silicone ring, each

A4385 Ostomy skin barrier, solid 4x4 or equivalent, extended wear, without built-in convexity, each

A4386 Ostomy skin barrier, with flange (solid, flexible or accordion), extended wear, without built-in convexity, any size, each

A4387 Ostomy pouch closed, with standard wear barrier attached, with built-in convexity (1 piece), each

A4388 Ostomy pouch, drainable, with extended wear barrier attached, without built-in convexity (1 piece)

A4389 Ostomy pouch, drainable, with standard wear barrier attached, with built-in convexity (1 piece), each

A4390 Ostomy pouch, drainable, with extended wear barrier attached, with built-in convexity (1 piece), each

A4391 Ostomy pouch, urinary, with extended wear barrier attached, without built-in convexity (1 piece), each

A4392 Ostomy pouch, urinary, with standard wear barrier attached, with built-in convexity (1 piece), each

A4393 Ostomy pouch, urinary, with extended wear barrier attached, with built-in convexity (1 piece), each

A4394 Ostomy deodorant for use in ostomy pouch, liquid, per fluid ounce

A4395 Ostomy deodorant for use in ostomy pouch, solid, per tablet

A4396 Ostomy belt with peristomal hernia support

A4397 Irrigation supply; sleeve, each

A4398 Ostomy irrigation supply; bag, each

A4399   cone/catheter, including brush

A4400 Ostomy irrigation set

A4402 Lubricant, per ounce

A4404 Ostomy ring, each

A4421 Ostomy supply; miscellaneous

SUPPLIES

A4454 Tape, all types, all sizes

A4455 Adhesive remover or solvent (for tape, cement or other adhesive), per ounce

A4460 Elastic bandage, per roll (e.g., compression bandage)

A4462 Abdominal dressing holder/binder, each

A4464 Joint supportive device/garment, elastic or equal, each

A4465 Non-elastic binder for extremity

A4470 Gravlee jet washer

A4480 Vabra aspirator

A4481 Thracheostoma filter, any type, any size, each

A4483 Moisture exchanger, disposable, for use with invasive mechanical ventilation

A4490 Surgical stockings; above knee length, each

A4495 thigh length, each

A4500 below knee length, each

A4510 full length, each

A4550 Surgical trays

A4554 Disposable underpads, all sizes, (e.g., chux's)

A4556 Electrodes, (e.g., apnea monitor), per pair

A4557 Lead wires, (e.g., apnea monitor), per pair

A4558 Conductive paste or gel

(A4560) Code deleted 2001

A4561 Pessary, rubber, any type

A4562 Pessary, non rubber, any type

A4565 Slings

A4570 Splint

A4572 Rib belt

A4575 Topical hyperbaric oxygen chamber, disposable

A4580 Cast supplies (e.g., plaster)

A4590 Special casting materials (e.g., fiberglass)

A4595 Tens supplies, 2 lead, per month

SUPPLIES FOR OXYGEN AND RELATED RESPIRATORY EQUIPMENT

A4608   Transtracheal oxygen catheter, each

A4611   Battery, heavy duty; replacement for patient-owned ventilator

A4612   Battery cables; replacement for patient-owned ventilator

A4613   Battery charger; replacement for patient-owned ventilator

A4614   Peak expiratory flow rate meter, hand held

A4615   Cannula, nasal

A4616   Tubing (oxygen), per foot

A4617   Mouth piece

A4618   Breathing circuits

A4619   Face tent

A4620   Variable concentration mask

A4621   Tracheotomy mask or collar

A4622   Tracheostomy or laryngectomy tube

A4623   Tracheostomy, inner cannula (replacement only)

A4624   Tracheal suction catheter, any type, each

A4625   Tracheostomy care kit for new tracheostomy

A4626   Tracheostomy cleaning brush, each

NOTE: All of the descriptions for tracheostomy supplies, codes A4622-A4626 are "per item". The correct number of items purchased must be entered in the days or units field (box 24-G) on the HCFA1500 claim form. The terms "items" and "units" are used interchangeably.

A4627   Spacer, bag or reservoir, with or without mask, for use with metered dose inhaler

---

A4628   Oropharyngeal suction catheter, each

A4629   Tracheostomy care kit for established tracheostomy

SUPPLIES FOR OTHER DURABLE MEDICAL EQUIPMENT

A4630   Replacement batteries for medically necessary T.E.N.S. owned by patient

A4631   Replacement batteries for medically necessary electronic wheelchair owned by patient

A4635   Underarm pad, crutch, replacement, each

A4636   Replacement, handgrip, cane, crutch, or walker, each

A4637   Replacement, tip, cane, crutch, walker, each

A4640   Replacement pad for use with medically necessary alternating pressure pad owned by patient

A4641   Supply of radiopharmaceutical diagnostic imaging agent, not otherwise classified

A4642   Supply of satumomab pendetide, radiopharmaceutical diagnostic imaging agent, per dose

A4643   Supply of additional high dose contrast material(s) during magnetic resonance imaging, e.g., gadoteridol injection

A4644   Supply of low osmolar contrast material (100-199 mgs of Iodine)

A4645   (200-299 mgs of Iodine)

A4646   (300-399 mgs of Iodine)

SUPPLIES FOR RADIOLOGICAL PROCEDURES

A4647   Supply of paramagnetic contrast material, e.g., gadolinium

A4649   Surgical supply, miscellaneous

SUPPLIES FOR ESRD

NOTE: For DME items for ESRD see procedure codes D1500-E1699. For dialysis Procedures, see M0900-M0999.

(A4650) Code deleted 2002

● **A4651** Calibrated microcapillary tube, each

● **A4652** Microcapillary tube sealant

(A4655) Code deleted 2002

● **A4656** Needle, any size, for dialysis, each

● **A4657** Syringe, with or without needle, for dialysis, each

▲ **A4660** Sphygmomanometer/blood pressure apparatus with cuff and stethoscope, for dialysis

▲ **A4663** Blood pressure cuff only, for dialysis

▲ **A4670** Automatic blood pressure monitor, for dialysis

▲ **A4680** Activated carbon filter for hemodialysis, each

▲ **A4690** Dialyzer (artificial kidneys), all types, all sizes, for hemodialysis, each

(A4700) Code deleted 2002

(A4705) Code deleted 2002

● **A4706** Bicarbonate concentrate, solution, for hemodialysis, per gallon

● **A4707** Bicarbonate concentrate, powder, for hemodialysis, per packet

● **A4708** Acetate concentrate solution, for hemodialysis, per gallon

● **A4709** Acid concentrate solution, for hemodialysis, per gallon

▲ **A4712** Water, sterile, for injection for dialysis, per 10 ml

▲ **A4714**   Treated water (deionized, distilled, or reverse osmosis) for peritoneal dialysis, per gallon

● **A4719**   Y set tubing for peritoneal dialysis

● **A4720**   Dialysate solution, any concentration of dextrose, fluid volume greater than 249cc, but less than or equal to 999cc, for peritoneal dialysis

● **A4721**   Dialysate solution, any concentration of dextrose, fluid volume greater than 999cc, but less than or equal to 1999cc, for peritoneal dialysis

● **A4722**   Dialysate solution, any concentration of dextrose, fluid volume greater than 1999cc, but less than or equal to 2999cc, for peritoneal dialysis

● **A4723**   Dialysate solution, any concentration of dextrose, fluid volume greater than 2999cc, but less than or equal to 3999cc, for peritoneal dialysis

● **A4724**   Dialysate solution, any concentration of dextrose, fluid volume greater than 3999cc, but less than or equal to 4999cc, for peritoneal dialysis

● **A4725**   Dialysate solution, any concentration of dextrose, fluid volume greater than 4999cc, but less than or equal to 5999cc, for peritoneal dialysis

● **A4726**   Dialysate solution, any concentration of dextrose, fluid volume greater than 5999cc, for peritoneal dialysis

▲ **A4730**   Fistula cannulation set for hemodialysis, each

(A4735)   Code deleted 2002

● **A4736**   Topical anesthetic, for dialysis, per gram

● **A4737**   Injectable anesthetic, for dialysis, per 10 ml

▲ **A4740**   Shunt accessory, for hemodialysis, any type, each

▲ **A4750**   Blood tubing, arterial or venous, for hemodialysis, each

▲ **A4755**   Blood tubing, arterial and venous combined, for hemodialysis, each

---

▲ **A4760** Dialysate solution test kit, for peritoneal dialysis, any type, each

▲ **A4765** Dialysate concentrate, powder, additive for peritoneal dialysis, per packet

● **A4766** Dialysate concentrate, solution, additive for peritoneal dialysis, per 10 ml

▲ **A4770** Blood collection tube, vacuum, for dialysis, per 50

▲ **A4771** Serum clotting time tube, for dialysis, per 50

▲ **A4772** Blood glucose test strips, for dialysis, per 50

▲ **A4773** Occult blood test strips, for dialysis, per 50

▲ **A4774** Ammonia test strips, for dialysis, per 50

(A4780) Code deleted 2002

(A4790) Code deleted 2002

(A4800) Code deleted 2002; use A4801

● **A4801** Heparin, any type, for hemodialysis, per 1000 units

● **A4802** Protamine sulfate, for hemodialysis, per 50 mg

(A4820) Code deleted 2002

(A4850) Code deleted 2002; use E1637

▲ **A4860** Disposable catheter tips for peritoneal dialysis, per 10

▲ **A4870** Plumbing and/or electrical work for home hemodialysis equipment

(A4880) Code deleted 2002

▲ **A4890** Contracts, repair and maintenance, for hemodialysis equipment

(A4900) Code deleted 2002

(A4901) Code deleted 2002

| | Not valid for Medicare | | Non-covered by Medicare | | Special coverage instructions | | Carrier discretion | **23** |

(A4905)   Code deleted 2002

(A4910)   Code deleted 2002

NOTE: The above procedure includes the following: scale, scissors, stopwatch, surgical brush, thermometer, tool kit, tourniquet, tube occluding forceps/clamps.

● A4911   Drain bag/bottle, for dialysis, each

(A4912)   Code deleted 2002; use A4911

▲ A4913   Miscellaneous dialysis supplies, not otherwise specified

(A4914)   Code deleted 2002

▲ A4918   Venous pressure clamp, for hemodialysis, each

(A4919)   Code deleted 2002

(A4920)   Code deleted 2002

(A4921)   Code deleted 2002

▲ A4927   Gloves, non-sterile, for dialysis, per 100

● A4928   Surgical mask, for dialysis, per 20

● A4929   Tourniquet for dialysis, each

ADDITIONAL OSTOMY SUPPLIES

A5051   Pouch, closed; with barrier attached (1 piece)

A5052   without barrier attached (1 piece)

A5053   for use on faceplate

A5054   for use on barrier with flange (2 piece)

A5055   Stoma cap

A5061   Pouch, drainable; with barrier attached (1 piece)

A5062   without barrier attached (1 piece)

A5063   for use on barrier with flange (2 piece)

(A5064) Code deleted 2002

(A5065) Code deleted 2001

A5071 Pouch, urinary; with barrier attached (1 piece)

A5072   without barrier attached (1 piece)

A5073   for use on barrier with flange (2 piece)

(A5074) Code deleted 2002

(A5075) Code deleted 2002

A5081 Continent device; plug for continent stoma

A5082   catheter for continent stoma

A5093 Ostomy accessory; convex insert

ADDITIONAL INCONTINENCE APPLIANCES/SUPPLIES

A5102 Bedside drainage bottle with or without tubing, rigid or expandable, each

A5105 Urinary suspensory; with leg bag, with or without tube

A5112 Urinary leg bag; latex

A5113 Leg strap; latex, replacement only, per set

A5114   foam or fabric, replacement only, per set

SUPPLIES FOR EITHER INCONTINENCE OR OSTOMY APPLIANCES

A5119 Skin barrier; wipes, box per 50

A5121   solid, 6 x 6 or equivalent, each

A5122   solid, 8 x 8 or equivalent, each

A5123   with flange (solid, flexible or accordion), any size, each

A5126 Adhesive or non-adhesive; disk or foam pad

| | Not valid for Medicare | | Non-covered by Medicare | | Special coverage instructions | | Carrier discretion | **25** |

A5131 Appliance cleaner, incontinence and ostomy appliances, per 16 oz.

(A5149) Code deleted 2001; use A4335, A4421

A5200 Percutaneous catheter/tube anchoring device, adhesive skin attachment

SHOE SUPPLIES FOR DIABETICS

A5500 For diabetics only, fitting (including follow-up), custom preparation and supply of off-the-shelf depth-inlay shoe manufactured to accommodate multi-density insert(s), per shoe

A5501 For diabetics only, fitting (including follow-up), custom preparation and supply of shoe molded from cast(s) of patient's foot (custom molded shoe), per shoe

(A5502) Code deleted 2002

A5503 For diabetics only, modification (including fitting) of off-the-shelf depth-inlay shoe or custom-molded shoe with roller or rigid rocker bottom, per shoe

A5504 For diabetics only, modification (including fitting) of off-the-shelf depth-inlay shoe or custom-molded shoe with wedge(s), per shoe

A5505 For diabetics only, modification (including fitting) of off-the-shelf depth-inlay shoe or custom-molded shoe with metatarsal bar, per shoe

A5506 For diabetics only, modification (including fitting) of off-the-shelf depth-inlay shoe or custom-molded shoe with off-set heel(s), per shoe

A5507 For diabetics only, not otherwise specified modification (including fitting) of off-the-shelf depth-inlay shoe or custom-molded shoe, per shoe

A5508 For diabetics only, deluxe feature of off-the-shelf depth-inlay shoe or custom-molded shoe, per shoe

● **A5509** For diabetics only, direct formed, molded to foot with external heat source (ie heat gun) multiple density insert(s), prefabricated, per shoe

●A5510   For diabetics only, direct formed, compression molded to patient's foot without external heat source, multiple-density insert(s), prefabricated, per shoe

●A5511   For diabetics only, custom-molded from model of patient's foot, multiple density insert(s), custom-fabricated, per shoe

●A6000   Non-contact wound warming wound cover for use with the non-contact wound warming device and warming card

●A6010   Collagen based wound filler, dry form, per gram of collagen

(A6020)   Code deleted 2000

A6021   Collagen dressing, pad size 16 sq. in. or less, each

A6022   Collagen dressing, pad size more than 16 sq. in. but less than or equal to 48 sq. in., each

A6023   Collagen dressing, pad size more than 48 sq. in., each

A6024   Collagen dressing wound filler, per 6 inches

A6025   Silicone gel sheet, each

A6154   Wound pouch, each

▲A6196   Alginate or other fiber gelling dressing, wound cover, pad size 16 sq. in. or less, each dressing

▲A6197   Alginate or other fiber gelling dressing, wound cover, pad size more than 16 sq. in. but less than or equal to 48 sq. in., each dressing

▲A6198   Alginate or other fiber gelling dressing, wound cover, pad size more than 48 sq. in., each dressing

▲A6199   Alginate or other fiber gelling dressing, wound filler, per 6 inches

A6200   Composite dressing, pad size 16 sq. in. or less, without adhesive border, each dressing

A6201 Composite dressing, pad size more than 16 sq. in. but less than or equal to 48 sq. in., without adhesive border, each dressing

A6202 Composite dressing, pad size more than 48 sq. in., without adhesive border, each dressing

A6203 Composite dressing, pad size 16 sq. in. or less, with any size adhesive border, each dressing

A6204 Composite dressing, pad size more than 16 sq. in. but less than or equal to 48 sq. in., with any size adhesive border, each dressing

A6205 Composite dressing, pad size more than 48 sq. in., with any size adhesive border, each dressing

A6206 Contact layer, 16 sq. in. or less, each dressing

A6207 Contact layer, more than 16 sq. in. but less than or equal to 48 sq. in., each dressing

A6208 Contact layer, more than 48 sq. in., each dressing

A6209 Foam dressing, wound cover, pad size 16 sq. in. or less, without adhesive border, each dressing

A6210 Foam dressing, wound cover, pad size more than 16 sq. in. but less than or equal to 48 sq. in., without adhesive border, each dressing

A6211 Foam dressing, wound cover, pad size more than 48 sq. in., without adhesive border, each dressing

A6212 Foam dressing, wound cover, pad size 16 sq. in. or less, with any size adhesive border, each dressing

A6213 Foam dressing, wound cover, pad size more than 16 sq. in. but less than or equal to 48 sq. in., with any size adhesive border, each dressing

A6214 Foam dressing, wound cover, pad size more than 48 sq. in., with any size adhesive border, each dressing

A6215 Foam dressing, wound filler, per gram

A6216 Gauze, non-impregnated, non-sterile, pad size 16 sq. in. or less, without adhesive border, each dressing

A6217 Gauze, non-impregnated, non-sterile, pad size more than 16 sq. in. but less than or equal to 48 sq. in., without adhesive border, each dressing

A6218 Gauze, non-impregnated, non-sterile, pad size more than 48 sq. in., without adhesive border, each dressing

A6219 Gauze, non-impregnated, pad size 16 sq. in. or less, with any size adhesive border, each dressing

A6220 Gauze, non-impregnated, pad size more than 16 sq. in. but less than or equal to 48 sq. in., with any size adhesive border, each dressing

A6221 Gauze, non-impregnated, pad size more than 48 sq. in., with any size adhesive border, each dressing

A6222 Gauze, impregnated with other than water, normal saline, or hydrogel, pad size 16 sq. in. or less, without adhesive border, each dressing

A6223 Gauze, impregnated with other than water, normal saline, or hydrogel, pad size more than 16 sq. in. but less than or equal to 48 sq. in., without adhesive border, each dressing

A6224 Gauze, impregnated with other than water, normal saline, or hydrogel, pad size more than 48 sq. in., without adhesive border, each dressing

A6228 Gauze, impregnated, water or normal saline, pad size 16 sq. in. or less, without adhesive border, each dressing

A6229 Gauze, impregnated, water or normal saline, pad size more than 16 sq. in. but less than or equal to 48 sq. in., without adhesive border, each dressing

A6230 Gauze, impregnated, water or normal saline, pad size more than 48 sq. in., without adhesive border, each dressing

A6231 Gauze, impregnated, hydrogel, for direct wound contact, pad size 16 sq. in. or less, each dressing

A6232 Gauze, impregnated, hydrogel, for direct wound contact, pad size greater than 16 sq. in., but less than or equal to 48 sq. in., each dressing

A6233 Gauze, impregnated, hydrogel, for direct wound contact, pad size more than 48 sq. in., each dressing

A6234 Hydrocolloid dressing, wound cover, pad size 16 sq. in. or less, without adhesive border, each dressing

A6235 Hydrocolloid dressing, wound cover, pad size more than 16 sq. in. but less than or equal to 48 sq. in., without adhesive border, each dressing

A6236 Hydrocolloid dressing, wound cover, pad size more than 48 sq. in., without adhesive border, each dressing

A6237 Hydrocolloid dressing, wound cover, pad size 16 sq. in. or less, with any size adhesive border, each dressing

A6238 Hydrocolloid dressing, wound cover, pad size more than 16 sq. in. but less than or equal to 48 sq. in., with any size adhesive border, each dressing

A6239 Hydrocolloid dressing, wound cover, pad size more than 48 sq. in., with any size adhesive border, each dressing

A6240 Hydrocolloid dressing, wound filler, paste, per fluid ounce

A6241 Hydrocolloid dressing, wound filler, dry form, per gram

A6242 Hydrogel dressing, wound cover, pad size 16 sq. in. or less, without adhesive border, each dressing

A6243 Hydrogel dressing, wound cover, pad size more than 16 sq. in. but less than or equal to 48 sq. in., without adhesive border, each dressing

A6244 Hydrogel dressing, wound cover, pad size more than 48 sq. in., without adhesive border, each dressing

A6245 Hydrogel dressing, wound cover, pad size 16 sq. in. or less, with any size adhesive border, each dressing

A6246 Hydrogel dressing, wound cover, pad size more than 16 sq. in. but less than or equal to 48 sq. in., with any size adhesive border, each dressing

A6247 Hydrogel dressing, wound cover, pad size more than 48 sq. in., with any size adhesive border, each dressing

A6248 Hydrogel dressing, wound filler, gel, per fluid ounce

A6250 Skin sealants, protectants, moisturizers, ointments, any type, any size

A6251 Specialty absorptive dressing, wound cover, pad size 16 sq. in. or less, without adhesive border, each dressing

A6252 Specialty absorptive dressing, wound cover, pad size more than 16 sq. in. but less than or equal to 48 sq. in., without adhesive border, each dressing

A6253 Specialty absorptive dressing, wound cover, pad size more than 48 sq. in., without adhesive border, each dressing

A6254 Specialty absorptive dressing, wound cover, pad size 16 sq. in. or less, with any size adhesive border, each dressing

A6255 Specialty absorptive dressing, wound cover, pad size more than 16 sq. in. but less than or equal to 48 sq. in., with any size adhesive border, each dressing

A6256 Specialty absorptive dressing, wound cover, pad size more than 48 sq. in., with any size adhesive border, each dressing

A6257 Transparent film, 16 sq. in. or less, each dressing

A6258 Transparent film, more than 16 sq. in. but less than or equal to 48 sq. in., each dressing

A6259 Transparent film, more than 48 sq. in., each dressing

A6260 Wound cleansers, any type, any size

A6261 Wound filler, gel/paste, per fluid ounce, not elsewhere classified

A6262 Wound filler, dry form, per gram, not elsewhere classified

A6263 Gauze, elastic, non-sterile, all types, per linear yard

A6264 Gauze, non-elastic, non-sterile, per linear yard

A6265 Tape, all types, per 18 square inches

A6266 Gauze, impregnated, other than water or normal saline, any width, per linear yard

A6402 Gauze, non-impregnated, sterile, pad size 16 sq. in. or less, without adhesive border, each dressing

A6403 Gauze, non-impregnated, sterile, pad size more than 16 sq. in. but less than or equal to 48 sq. in., without adhesive border, each dressing

A6404 Gauze, non-impregnated, sterile, pad size more than 48 sq. in., without adhesive border, each dressing

A6405 Gauze, elastic, sterile, all types, per linear yard

A6406 Gauze, non-elastic, sterile, all types, per linear yard

A7000 Canister, disposable, used with suction pump, each

A7001 Canister, non-disposable, used with suction pump, each

A7002 Tubing, used with suction pump, each

A7003 Administration set, with small volume nonfiltered pneumatic nebulizer, disposable

A7004 Small volume nonfiltered pneumatic nebulizer, disposable

A7005 Administration set, with small volume nonfiltered pneumatic nebulizer, non-disposable

A7006 Administration set, with small volume filtered pneumatic nebulizer

A7007 Large volume nebulizer, disposable, unfilled, used with aerosol compressor

A7008 Large volume nebulizer, disposable, prefilled, used with aerosol compressor

A7009 Reservoir bottle, non-disposable, used with large volume ultrasonic nebulizer

A7010 Corrugated tubing, disposable, used with large volume nebulizer, 100 feet

A7011 Corrugated tubing, non-disposable, used with large volume nebulizer, 10 feet

A7012 Water collection device, used with large volume nebulizer

A7013 Filter, disposable, used with aerosol compressor

A7014 Filter, non-disposable, used with aerosol compressor or ultrasonic generator

A7015 Aerosol mask, used with DME nebulizer

A7016 Dome and mouthpiece, used with small volume ultrasonic nebulizer

A7017 Nebulizer, durable, glass or autoclavable plastic, bottle type, not used with oxygen

A7018 Water, distilled, used with large volume nebulizer, 1000 ml

A7019 Saline solution, per 10 ml, metered dose dispenser, for use with inhalation drugs

A7020 Sterile water or sterile saline, 1000 ml, used with large volume nebulizer

A7501 Tracheostoma valve, including diaphram, each

A7502 Replacement diaphram/faceplate for tracheostoma valve, each

A7503 Filter holder or filter cap, reusable, for use in a tracheostoma heat and moisture exchange system, each

A7504 Filter for use in a tracheostoma heat and moisture exchange system, each

A7505 Housing, reusable without adhesive, for use in a heat and moisture exchange system and/or with a tracheostoma valve, each

A7506 Adhesive disc for use in a heat and moisture exchange system and/or with tracheostoma valve, any type, each

A7507 Filter holder and integrated filter without adhesive, for use in a tracheostoma heat and moisture exchange system, each

A7508 Housing and integrated adhesive, for use in a tracheostoma heat and moisture exchange system and/or with a tracheostoma valve, each

A7509 Filter holder and integrated filter housing, and adhesive, for use as a tracheostoma heat and moisture exchange system, each

ADMINISTRATIVE, MISCELLANEOUS AND INVESTIGATIONAL

NOTE: The following codes do not imply that codes in other sections are necessarily covered.

Guidelines

In addition to the information presented in the INTRODUCTION, several other items unique to this section are defined or identified here:

1. **SPECIAL REPORT:** A service, material or supply that is rarely provided, unusual, variable or new may require a special report in determining medical appropriateness for reimbursement purposes. Pertinent information should include an adequate definition or description of the nature, extent, and need for the service, material or supply.

2. **CPT CODE CROSS-REFERENCE:** Unless specified otherwise, there is no equivalent CPT code for listings in this section.

Miscellaneous And Experimental

A9150 Non-prescription drugs

(A9160) Code deleted 2002

(A9170) Code deleted 2001

(A9190) Code deleted 2001

A9270 Non-covered item or service

A9300 Exercise equipment

A9500 Supply of radiopharmaceutical diagnostic imaging agent, technetium Tc 99m sestamibi, per dose

A9502 Supply of radiopharmaceutical diagnostic imaging agent, technetium Tc 99m tetrofosim, per unit dose

---

A9503 Supply of radiopharmaceutical diagnostic imaging agent, technetium Tc 99m, medronate, up to 30 mci

A9504 Supply of radiopharmaceutical diagnostic imaging agent, technetium Tc 99m apcitide

A9505 Supply of radiopharmaceutical diagnostic imaging agent, thallous chloride Tl 201, per mci

A9507 Supply of radiopharmaceutical diagnostic imaging agent, indium In 111 capromab pendetide, per dose

A9508 Supply of radiopharmaceutical diagnostic imaging agent, iobenguane sulfate I-131, per 0.5 mci

A9510 Supply of radiopharmaceutical diagnostic imaging agent, technetium TC99M disofenin, per vial

●**A9511** Supply of radiopharmaceutical diagnostic imaging agent, technetium tc 99m, depreotide, per mci

A9600 Supply of therapeutic radiopharmaceutical, strontium-89 chloride, per mci

A9605 Supply of therapeutic radiopharmaceutical, samarium Sm 153 Lexidronamm, 50 mci

A9700 Supply of injectable contrast material for use in echocardiography, per study

A9900 Miscellaneous DME supply, accessory, and/or service component of another HCPCS code

A9901 DME delivery, set up, and/or dispensing service component of another HCPCS code

ENTERAL AND PARENTERAL THERAPY

Guidelines

In addition to the information presented in the INTRODUCTION, several other items unique to this section are defined or identified here:

1. **SUBSECTION INFORMATION:** Some of the listed subheadings or subsections have special needs or instructions unique to that section. Where these are indicated, special "notes" will be presented preceding or following the listings. Those subsections within the ENTERAL AND PARENTERAL THERAPY section that have "notes" are as follows:

Subsection	Code Numbers
Enteral formulae and enteral medical supplies	B4034-B5200

2. **UNLISTED SERVICE OR PROCEDURE:** A service or procedure may be provided that is not listed in this edition of HCPCS. When reporting such a service, the appropriate "unlisted procedure" code may be used to indicate the service, identifying it by "special report" as defined below. HCPCS terminology is inconsistent in defining unlisted procedures. The procedure definition may include the term(s) "unlisted", "not otherwise classified", "unspecified", "unclassified", "other" and "miscellaneous". Prior to using these codes, try to determine if a Local Level III code or CPT code is available. The "unlisted procedures" and accompanying codes for ENTERAL AND PARENTERAL THERAPY are as follows:

    B9998   NOC for enteral supplies
    B9999   NOC for parenteral supplies

3. **SPECIAL REPORT:** A service, material or supply that is rarely provided, unusual, variable or new may require a special report in determining medical appropriateness for reimbursement purposes. Pertinent information should include an adequate definition or description of the nature, extent, and need for the service, material or supply.

4. **MODIFIERS:** Listed services may be modified under certain circumstances. When appropriate, the modifying circumstance is identified by adding a modifier to the basic procedure code. CPT and HCPCS National Level II modifiers may be used with CPT and

Not valid   Non-covered   Special   Carrier
for Medicare   by Medicare   coverage   discretion
                                    instructions

HCPCS National Level II procedure codes. Modifiers commonly used with ENTERAL AND PARENTERAL THERAPY are as follows:

-CC   Procedure code change (used when the procedure code submitted was changed either for administrative reasons or because an incorrect code was filed)

5. **CPT CODE CROSS-REFERENCE:** Unless specified otherwise, the equivalent CPT code for all listings in this section is 99070.

Enteral Formulae And Enteral Medical Supplies

B4034   Enteral feeding supply kit; syringe, per day

B4035   pump fed, per day

B4036   gravity fed, per day

B4081   Nasogastric tubing; with stylet

B4082   without stylet

B4083   Stomach tube - levine type

(B4084)   Code deleted 2002

(B4085)   Code deleted 2002

● **B4086**   Gastrostomy / jejunostomy tube, any material, any type, (standard or low profile), each

B4150   Enteral formulae; category I; semi-synthetic intact protein/protein isolates, administered through an enteral feeding tube, 100 calories = 1 unit

B4151   category I; natural intact protein/protein isolates, administered through an enteral feeding tube, 100 calories = 1 unit

B4152   category II; intact protein/protein isolates (calorically dense), administered through an enteral feeding tube, 100 calories = 1 unit

B4153   category III; hydrolyzed protein/amino acids, administered through an enteral feeding tube, 100 calories = 1 unit

B4154   category IV; defined formula for special metabolic need, administered through an enteral feeding tube, 100 calories = 1 unit

B4155   category V; modular components, administered through an enteral feeding tube, 100 calories = 1 unit

B4156   category VI; standardized nutrients, administered through an enteral feeding tube, 100 calories = 1 unit

NOTE: For solution codes for other than parenteral nutrition therapy use, see J7060, J7070 and J7042.

PARENTERAL NUTRITION

B4164   Parenteral nutrition solution; carbohydrates (dextrose), 50% or less (500 ml = 1 unit)—homemix

B4168   amino acid, 3.5% (500 ml = 1 unit)—homemix

B4172   amino acid, 5.5% Thru 7%, (500 ml = 1 unit)—homemix

B4176   amino acid, 7% thru 8.5% (500 ml = 1 unit)—homemix

B4178   amino acid, greater than 8.5% (500 ml = 1 unit)—homemix

B4180   carbohydrates (dextrose), greater than 50% (500 ml = 1 unit)—homemix

B4184   lipids, 10% with administration set (500 ml = 1 unit)

B4186   lipids, 20% with administration set (500 ml = 1 unit)

B4189   compounded amino acids and carbohydrates with electrolytes, trace elements, and vitamins, including preparation, any strength, 10 to 51 grams of protein-premix

B4193   compounded amino acid and carbohydrates with electrolytes, trace elements, and vitamins, including preparation, any strength, 52 to 73 grams of protein-premix

B4197   compounded amino acid and carbohydrates with electrolytes, trace elements and vitamins, including preparation, any strength, 74 to 100 grams of protein - premix

B4199   compounded amino acid and carbohydrates with electrolytes, trace elements and vitamins, including preparation, any strength, over 100 grams of protein - premix

B4216   Parenteral nutrition; additives (vitamins, trace elements, heparin, electrolytes) homemix per day

B4220   Parenteral nutrition supply kit; premix, per day

B4222   home mix, per day

B4224   Parenteral nutrition administration kit, per day

B5000   Parenteral nutrition solution: compounded amino acid and carbohydrates with electrolytes, trace elements, and vitamins, including preparation, any strength; renal - amirosyn RF, nephramine, renamine - premix

B5100   hepatic - freamine HBC, hepatamine - premix

B5200   stress - branch chain amino acids - premix

ENTERAL AND PARENTERAL PUMPS

B9000   Enteral nutrition infusion pump; without alarm

B9002   with alarm

B9004   Parenteral nutrition infusion pump; portable

B9006   stationary

B9998   NOC for enteral supplies

B9999   NOC for parenteral supplies

HOSPITAL OUTPATIENT PPS CODES

Guidelines

The "C" codes are unique temporary codes established by HCFA for use under the Hospital Outpatient Prospective Payment System (OPPS). Non-OPPS use of these codes for Medicare is not valid.

The purpose of the "C" codes is to provide hospitals with a list of codes and long descriptors for drugs, biologicals and devices eligible for transitional pass-through payments, and for items classified in "new technology" ambulatory payment classifications (APCs) under the new Hospital Outpatient Prospective Payment System (OPPS).

The listing of HCPCS codes in this section does not assure coverage of the specific item or service in a given case. To be eligible for pass-through and new technology payments, the items reported with "C" codes must be considered reasonable and necessary.

All of the "C" codes are used exclusively for services paid under the Hospital Outpatient Prospective Payment System and **may not be used to bill for services paid under other Medicare payment systems.**

In addition to the information presented above, several other items unique to this section are defined here:

1. **SPECIAL REPORT:** A service, material or supply that is rarely provided, unusual, variable or new may require a special report in determining medical appropriateness for reimbursement purposes. Pertinent information should include an adequate definition or description of the nature, extent, and need for the service, material or supply.

2. **MODIFIERS:** Listed services may be modified under certain circumstances. When appropriate, the modifying circumstance is identified by adding a modifier to the basic procedure code. CPT and HCPCS National Level II modifiers may be used with CPT and HCPCS National Level II procedure codes.

Hospital Outpatient PPS Codes

(C1000) Code deleted 2001

(C1001) Code deleted 2001

(C1003) Code deleted 2001

(C1004) Code deleted 2001

● C1005 Intraocular lens, sensar soft acrylic ultraviolet light absorbing posterior chamber intraocular lens

(C1006) Code deleted 2001

(C1007) Code deleted 2001

(C1008) Code deleted 2001

(C1009) Code deleted 2001

C1010 Blood, leukoreduced, cmv-negative, each unit

C1011 Platelet, HLA-matched leukoreduced, apheresis/pheresis, each unit

C1012 Platelet concentrate, leukoreduced, irradiated, each unit

C1013 Platelet concentrate, leukoreduced, each unit

C1014 Platelet, leukoreduced, apheresis/pheresis, each unit

C1016 Blood, leukoreduced, frozen/deglycerol/washed, each unit

C1017 Platelet, leukoreduced, cmv-negative, apheresis/pheresis, each unit

C1018 Blood, leukoreduced, irradiated, each unit

(C1019) Code deleted 2002

(C1024) Code deleted 2001

(C1025) Code deleted 2001

(C1026) Code deleted 2001

(C1027)   Code deleted 2001

(C1028)   Code deleted 2001

(C1029)   Code deleted 2001

(C1030)   Code deleted 2001

C1031   Electrode, needle, ablation, mr compatible leveen, modified leveen needle electrode

(C1033)   Code deleted 2001

(C1034)   Code deleted 2001

(C1035)   Code deleted 2001

(C1036)   Code deleted 2001

(C1037)   Code deleted 2001

(C1038)   Code deleted 2001

(C1039)   Code deleted 2001

(C1040)   Code deleted 2001

(C1042)   Code deleted 2001

(C1043)   Code deleted 2001

(C1045)   Code deleted 2001

(C1047)   Code deleted 2001

(C1048)   Code deleted 2001

(C1050)   Code deleted 2002

(C1051)   Code deleted 2001

(C1053)   Code deleted 2001

(C1054)   Code deleted 2001

(C1055)   Code deleted 2001

Not valid for Medicare   Non-covered by Medicare   Special coverage instructions   Carrier discretion   **43**

(C1056) Code deleted 2001

(C1057) Code deleted 2001

● C1058 Supply of radiopharmaceutical diagnostic imaging agent, technetium Tc 99m oxidronate, per vial

(C1059) Code deleted 2001

(C1060) Code deleted 2001

(C1061) Code deleted 2001

(C1063) Code deleted 2001

● C1064 Supply of radiopharmaceutical therapeutic imaging agent, sodium iodide i-131, capsule, each additional mci

● C1065 Supply of radiopharmaceutical therapeutic imaging agent, sodium iodide i-131, solution, each additional mci

● C1066 Supply of radiopharmaceutical diagnostic imaging agent, indium 111 satumomab pendetide, per vial

(C1067) Code deleted 2001

(C1068) Code deleted 2001

(C1069) Code deleted 2001

(C1071) Code deleted 2001

(C1072) Code deleted 2001

(C1073) Code deleted 2001

(C1074) Code deleted 2001

(C1075) Code deleted 2001

(C1076) Code deleted 2001

(C1077) Code deleted 2001

(C1078) Code deleted 2001

▲**C1079** Supply of radiopharmaceutical diagnostic imaging agent, cyanocobalamin CO 57/58, per 0.5 microcurie

(**C1084**) Code deleted 2001

(**C1086**) Code deleted 2001

▲**C1087** Supply of radiopharmaceutical diagnostic imaging agent, sodium iodide I-123 per 100 microcuries

C1088 Laser optic treatment system, indigo laseroptic treatment system

(**C1089**) Code deleted 2001

(**C1090**) Code deleted 2002

▲**C1091** Supply of radiopharmaceutical diagnostic imaging agent, indium 111 oxyquinoline, per 0.5 millicurie

▲**C1092** Supply of radiopharmaceutical diagnostic imaging agent, indium 111 pentetate, per 0.5 millicurie

▲**C1094** Supply of radiopharmaceutical diagnostic imaging agent, technetium Tc 99m albumin aggregated, per 1.0 millicurie

(**C1095**) Code deleted 2002

C1096 Supply of radiopharmaceutical diagnostic imaging agent, technetium Tc 99m exametazime, per dose

C1097 Supply of radiopharmaceutical diagnostic imaging agent, technetium Tc 99m mebrofenin, per vial

C1098 Supply of radiopharmaceutical diagnostic imaging agent, technetium Tc 99m pentetate, per vial

C1099 Supply of radiopharmaceutical diagnostic imaging agent, technetium Tc 99m pyrophosphate, per vial

(**C1100**) Code deleted 2001

(**C1101**) Code deleted 2001

(**C1102**) Code deleted 2001

(**C1103**) Code deleted 2001

(C1104) Code deleted 2001

(C1105) Code deleted 2001

(C1106) Code deleted 2001

(C1107) Code deleted 2001

(C1109) Code deleted 2001

(C1110) Code deleted 2001

(C1111) Code deleted 2001

(C1112) Code deleted 2001

(C1113) Code deleted 2001

(C1114) Code deleted 2001

(C1115) Code deleted 2001

(C1116) Code deleted 2001

(C1117) Code deleted 2001

(C1118) Code deleted 2001

(C1119) Code deleted 2001

(C1120) Code deleted 2001

(C1121) Code deleted 2001

C1122 Supply of radiopharmaceutical diagnostic imaging agent, technetium Tc 99m arcitumomab, per vial

(C1123) Code deleted 2001

(C1124) Code deleted 2001

(C1125) Code deleted 2001

(C1126) Code deleted 2001

(C1127) Code deleted 2001

(C1128)   Code deleted 2001

(C1129)   Code deleted 2001

(C1130)   Code deleted 2001

(C1131)   Code deleted 2001

(C1132)   Code deleted 2001

(C1133)   Code deleted 2001

(C1134)   Code deleted 2001

(C1135)   Code deleted 2001

(C1136)   Code deleted 2001

(C1137)   Code deleted 2001

(C1143)   Code deleted 2001

(C1144)   Code deleted 2001

(C1145)   Code deleted 2001

C1146   Endotracheal tube, vett tracheobronchial tube

(C1147)   Code deleted 2001

(C1148)   Code deleted 2001

(C1149)   Code deleted 2001

(C1151)   Code deleted 2001

(C1152)   Code deleted 2001

(C1153)   Code deleted 2001

(C1154)   Code deleted 2001

(C1155)   Code deleted 2001

(C1156)   Code deleted 2001

(C1157)   Code deleted 2001

(C1158) Code deleted 2001

(C1159) Code deleted 2001

(C1160) Code deleted 2001

(C1161) Code deleted 2001

(C1162) Code deleted 2001

(C1163) Code deleted 2001

(C1164) Code deleted 2001

C1166 Injection, cytarabine liposome, 10 mg, depocyt/liposomal cytarabine

C1167 Injection, epirubicin hydrochloride, 2 mg

C1170 Biopsy device, breast, abbi device

(C1171) Code deleted 2001

(C1172) Code deleted 2001

(C1173) Code deleted 2001

(C1174) Code deleted 2001

C1175 Biopsy device, mibb device

C1176 Biopsy device, mammotome hh hand-held probe with smartvac vacuum system

C1177 Biopsy device, 11-gauge mammotome probe with vacuum cannister

C1178 Injection, busulfan (busulfex iv) per 6 mg

C1179 Biopsy device, 14-gauge mammotome probe with vacuum cannister

(C1180) Code deleted 2001

(C1181) Code deleted 2001

(C1182) Code deleted 2001

(C1183)   Code deleted 2001

(C1184)   Code deleted 2001

▲ C1188   Supply of radiopharmaceutical therapeutic imaging agent, sodium iodide i-131, capsule, per initial 1-5 mci

C1200   Supply of radiopharmaceutical diagnostic imaging agent, technetium Tc 99m sodium glucoheptonate, per vial

C1201   Supply of radiopharmaceutical diagnostic imaging agent, technetium Tc 99m succimer, per vial

C1202   Supply of radiopharmaceutical diagnostic imaging agent, technetium Tc 99m sulfur colloid, per dose

(C1203)   Code deleted 2001

(C1205)   Code deleted 2001

C1207   Octreotide acetate, 1 mg

C1300   Hyperbaric oxygen under pressure, full body chamber, per 30 minute interval

(C1302)   Code deleted 2001

(C1303)   Code deleted 2001

(C1304)   Code deleted 2001

C1305   Apligraf, per 44 square centimeters

(C1306)   Code deleted 2001

(C1311)   Code deleted 2001

(C1312)   Code deleted 2001

(C1313)   Code deleted 2001

(C1314)   Code deleted 2001

(C1315)   Code deleted 2001

(C1316)   Code deleted 2001

(C1317) Code deleted 2001

(C1318) Code deleted 2001

(C1319) Code deleted 2001

(C1320) Code deleted 2001

C1321 Electrode, disposable, palate somnoplasty coagulating electrode, base of tongue somnoplasty coagulating electrode

C1322 Electrode, disposable, turbinate somnoplasty coagulating electrode

C1323 Electrode, disposable, vapr electrode, vapr t thermal electrode

C1324 Electrode, disposable, ligasure disposable electrode

(C1325) Code deleted 2001

(C1326) Code deleted 2001

(C1328) Code deleted 2001

C1329 Electrode, disposable, gynecare versapoint resectoscopic system bipolar electrode

(C1333) Code deleted 2001

(C1334) Code deleted 2001

(C1335) Code deleted 2001

(C1336) Code deleted 2001

(C1337) Code deleted 2001

▲**C1348** Supply of radiopharmaceutical therapeutic imaging agent, sodium iodide i-131, solution, per initial 1-6 mci

(C1350) Code deleted 2001

(C1351) Code deleted 2001

(C1352) Code deleted 2001

(C1353)   Code deleted 2001

(C1354)   Code deleted 2001

(C1355)   Code deleted 2001

(C1356)   Code deleted 2001

(C1357)   Code deleted 2001

(C1358)   Code deleted 2001

(C1359)   Code deleted 2001

(C1360)   Code deleted 2001

(C1361)   Code deleted 2001

(C1362)   Code deleted 2001

(C1363)   Code deleted 2001

(C1364)   Code deleted 2001

(C1365)   Code deleted 2001

(C1366)   Code deleted 2001

(C1367)   Code deleted 2001

C1368   Infusion system, on-q pain management system, on-q soaker pain management system, and painbuster pain management system. NOTE: the on-q pain management system, on-q soaker pain management system, and painbuster pain management system are effective August 1, 2000.

(C1369)   Code deleted 2001

(C1370)   Code deleted 2001

(C1371)   Code deleted 2001

(C1372)   Code deleted 2001

(C1375)   Code deleted 2001

(C1376) Code deleted 2001

(C1377) Code deleted 2001

(C1378) Code deleted 2001

(C1379) Code deleted 2001

(C1420) Code deleted 2001

(C1421) Code deleted 2001

(C1450) Code deleted 2001

(C1451) Code deleted 2001

(C1500) Code deleted 2001

● C1531   Stent, colorectal, Bard Memotherm colorectal stent model S30R060

(C1700) Code deleted 2001

(C1701) Code deleted 2001

(C1702) Code deleted 2001

(C1703) Code deleted 2001

(C1704) Code deleted 2001

(C1705) Code deleted 2001

(C1706) Code deleted 2001

(C1707) Code deleted 2001

(C1708) Code deleted 2001

(C1709) Code deleted 2001

(C1710) Code deleted 2001

(C1711) Code deleted 2001

(C1712) Code deleted 2001

● **C1713** Anchor/screw for opposing bone-to-bone or soft tissue-to bone (implantable)

● **C1714** Catheter, transluminal atherectomy, directional

● **C1715** Brachytherapy needle

● **C1716** Brachytherapy seed, gold 198

● **C1717** Brachytherapy seed, high dose rate iridium 192

● **C1718** Brachytherapy seed, iodine 125

● **C1719** Brachytherapy seed, non-high dose rate iridium 192

● **C1720** Brachytherapy seed, palladium 103

● **C1721** Cardioverter-defibrillator, dual chamber (implantable)

● **C1722** Cardioverter-defibrillator, single chamber (implantable)

(C1723) Code deleted 2002

● **C1724** Catheter, transluminal atherectomy, rotational

● **C1725** Catheter, transluminal angioplasty, non-laser (may include guidance, infusion/perfusion capability)

● **C1726** Catheter, balloon dilatation, non-vascular

● **C1727** Catheter, balloon tissue dissector, non-vascular (insertable)

● **C1728** Catheter, brachytherapy seed administration

● **C1729** Catheter, drainage

● **C1730** Catheter, electrophysiology, diagnostic, other than 3D mapping (19 or fewer electrodes)

● **C1731** Catheter, electrophysiology, diagnostic, other than 3D mapping (20 or more electrodes)

● **C1732** Catheter, electrophysiology, diagnostic/ablation, 3D or vector mapping

● **C1733** Catheter, electrophysiology, diagnostic/ablation, other than 3D or vector mapping, other than cool-tip

● **C1750**   Catheter, hemodialysis, long-term

● **C1751**   Catheter, infusion, inserted peripherally, centrally or midline (other than hemodialysis)

● **C1752**   Catheter, hemodialysis, short-term

● **C1753**   Catheter, intravascular ultrasound

● **C1754**   Catheter, intradiscal

● **C1755**   Catheter, intraspinal

● **C1756**   Catheter, pacing, transesophageal

● **C1757**   Catheter, thrombectomy/embolectomy

● **C1758**   Catheter, ureteral

● **C1759**   Catheter, intracardiac echocardiography

● **C1760**   Closure device, vascular (implantable/insertable)

● **C1762**   Connective tissue, human (includes fascia lata)

● **C1763**   Connective tissue, non-human (includes synthetic)

● **C1764**   Event recorder, cardiac (implantable)

● **C1765**   Adhesion barrier

● **C1766**   Introducer/sheath, guiding, intracardiac electrophysiological, steerable, other than peel-away

● **C1767**   Generator, neurostimulator (implantable)

● **C1768**   Graft, vascular

● **C1769**   Guide wire

● **C1770**   Imaging coil, magnetic resonance (insertable)

● **C1771**   Repair device, urinary, incontinence, with sling graft

● **C1772**   Infusion pump, programmable (implantable)

---

54   ● New code   ▲ Revised code   ( ) Deleted code

● **C1773** Retrieval device, insertable (used to retrieve fractured medical devices)

● **C1776** Joint device (implantable)

● **C1777** Lead, cardioverter-defibrillator, endocardial single coil (implantable)

● **C1778** Lead, neurostimulator (implantable)

● **C1779** Lead, pacemaker, transvenous vdd single pass

● **C1780** Lens, intraocular (new technology)

● **C1781** Mesh (implantable)

● **C1782** Morcellator

● **C1784** Ocular device, intraoperative, detached retina

● **C1785** Pacemaker, dual chamber, rate-responsive (implantable)

● **C1786** Pacemaker, single chamber, rate-responsive (implantable)

● **C1787** Patient programmer, neurostimulator

● **C1788** Port, indwelling (implantable)

● **C1789** Prosthesis, breast (implantable)

  (C1790) Code deleted 2001

  (C1791) Code deleted 2001

  (C1792) Code deleted 2001

  (C1793) Code deleted 2001

  (C1794) Code deleted 2001

  (C1795) Code deleted 2001

  (C1796) Code deleted 2001

  (C1797) Code deleted 2001

  (C1798) Code deleted 2001

Not valid for Medicare   Non-covered by Medicare   Special coverage instructions   Carrier discretion   **55**

(C1799) Code deleted 2001

(C1800) Code deleted 2001

(C1801) Code deleted 2001

(C1802) Code deleted 2001

(C1803) Code deleted 2001

(C1804) Code deleted 2001

(C1805) Code deleted 2001

(C1806) Code deleted 2001

(C1810) Code deleted 2001

(C1811) Code deleted 2001

(C1812) Code deleted 2001

● **C1813** Prosthesis, penile, inflatable

● **C1815** Prosthesis, urinary sphincter (implantable)

● **C1816** Receiver and/or transmitter, neurostimulator (implantable)

● **C1817** Septal defect implant system, intracardiac

(C1850) Code deleted 2001

(C1851) Code deleted 2001

(C1852) Code deleted 2001

(C1853) Code deleted 2001

(C1854) Code deleted 2001

(C1855) Code deleted 2001

(C1856) Code deleted 2001

(C1857) Code deleted 2001

(C1858) Code deleted 2001

(C1859) Code deleted 2001

(C1860) Code deleted 2001

(C1861) Code deleted 2001

(C1862) Code deleted 2001

(C1863) Code deleted 2001

(C1864) Code deleted 2001

(C1865) Code deleted 2001

(C1866) Code deleted 2001

(C1867) Code deleted 2001

(C1868) Code deleted 2001

(C1869) Code deleted 2001

(C1870) Code deleted 2001

(C1871) Code deleted 2001

(C1872) Code deleted 2001

(C1873) Code deleted 2001

● **C1874** Stent, coated/covered, with delivery system

● **C1875** Stent, coated/covered, without delivery system

● **C1876** Stent, non-coated/non-covered, with delivery system

● **C1877** Stent, non-coated/non-covered, without delivery system

● **C1878** Material for vocal cord medialization, synthetic (implantable)

● **C1879** Tissue marker (implantable)

● **C1880** Vena cava filter

● **C1881** Dialysis access system (implantable)

● **C1882**   Cardioverter-defibrillator, other than single or dual chamber (implantable)

● **C1883**   Adaptor/extension, pacing lead or neurostimulator lead (implantable)

● **C1885**   Catheter, transluminal angioplasty, laser

● **C1887**   Catheter, guiding (may include infusion/perfusion capability)

● **C1891**   Infusion pump, non-programmable, permanent (implantable)

● **C1892**   Introducer/sheath, guiding, intracardiac electrophysiological, fixed-curve, peel-away

● **C1893**   Introducer/sheath, guiding, intracardiac electrophysiological, fixed-curve, other than peel-away

● **C1894**   Introducer/sheath, other than guiding, intracardiac electrophysiological, non-laser

● **C1895**   Lead, cardioverter-defibrillator, endocardial dual coil (implantable)

● **C1896**   Lead, cardioverter-defibrillator, other than endocardial single or dual coil (implantable)

● **C1897**   Lead, neurostimulator test kit (implantable)

● **C1898**   Lead, pacemaker, other than transvenous vdd single pass

● **C1899**   Lead, pacemaker/cardioverter-defibrillator combination (implantable)

(C1929)   Code deleted 2001

(C1930)   Code deleted 2001

(C1931)   Code deleted 2001

(C1932)   Code deleted 2001

(C1933)   Code deleted 2001

(C1934)   Code deleted 2001

(C1935) Code deleted 2001

(C1936) Code deleted 2001

(C1937) Code deleted 2001

(C1938) Code deleted 2001

(C1939) Code deleted 2001

(C1940) Code deleted 2001

(C1941) Code deleted 2001

(C1942) Code deleted 2001

(C1943) Code deleted 2001

(C1944) Code deleted 2001

(C1945) Code deleted 2001

(C1946) Code deleted 2001

(C1947) Code deleted 2001

(C1948) Code deleted 2001

(C1949) Code deleted 2001

(C1979) Code deleted 2001

(C1980) Code deleted 2001

(C1981) Code deleted 2001

(C2000) Code deleted 2001

(C2001) Code deleted 2001

(C2002) Code deleted 2001

(C2003) Code deleted 2001

(C2004) Code deleted 2001

(C2005) Code deleted 2001

(C2006) Code deleted 2001

(C2007) Code deleted 2001

(C2008) Code deleted 2001

(C2009) Code deleted 2001

(C2010) Code deleted 2001

(C2011) Code deleted 2001

(C2012) Code deleted 2001

(C2013) Code deleted 2001

(C2014) Code deleted 2001

(C2015) Code deleted 2001

(C2016) Code deleted 2001

(C2017) Code deleted 2001

(C2018) Code deleted 2001

(C2019) Code deleted 2001

(C2020) Code deleted 2001

(C2021) Code deleted 2001

(C2022) Code deleted 2001

(C2023) Code deleted 2001

(C2100) Code deleted 2001

(C2101) Code deleted 2001

(C2102) Code deleted 2001

(C2103) Code deleted 2001

(C2104) Code deleted 2001

(C2151) Code deleted 2001

(C2152)   Code deleted 2001

(C2153)   Code deleted 2001

(C2200)   Code deleted 2001

(C2300)   Code deleted 2001

(C2597)   Code deleted 2001

(C2598)   Code deleted 2001

(C2599)   Code deleted 2001

C2600   Catheter, gold probe single-use electrohemostasis catheter

(C2601)   Code deleted 2001

(C2602)   Code deleted 2001

(C2603)   Code deleted 2001

(C2604)   Code deleted 2001

(C2605)   Code deleted 2001

(C2606)   Code deleted 2001

(C2607)   Code deleted 2001

(C2608)   Code deleted 2001

(C2609)   Code deleted 2001

(C2610)   Code deleted 2001

(C2611)   Code deleted 2001

(C2612)   Code deleted 2001

● **C2615**   Sealant, pulmonary, liquid

● **C2616**   Brachytherapy seed, yttrium-90

● **C2617**   Stent, non-coronary, without delivery system

● **C2618**   Probe, cryoablation

| | Not valid for Medicare | | Non-covered by Medicare | | Special coverage instructions | | Carrier discretion | **61** |

● **C2619**   Pacemaker, dual chamber, non rate-responsive (implantable)

● **C2620**   Pacemaker, single chamber, non rate-responsive (implantable)

● **C2621**   Pacemaker, other than single or dual chamber (implantable)

● **C2622**   Prosthesis, penile, non-inflatable

● **C2625**   Stent, non-coronary, temporary, with delivery system

● **C2626**   Infusion pump, non-programmable, temporary (implantable)

● **C2627**   Catheter, suprapubic/cystoscopic

● **C2628**   Catheter, occlusion

● **C2629**   Introducer/sheath, other than guiding, intracardiac electrophysiological, laser

● **C2630**   Catheter, electrophysiology, diagnostic/ablation, other than 3D or vector mapping, cool-tip

● **C2631**   Repair device, urinary, incontinence, without sling graft

(C2676)   Code deleted 2001

(C2700)   Code deleted 2001

(C2701)   Code deleted 2001

(C2702)   Code deleted 2001

(C2703)   Code deleted 2001

(C2704)   Code deleted 2001

(C2801)   Code deleted 2001

(C2802)   Code deleted 2001

(C2803)   Code deleted 2001

(C2804)   Code deleted 2001

(C2805) Code deleted 2001

(C2806) Code deleted 2001

(C2807) Code deleted 2001

(C2808) Code deleted 2001

(C3001) Code deleted 2001

(C3002) Code deleted 2001

(C3003) Code deleted 2001

(C3004) Code deleted 2001

(C3400) Code deleted 2001

(C3401) Code deleted 2001

(C3500) Code deleted 2001

(C3510) Code deleted 2001

(C3551) Code deleted 2001

(C3552) Code deleted 2001

(C3553) Code deleted 2001

(C3554) Code deleted 2001

(C3555) Code deleted 2001

(C3556) Code deleted 2001

(C3557) Code deleted 2001

(C3800) Code deleted 2001

(C3801) Code deleted 2001

(C3851) Code deleted 2001

(C4000) Code deleted 2001

(C4001) Code deleted 2001

(C4002) Code deleted 2001

(C4003) Code deleted 2001

(C4004) Code deleted 2001

(C4005) Code deleted 2001

(C4006) Code deleted 2001

(C4007) Code deleted 2001

(C4008) Code deleted 2001

(C4009) Code deleted 2001

(C4300) Code deleted 2001

(C4301) Code deleted 2001

(C4302) Code deleted 2001

(C4303) Code deleted 2001

(C4304) Code deleted 2001

(C4305) Code deleted 2001

(C4306) Code deleted 2001

(C4307) Code deleted 2001

(C4308) Code deleted 2001

(C4309) Code deleted 2001

(C4310) Code deleted 2001

(C4311) Code deleted 2001

(C4312) Code deleted 2001

(C4313) Code deleted 2001

(C4314) Code deleted 2001

(C4315) Code deleted 2001

(**C4316**)   Code deleted 2001

(**C4317**)   Code deleted 2001

(**C4600**)   Code deleted 2001

(**C4601**)   Code deleted 2001

(**C4602**)   Code deleted 2001

(**C4603**)   Code deleted 2001

(**C4604**)   Code deleted 2001

(**C4605**)   Code deleted 2001

(**C4606**)   Code deleted 2001

(**C4607**)   Code deleted 2001

(**C5000**)   Code deleted 2001

(**C5001**)   Code deleted 2001

(**C5002**)   Code deleted 2001

(**C5003**)   Code deleted 2001

(**C5004**)   Code deleted 2001

(**C5005**)   Code deleted 2001

(**C5006**)   Code deleted 2001

(**C5007**)   Code deleted 2001

(**C5008**)   Code deleted 2001

(**C5009**)   Code deleted 2001

(**C5010**)   Code deleted 2001

(**C5011**)   Code deleted 2001

(**C5012**)   Code deleted 2001

(**C5013**)   Code deleted 2001

(C5014) Code deleted 2001

(C5015) Code deleted 2001

(C5016) Code deleted 2001

(C5017) Code deleted 2001

(C5018) Code deleted 2001

(C5019) Code deleted 2001

(C5020) Code deleted 2001

(C5021) Code deleted 2001

(C5022) Code deleted 2001

(C5023) Code deleted 2001

(C5024) Code deleted 2001

(C5025) Code deleted 2001

(C5026) Code deleted 2001

(C5027) Code deleted 2001

(C5028) Code deleted 2001

(C5029) Code deleted 2001

(C5030) Code deleted 2001

(C5031) Code deleted 2001

(C5032) Code deleted 2001

(C5033) Code deleted 2001

(C5034) Code deleted 2001

(C5035) Code deleted 2001

(C5036) Code deleted 2001

(C5037) Code deleted 2001

(C5038) Code deleted 2001

(C5039) Code deleted 2001

(C5040) Code deleted 2001

(C5041) Code deleted 2001

(C5042) Code deleted 2001

(C5043) Code deleted 2001

(C5044) Code deleted 2001

(C5045) Code deleted 2001

(C5046) Code deleted 2001

(C5047) Code deleted 2001

(C5048) Code deleted 2001

(C5130) Code deleted 2001

(C5131) Code deleted 2001

(C5132) Code deleted 2001

(C5133) Code deleted 2001

(C5134) Code deleted 2001

(C5279) Code deleted 2001

(C5280) Code deleted 2001

(C5281) Code deleted 2001

(C5282) Code deleted 2001

(C5283) Code deleted 2001

(C5284) Code deleted 2001

(C5600) Code deleted 2001

(C5601) Code deleted 2001

(C6001) Code deleted 2001

(C6002) Code deleted 2001

(C6003) Code deleted 2001

(C6004) Code deleted 2001

(C6005) Code deleted 2001

(C6006) Code deleted 2001

(C6012) Code deleted 2001

(C6013) Code deleted 2001

(C6014) Code deleted 2001

(C6015) Code deleted 2001

(C6016) Code deleted 2001

(C6017) Code deleted 2001

(C6018) Code deleted 2001

(C6019) Code deleted 2001

(C6020) Code deleted 2001

(C6021) Code deleted 2001

(C6022) Code deleted 2001

(C6023) Code deleted 2001

(C6024) Code deleted 2001

(C6025) Code deleted 2001

(C6026) Code deleted 2001

(C6027) Code deleted 2001

(C6028) Code deleted 2001

(C6029) Code deleted 2001

(**C6030**) Code deleted 2001

(**C6031**) Code deleted 2001

(**C6032**) Code deleted 2001

(**C6033**) Code deleted 2001

(**C6034**) Code deleted 2001

(**C6035**) Code deleted 2001

(**C6036**) Code deleted 2001

(**C6037**) Code deleted 2001

(**C6038**) Code deleted 2001

(**C6039**) Code deleted 2001

(**C6040**) Code deleted 2001

(**C6041**) Code deleted 2001

(**C6050**) Code deleted 2001

(**C6051**) Code deleted 2001

(**C6052**) Code deleted 2001

(**C6053**) Code deleted 2001

(**C6054**) Code deleted 2001

(**C6055**) Code deleted 2001

(**C6056**) Code deleted 2001

(**C6057**) Code deleted 2001

(**C6058**) Code deleted 2001

(**C6080**) Code deleted 2001

(**C6200**) Code deleted 2001

(**C6201**) Code deleted 2001

Not valid
for Medicare

Non-covered
by Medicare

Special
coverage
instructions

Carrier
discretion

69

(C6202) Code deleted 2001

(C6203) Code deleted 2001

(C6204) Code deleted 2001

(C6205) Code deleted 2001

(C6206) Code deleted 2001

(C6207) Code deleted 2001

(C6208) Code deleted 2001

(C6209) Code deleted 2001

(C6210) Code deleted 2001

(C6300) Code deleted 2001

(C6500) Code deleted 2001

(C6501) Code deleted 2001

(C6502) Code deleted 2001

(C6525) Code deleted 2001

(C6600) Code deleted 2001

(C6650) Code deleted 2001

(C6651) Code deleted 2001

(C6652) Code deleted 2001

(C6700) Code deleted 2001

(C8099) Code deleted 2001

(C8100) Code deleted 2001

(C8102) Code deleted 2001

(C8103) Code deleted 2001

(C8500) Code deleted 2001

(C8501) Code deleted 2001

(C8502) Code deleted 2001

(C8503) Code deleted 2001

(C8504) Code deleted 2001

(C8505) Code deleted 2001

(C8506) Code deleted 2001

(C8507) Code deleted 2001

(C8508) Code deleted 2001

(C8509) Code deleted 2001

(C8510) Code deleted 2001

(C8511) Code deleted 2001

(C8512) Code deleted 2001

(C8513) Code deleted 2001

(C8514) Code deleted 2001

● **C8515** Prosthesis, penile, Mentor Alpha I narrow-base inflatable penile prosthesis

(C8516) Code deleted 2001

● **C8517** Prosthesis, penile, Ambicor penile prosthesis

(C8518) Code deleted 2001

(C8519) Code deleted 2001

(C8520) Code deleted 2001

(C8521) Code deleted 2001

(C8522) Code deleted 2001

(C8523) Code deleted 2001

(C8524)   Code deleted 2001

(C8525)   Code deleted 2001

(C8526)   Code deleted 2001

(C8528)   Code deleted 2001

(C8529)   Code deleted 2001

(C8530)   Code deleted 2001

(C8531)   Code deleted 2001

(C8532)   Code deleted 2001

(C8533)   Code deleted 2001

(C8534)   Code deleted 2001

(C8535)   Code deleted 2001

(C8536)   Code deleted 2001

(C8539)   Code deleted 2001

(C8540)   Code deleted 2001

(C8541)   Code deleted 2001

(C8542)   Code deleted 2001

(C8543)   Code deleted 2001

(C8550)   Code deleted 2001

(C8551)   Code deleted 2001

(C8552)   Code deleted 2001

(C8597)   Code deleted 2001

(C8598)   Code deleted 2001

(C8599)   Code deleted 2001

(C8600)   Code deleted 2001

(C8650) Code deleted 2001

(C8724) Code deleted 2001

(C8725) Code deleted 2001

(C8748) Code deleted 2001

(C8749) Code deleted 2001

(C8750) Code deleted 2001

(C8775) Code deleted 2001

(C8776) Code deleted 2001

(C8777) Code deleted 2001

(C8800) Code deleted 2001

(C8801) Code deleted 2001

(C8802) Code deleted 2001

(C8830) Code deleted 2001

(C8890) Code deleted 2001

(C8891) Code deleted 2001

● **C8900** Magnetic resonance angiography with contrast, abdomen

● **C8901** Magnetic resonance angiography without contrast, abdomen

● **C8902** Magnetic resonance angiography without contrast followed by with contrast, abdomen

● **C8903** Magnetic resonance imaging with contrast, breast; unilateral

● **C8904** Magnetic resonance imaging without contrast, breast; unilateral

● **C8905** Magnetic resonance imaging without contrast followed by with contrast, breast; unilateral

● **C8906** Magnetic resonance imaging with contrast, breast; bilateral

● **C8907** Magnetic resonance imaging without contrast, breast; bilateral

● **C8908** Magnetic resonance imaging without contrast followed by with contrast, breast; bilateral

● **C8909** Magnetic resonance angiography with contrast, chest (excluding myocardium)

● **C8910** Magnetic resonance angiography without contrast, chest (excluding myocardium)

● **C8911** Magnetic resonance angiography without contrast followed by with contrast, chest (excluding myocardium)

● **C8912** Magnetic resonance angiography with contrast, lower extremity

● **C8913** Magnetic resonance angiography without contrast, lower extremity

● **C8914** Magnetic resonance angiography without contrast followed by with contrast, lower extremity

C9000 Injection, sodium chromate cr51, per 0.25 mci

(C9001) Code deleted 2002

(C9002) Code deleted 2002

C9003 Palivizumab-rsv-igm, per 50 mg

(C9004) Code deleted 2002

(C9005) Code deleted 2001

(C9006) Code deleted 2002

C9007 Baclofen intrathecal screening kit (1 amp)

C9008 Baclofen intrathecal refill kit, per 500 mcg

C9009 Baclofen refill kit, per 2000 mcg

C9010 Baclofen intrathecal refill kit, per 4000 mcg

(C9011)   Code deleted 2002

(C9012)   Code deleted 2002

● **C9013**   Supply of co 57 cobaltous chloride, radiopharmaceutical diagnostic imaging agent

(C9017)   Code deleted 2001

(C9018)   Code deleted 2002

● **C9019**   Injection, caspofungin acetate, 5 mg

● **C9020**   Sirolimus tablet, 1 mg

C9100   Supply of radiopharmaceutical diagnostic imaging agent, iodinated i-131 Albumin, per mci

C9102   Supply of radiopharmaceutical diagnostic imaging agent, 51 sodium chromate, per 50 mci

C9103   Supply of radiopharmaceutical diagnostic imaging agent, sodium iothalamate i-125 injection, per 10 uci

(C9104)   Code deleted 2002

C9105   Injection, hepatitis B immune globulin, per 1 ml

(C9106)   Code deleted 2001

(C9107)   Code deleted 2001

● **C9108**   Injection, thyrotropin alpha, 1.1 mg

● **C9109**   Injection, tirofiban hydrochloride, 6.25 mg

● **C9110**   Alemtuzumab, per 10 mg/ml

● **C9111**   Injection, bivalirudin, 250 mg per vial

● **C9112**   Injection, perflutren lipid microsphere, per 2 ml vial

● **C9113**   Injection, pantoprazole sodium, per vial

● **C9114**   Injection, nesiritide, per 1.5 mg vial

● **C9115**   Injection, zoledronic acid, per 2 mg

● **C9200**   Orcel, per 36 square centimeters

● **C9201**   Dermagraft, per 37.5 square centimeters

  (C9500)   Code deleted 2001

  (C9501)   Code deleted 2001

  (C9502)   Code deleted 2001

  C9503   Fresh frozen plasma, donor retested, each unit

  (C9504)   Code deleted 2001

  (C9505)   Code deleted 2001

  (C9506)   Code deleted 2002

  (C9700)   Code deleted 2002

  C9701   Stretta system

  (C9702)   Code deleted 2002

● **C9703**   Bard endoscopic suturing system

● **C9708**   Preview treatment planning software

● **C9711**   H.E.L.P. apheresis system

DENTAL PROCEDURES

Guidelines

In addition to the information presented in the INTRODUCTION, several other items unique to this section are defined or identified here:

1. **SUBSECTION INFORMATION:** Some of the listed subheadings or subsections have special needs or instructions unique to that section. Where these are indicated, special "notes" will be presented preceding or following the listings. Those subsections within the DENTAL PROCEDURES section that have "notes" are as follows:

Subsection	Code Numbers
Root canal therapy	D3310-D3350
Surgical services	D4210-D4274
Complete dentures	D5110-D5140
Partial dentures	D5211-D5281
Extraoral prostheses	D5911-D5921
Prosthodontics, fixed	D6200-D6999
Oral surgery	D7000-D7999
Complicated suturing	D7911-D7912
Professional consultation	D9310

2. **UNLISTED SERVICE OR PROCEDURE:** A service or procedure may be provided that is not listed in this edition of HCPCS. When reporting such a service, the appropriate "unlisted procedure" code may be used to indicate the service, identifying it by "special report" as defined below. HCPCS terminology is inconsistent in defining unlisted procedures. The procedure definition may include the term(s) "unlisted", "not otherwise classified", "unspecified", "unclassified", "other" and "miscellaneous". Prior to using these codes, try to determine if a Local Level III code or CPT code is available. The "unlisted procedures" and accompanying codes for DENTAL PROCEDURES are as follows:

D0502	Other oral pathology procedures, by report
D0999	Unspecified diagnostic procedure, by report
D2999	Unspecified restorative procedure, by report
D3999	Unspecified endodontic procedure, by report
D4999	Unspecified periodontal procedure, by report
D5899	Unspecified removable prosthodontic procedure, by report
D5999	Unspecified maxillofacial prosthesis, by report
D6199	Unspecified implant procedure, by report

D CODES

Not valid for Medicare   Non-covered by Medicare   Special coverage instructions   Carrier discretion

D6999	Unspecified, fixed prosthodontic procedure, by report
D7899	Unspecified TMD therapy, by report
D7999	Unspecified oral surgery procedure, by report
D8999	Unspecified orthodontic procedure, by report
D9999	Unspecified adjunctive procedure, by report

3. **SPECIAL REPORT:** A service, material or supply that is rarely provided, unusual, variable or new may require a special report in determining medical appropriateness for reimbursement purposes. Pertinent information should include an adequate definition or description of the nature, extent, and need for the service, material or supply.

4. **MODIFIERS:** Listed services may be modified under certain circumstances. When appropriate, the modifying circumstance is identified by adding a modifier to the basic procedure code. CPT and HCPCS National Level II modifiers may be used with CPT and HCPCS National Level II procedure codes. Modifiers commonly used with DENTAL PROCEDURES are as follows:

-CC Procedure code change (use "CC" when the procedure code submitted was changed either for administrative reasons or because an incorrect code was filed)

-ET Emergency services (dental procedures performed in emergency situations should show the modifier -ET)

-LT Left side (used to identify procedures performed on the left side of the body)

-QB Physician providing service in a rural HPSA

-QU Physician providing service in an urban HPSA

-RT Right side (used to identify procedures performed on the right side of the body)

-TC Technical component. Under certain circumstances, a charge may be made for the technical component alone. Under these circumstances, the technical component charge is identified by adding the modifier -TC to the usual procedure number. Technical component charges are institutional charges and not billed separately by physicians. However, portable x-ray suppliers only bill for technical component and should utilize modifier -TC. The charge data from portable x-ray suppliers will then be used to build customary and prevailing profiles.

5. **CPT CODE CROSS-REFERENCE:** Unless specified otherwise, there are no equivalent CPT codes for listings in this section.

6. **CDT CODES:** Dental procedures are reported to non-Medicare carriers using Common Dental Terminology (CDT), published by the American Dental Association (ADA).

Dental Procedures

I. DIAGNOSTIC PROCEDURES (D0100-D0999)

CLINICAL ORAL EXAMINATIONS

D0120 Periodic oral evaluation

D0140 Limited oral evaluation - problem focused

D0150 Comprehensive oral evaluation

D0160 Detailed and extensive oral evaluation - problem focused, by report

D0170 Re-evaluation - limited, problem focused (established patient; not post-operative visit)

RADIOGRAPHS/DIAGNOSTIC IMAGING

D0210 Intraoral; complete series (including bitewings)

D0220 periapical - first film

D0230 periapical - each additional film

D0240 occlusal film

D0250 Extraoral; first film

D0260 each additional film

D0270 Bitewing(s); single film

D0272 two films

D0274 four films

D0277 Vertical bitewings; 7 to 8 films

Not valid for Medicare	Non-covered by Medicare	Special coverage instructions	Carrier discretion

D0290 Posterior-anterior or lateral skull and facial bone, survey film

D0310 Sialography

D0320 Temporomandibular joint arthrogram, including injection

D0321 Other temporomandibular joint films, by report

D0322 Tomographic survey

D0330 Panoramic film

D0340 Cephalometric film

D0350 Oral/facial images (includes intra and extraoral images)

TESTS AND LABORATORY EXAMINATIONS

D0415 Bacteriologic studies for determination of pathologic agents

D0425 Caries susceptibility tests

D0460 Pulp vitality tests

D0470 Diagnostic casts

(D0471) Code deleted 2000

ORAL PATHOLOGY LABORATORY (USE CODES D0472-D0474)

D0472 Accession of tissue; gross examination, preparation and transmission of written report

D0473 gross and microscopic examination, preparation and transmission of written report

D0474 gross and microscopic examination, including assessment of surgical margins for presence of disease, preparation and transmission of written report

D0480 Processing and interpretation of cytologic smears, including the preparation and transmission of written report

D0501 Histopathologic examinations

D0502 Other oral pathology procedures, by report

D0999 Unspecified diagnostic procedure, by report

II. PREVENTIVE (D1000-D1999)

DENTAL PROPHYLAXIS

D1110 Prophylaxis; adult

D1120 child

TOPICAL FLUORIDE TREATMENT (OFFICE PROCEDURE)

D1201 Topical application of fluoride (including prophylaxis); child

D1203 Topical application of fluoride (prophylaxis not included); child

D1204 adult

D1205 Topical application of fluoride (including prophylaxis); adult

OTHER PREVENTIVE SERVICES

D1310 Nutritional counseling for control of dental disease

D1320 Tobacco counseling for the control and prevention of oral disease

D1330 Oral hygiene instructions

D1351 Sealant - per tooth

SPACE MAINTENANCE (PASSIVE APPLIANCES)

D1510 Space maintainer; fixed-unilateral

D1515 fixed-bilateral

D1520 removable-unilateral

D1525   removable-bilateral

D1550   Recementation of space maintainer

III. RESTORATIVE PROCEDURES (D2000-D2999)

AMALGAM RESTORATIONS (INCLUDING POLISHING)

D2110   Amalgam; one surface, primary

D2120   two surfaces, primary

D2130   three surfaces, primary

D2131   four or more surfaces, primary

D2140   one surface, permanent

D2150   two surfaces, permanent

D2160   three surfaces, permanent

D2161   four or more surfaces, permanent

SILICATE RESTORATIONS

(D2210)   Code deleted 2000

RESIN-BASED COMPOSITE RESTORATIONS

D2330   Resin-based composite; one surface, anterior

D2331   two surfaces, anterior

D2332   three surfaces, anterior

D2335   four or more surfaces or involving incisal angle (anterior)

D2336   Resin-based composite crown; anterior-primary

D2337   Resin-based composite crown; anterior-permanent

D2380   Resin-based composite; one surface, posterior-primary

D2381   two surfaces, posterior-primary

D2382	three or more surfaces, posterior-primary
D2385	one surface, posterior-permanent
D2386	two surfaces, posterior-permanent
D2387	three surfaces, posterior-permanent
D2388	four or more surfaces, posterior-permanent

GOLD FOIL RESTORATIONS

D2410	Gold foil; one surface
D2420	two surfaces
D2430	three surfaces

INLAY/ONLAY RESTORATIONS

D2510	Inlay - metallic; one surface
D2520	two surfaces
D2530	three or more surfaces
D2542	Onlay - metallic; two surfaces
D2543	three surfaces
D2544	four or more surfaces
D2610	Inlay - porcelain/ceramic; one surface
D2620	two surfaces
D2630	three or more surfaces
D2642	Onlay - porcelain/ceramic; two surfaces
D2643	three surfaces
D2644	four or more surfaces
D2650	Inlay - resin-based composite; one surface

D2651   two surfaces

D2652   three or more surfaces

D2662   Onlay - resin-based composite; two surfaces

D2663   three surfaces

D2664   four or more surfaces

CROWNS - SINGLE RESTORATIONS ONLY

D2710   Crown; resin (laboratory)

D2720   resin with high noble metal

D2721   resin with predominantly base metal

D2722   resin with noble metal

D2740   porcelain/ceramic substrate

D2750   porcelain fused to high noble metal

D2751   porcelain fused to predominantly base metal

D2752   porcelain fused to noble metal

D2780   3/4 cast high noble metal

D2781   3/4 cast predominantly base metal

D2782   3/4 cast noble metal

D2783   3/4 porcelain/ceramic

D2790   full cast high noble metal

D2791   full cast predominantly base metal

D2792   full cast noble metal

D2799   Provisional crown

(D2810)   Code deleted 2000

OTHER RESTORATIVE SERVICES

D2910   Recement inlay

D2920   Recement crown

D2930   Prefabricated stainless steel crown; primary tooth

D2931   permanent tooth

D2932   Prefabricated resin crown

D2933   Prefabricated stainless steel crown with resin window

D2940   Sedative filling

D2950   Crown build-up, including any pins

D2951   Pin retention - per tooth, in addition to restoration

D2952   Cast post and core in addition to crown

D2953   Each additional cast post - same tooth

D2954   Prefabricated post and core in addition to crown

D2955   Post removal (not in conjunction with endodontic therapy)

D2957   Each additional prefabricated post — same tooth (to be used with D2954)

D2960   Labial veneer (resin laminate); chairside

D2961   Labial veneer (resin laminate); laboratory

D2962   Labial veneer (porcelain laminate); laboratory

D2970   Temporary crown (fractured tooth)

D2980   Crown repair, by report

D2999   Unspecified restorative procedure, by report

IV. ENDODONTICS (D3000-D3999)

PULP CAPPING

D3110 Pulp cap; direct (excluding final restoration)

D3120   indirect (excluding final restoration)

PULPOTOMY

D3220 Therapeutic pulpotomy (excluding final restoration); removal of pulp coronal to the dentinocemental junction and application of medicament

D3221 Gross pulpal debridement, primary and permanent teeth

ENDODONTIC THERAPY ON PRIMARY TEETH

D3230 Pulpal therapy (resorbable filling); anterior, primary tooth (excluding final restoration)

D3240   posterior, primary tooth (excluding final restoration)

ENDODONTIC THERAPY (INCLUDING TREATMENT PLAN, CLINICAL PROCEDURES AND FOLLOW-UP CARE)

D3310 Anterior (excluding final restoration)

D3320 Bicuspid (excluding final restoration)

D3330 Molar (excluding final restoration)

D3331 Treatment of root canal obstruction; non-surgical access

D3332 Incomplete endodontic therapy; inoperable or fractured tooth

D3333 Internal root repair of perforation defects

ENDODONTIC RETREATMENT

D3346 Retreatment of previous root canal therapy; anterior

D3347   bicuspid

D3348 molar

APEXICATION/RECALCIFICATION PROCEDURES

D3351 Apexification/recalcification; initial visit (apical closure/calcific repair of perforations, root resorption, etc.)

D3352 interim medication replacement (apical closure/calcific repair of perforations, root resorption, etc.)

D3353 final visit (includes completed root canal therapy, apical closure/calcific repair of perforations, root resorption, etc.)

APICOECTOMY/PERIRADICULAR SERVICES

D3410 Apicoectomy/periradicular surgery; anterior

D3421 bicuspid (first root)

D3425 molar (first root)

D3426 (each additional root)

D3430 Retrograde filling - per root

D3450 Root amputation - per root

D3460 Endodontic endosseous implant

D3470 Intentional reimplantation (including necessary splinting)

OTHER ENDODONTIC PROCEDURES

D3910 Surgical procedure for isolation of tooth with rubber dam

D3920 Hemisection (including any root removal), not including root canal therapy

D3950 Canal preparation and fitting of preformed dowel or post

(D3960) Code deleted 2000

D3999 Unspecified endodontic procedure, by report

Not valid for Medicare   Non-covered by Medicare   Special coverage instructions   Carrier discretion

V. PERIODONTICS (D4000-D4999)

SURGICAL SERVICES (INCLUDING USUAL POSTOPERATIVE CARE)

D4210   Gingivectomy or gingivoplasty; per quadrant

D4211   per tooth

D4220   Gingival curettage, per quadrant, by report

D4240   Gingival flap procedure, including root planing, per quadrant

D4245   Apically positioned flap

D4249   Clinical crown lengthening; hard tissue

(D4250)   Code deleted 2000

D4260   Osseous surgery (including flap entry and closure) - per quadrant

D4263   Bone replacement graft; first site in quadrant

D4264   each additional site in quadrant

D4266   Guided tissue regeneration; resorbable barrier, per site

D4267   non-resorbable barrier, per site (includes membrane removal)

D4268   Surgical revision procedure, per tooth

D4270   Pedicle soft tissue graft procedure

D4271   Free soft tissue graft procedure (including donor site surgery)

D4273   Subepithelial connective tissue graft procedure (including donor site surgery)

D4274   Distal or proximal wedge procedure (when not performed in conjunction with surgical procedures in the same anatomical area)

NON-SURGICAL PERIODONTAL SERVICES

D4320 Provisional splinting; intracoronal

D4321   extracoronal

D4341 Periodontal scaling and root planing; per quadrant

D4355 Full mouth debridement to enable comprehensive periodontal evaluation and diagnosis

D4381 Localized delivery of chemotherapeutic agents via a controlled-release vehicle into diseased crevicular tissue, per tooth, by report

OTHER PERIODONTIC SERVICES

D4910 Periodontal maintenance procedures (following active therapy)

D4920 Unscheduled dressing change (by someone other than treating dentist)

D4999 Unspecified periodontal procedure, by report

VI. PROSTHODONTICS (REMOVABLE) (D5000-D5899)

COMPLETE DENTURES (INCLUDING ROUTINE POST-DELIVERY CARE)

D5110 Complete denture; maxillary

D5120   mandibular

D5130 Immediate denture; maxillary

D5140   mandibular

PARTIAL DENTURES (INCLUDING ROUTINE POST-DELIVERY CARE)

D5211 Maxillary (upper) partial denture; resin base (including any conventional clasps, rests and teeth)

D5212 Mandibular (lower) partial denture; resin base (including any conventional clasps, rests and teeth)

| | Not valid for Medicare | | Non-covered by Medicare | | Special coverage instructions | | Carrier discretion | **89** |

D5213 Maxillary partial denture; cast metal framework with resin denture bases (including any conventional clasps, rests and teeth)

D5214 Mandibular partial denture; cast metal framework with resin denture bases (including any conventional clasps, rests and teeth)

D5281 Removable unilateral partial denture; one piece cast metal (including clasps and teeth)

ADJUSTMENTS TO DENTURES

D5410 Adjust complete denture; maxillary

D5411   mandibular

D5421 Adjust partial denture; maxillary

D5422   mandibular

REPAIRS TO COMPLETE DENTURES

D5510 Repair broken complete denture base

D5520 Replace missing or broken teeth - complete denture (each tooth)

REPAIRS TO PARTIAL DENTURES

D5610 Repair resin denture base

D5620 Repair cast framework

D5630 Repair or replace broken clasp

D5640 Replace broken teeth - per tooth

D5650 Add tooth to existing partial denture

D5660 Add clasp to existing partial denture

DENTURE REBASE PROCEDURES

D5710 Rebase complete maxillary denture

D5711 Rebase complete mandibular denture

D5720 Rebase maxillary partial denture

D5721 Rebase mandibular partial denture

DENTURE RELINE PROCEDURES

D5730 Reline complete maxillary denture (chairside)

D5731 Reline complete mandibular denture (chairside)

D5740 Reline maxillary partial denture (chairside)

D5741 Reline mandibular partial denture (chairside)

D5750 Reline complete maxillary denture (laboratory)

D5751 Reline complete mandibular denture (laboratory)

D5760 Reline maxillary partial denture (laboratory)

D5761 Reline mandibular partial denture (laboratory)

INTERIM PROSTHESIS

D5810 Interim complete denture (maxillary)

D5811 Interim complete denture (mandibular)

D5820 Interim partial denture (maxillary)

D5821 Interim partial denture (mandibular)

OTHER REMOVABLE PROSTHETIC SERVICES

D5850 Tissue conditioning; maxillary

D5851 mandibular

D5860 Overdenture; complete, by report

D5861 partial, by report

D5862 Precision attachment, by report

D5867 Replacement of replaceable part of semi-precision or precision attachment (male or female component)

Not valid for Medicare   Non-covered by Medicare   Special coverage instructions   Carrier discretion

D5875 Modification of removable prosthesis following implant surgery

D5899 Unspecified removable prosthodontic procedure, by report

VII. MAXILLOFACIAL PROSTHETICS (D5900-D5999)

D5911 Facial moulage (sectional)

D5912 Facial moulage (complete)

D5913 Nasal prosthesis

D5914 Auricular prosthesis

D5915 Orbital prosthesis

D5916 Ocular prosthesis

D5919 Facial prosthesis

D5922 Nasal septal prosthesis

D5923 Ocular prosthesis, interim

D5924 Cranial prosthesis

D5925 Facial augmentation implant prosthesis

D5926 Nasal prosthesis, replacement

D5927 Auricular prosthesis, replacement

D5928 Orbital prosthesis, replacement

D5929 Facial prosthesis, replacement

D5931 Obturator prosthesis; surgical

D5932 definitive

D5933 modification

D5934 Mandibular resection prosthesis with guide flange

D5935 Mandibular resection prosthesis without guide flange

D5936	Obturator prosthesis, interim
D5937	Trismus appliance (not for TM treatment)
D5951	Feeding aid
D5952	Speech aid prosthesis; pediatric
D5953	adult
D5954	Palatal augmentation prosthesis
D5955	Palatal lift prosthesis, definitive
D5958	interim
D5959	modification
D5960	Speech aid prosthesis, modification
D5982	Surgical stent
D5983	Radiation carrier
D5984	Radiation shield
D5985	Radiation cone locator
D5986	Fluoride gel carrier
D5987	Commissure splint
D5988	Surgical splint
D5999	Unspecified maxillofacial prosthesis, by report

VIII. IMPLANT SERVICES (D6000-D6199)

D6010	Surgical placement of implant body: endosteal implant
D6020	Abutment placement or substitution: endosteal implant
D6040	Surgical placement: eposteal implant
D6050	Surgical placement: transosteal implant

IMPLANT SUPPORTED PROSTHETICS

D6055   Dental implant supported connection bar

D6056   Prefabricated abutment

D6057   Custom abutment

D6058   Abutment supported porcelain/ceramic crown

D6059   Abutment supported porcelain fused to metal crown (high noble metal)

D6060   Abutment supported porcelain fused to metal crown (predominantly base metal)

D6061   Abutment supported porcelain fused to metal crown (noble metal)

D6062   Abutment supported cast metal crown (high noble metal)

D6063   Abutment supported cast metal crown (predominantly base metal)

D6064   Abutment supported cast metal crown (noble metal)

D6065   Implant supported porcelain/ceramic crown

D6066   Implant supported porcelain fused to metal crown (titanium, titanium alloy, high noble metal)

D6067   Implant supported metal crown (titanium, titanium alloy, high noble metal)

D6068   Abutment supported retainer for porcelain/ceramic FPD

D6069   Abutment supported retainer for porcelain fused to metal FPD (high noble metal)

D6070   Abutment supported retainer for porcelain fused to metal FPD (predominantly base metal)

D6071   Abutment supported retainer for porcelain fused to metal FPD (noble metal)

D6072   Abutment supported retainer for cast metal FPD (high noble metal)

D6073 Abutment supported retainer for cast metal FPD (predominantly base metal)

D6074 Abutment supported retainer for cast metal FPD (noble metal)

D6075 Implant supported retainer for ceramic FPD

D6076 Implant supported retainer for porcelain fused to metal FPD (titanium, titanium alloy, or high noble metal)

D6077 Implant supported retainer for cast metal FPD (titanium, titanium alloy, or high noble metal)

D6078 Implant/abutment supported fixed denture for completely edentulous arch

D6079 Implant/abutment supported fixed denture for partially edentulous arch

OTHER IMPLANT SERVICES

D6080 Implant maintenance procedures, including; removal of prosthesis, cleansing of prosthesis and abutment reinsertion of prosthesis

D6090 Repair implant supported prosthesis, by report.

D6095 Repair implant abutment, by report

D6100 Implant removal, by report.

D6199 Unspecified implant procedure, by report.

IX. PROSTHODONTICS, FIXED (EACH RETAINER AND EACH PONTIC CONSTITUTES A UNIT IN A FIXED PARTIAL DENTURE) (D6200-D6999)

FIXED PARTIAL DENTURE PONTICS

D6210 Pontic; cast high noble metal

D6211 cast predominantly base metal

D6212 cast noble metal

| | Not valid for Medicare | | Non-covered by Medicare | | Special coverage instructions | | Carrier discretion |

D6240	porcelain fused to high noble metal
D6241	porcelain fused to predominantly base metal
D6242	porcelain fused to noble metal
D6245	porcelain/ceramic
D6250	resin with high noble metal
D6251	resin base predominantly base metal
D6252	resin with noble metal

FIXED PARTIAL DENTURE RETAINERS - INLAYS/ONLAYS

D6519	Inlay/onlay - porcelain/ceramic
D6520	Inlay - metallic; two surfaces
D6530	three or more surfaces
D6543	Onlay - metallic; three surfaces
D6544	four or more surfaces
D6545	Retainer; cast metal for resin bonded fixed prosthesis
D6548	porcelain/ceramic for resin bonded fixed prosthesis

FIXED PARTIAL DENTURE RETAINERS - CROWNS

D6720	Crown; resin with high noble metal
D6721	resin with predominantly base metal
D6722	resin with noble metal
D6740	porcelain/ceramic
D6750	porcelain fused to high noble metal
D6751	porcelain fused to predominantly base metal
D6752	porcelain fused to noble metal

D6780   3/4 cast high noble metal

D6781   3/4 cast predominantly base metal

D6782   3/4 cast noble metal

D6783   3/4 porcelain/ceramic

D6790   full cast high noble metal

D6791   full cast predominantly base metal

D6792   full cast noble metal

OTHER FIXED PARTIAL DENTURE SERVICES

D6920   Connector bar

D6930   Recement fixed partial denture

D6940   Stress breaker

D6950   Precision attachment

D6970   Cast post and core in addition to fixed partial denture retainer

D6971   Cast post as part of fixed partial denture retainer

D6972   Prefabricated post and core in addition to fixed partial denture retainer

D6973   Core build up for retainer, including any pins

D6975   Coping; metal

D6976   Each additional cast post - same tooth

D6977   Each additional prefabricated post - same tooth

D6980   Fixed partial denture repair, by report

D6999   Unspecified, fixed prosthodontic procedure, by report

X. ORAL AND MAXILLOFACIAL SURGERY (D7000-D7999)

EXTRACTIONS (INCLUDES LOCAL ANESTHESIA, SUTURING, IF NEEDED, AND ROUTINE POSTOPERATIVE CARE)

D7110 Single tooth

D7120 Each additional tooth

D7130 Root removal - exposed roots

SURGICAL EXTRACTIONS (INCLUDES LOCAL ANESTHESIA, SUTURING, IF NEEDED, AND ROUTINE POSTOPERATIVE CARE)

D7210 Surgical removal of erupted tooth requiring elevation of mucoperiosteal flap and removal of bone and/or section of tooth

D7220 Removal of impacted tooth; soft tissue

D7230   partially bony

D7240   completely bony

D7241   completely bony, with unusual surgical complications

D7250 Surgical removal of residual tooth roots (cutting procedure)

OTHER SURGICAL PROCEDURES

D7260 Oroantral fistula closure

D7270 Tooth re-implantation and/or stabilization of accidentally evulsed or displaced tooth and/or alveolus

D7272 Tooth transplantation (includes reimplantation from one site to another and splinting and/or stabilization)

D7280 Surgical exposure of impacted or unerupted tooth for orthodontic reasons (including orthodontic attachments)

D7281 Surgical exposure of impacted or unerupted tooth to aid eruption

D7285   Biopsy of oral tissue; hard (bone, tooth)

D7286   soft (all others)

D7290   Surgical repositioning of teeth

D7291   Transseptal fiberotomy, by report

ALVEOLOPLASTY-SURGICAL PREPARATION OF RIDGE FOR DENTURES

D7310   Alveoloplasty in conjunction with extractions - per quadrant

D7320   Alveoloplasty not in conjunction with extractions - per quadrant

VESTIBULOPLASTY

D7340   Vestibuloplasty; ridge extension (secondary epithelialization)

D7350   ridge extension (including soft tissue grafts, muscle reattachments, revision of soft tissue attachment and management of hypertrophied and hyperplastic tissue)

SURGICAL EXCISION OF REACTIVE INFLAMMATORY LESIONS (SCAR TISSUE OR LOCALIZED CONGENITAL LESIONS)

D7410   Radical excision; lesion diameter up to 1.25 cm

D7420   lesion diameter greater than 1.25 cm

REMOVAL OF TUMORS, CYSTS, AND NEOPLASMS

D7430   Excision of benign tumor; lesion diameter up to 1.25 cm

D7431   lesion diameter greater than 1.25 cm

D7440   Excision of malignant tumor; lesion diameter up to 1.25 cm

D7441   lesion diameter greater than 1.25 cm

D7450   Removal of odontogenic cyst or tumor; lesion diameter up to 1.25 cm

D7451   lesion diameter greater than 1.25 cm

D7460   Removal of nonodontogenic cyst or tumor; lesion diameter up to 1.25 cm

D7461   lesion diameter greater than 1.25 cm

D7465   Destruction of lesion(s) by physical methods, by report

EXCISION OF BONE TISSUE

(D7470)   Code deleted 2000

D7471   Removal of exostosis, per site

D7480   Partial ostectomy (guttering or saucerization)

D7490   Radical resection of mandible with bone graft

SURGICAL INCISION

D7510   Incision and drainage of abscess; intraoral soft tissue

D7520   extraoral soft tissue

D7530   Removal of foreign body, skin, or subcutaneous alveolar tissue

D7540   Removal of reaction-producing foreign bodies, musculoskeletal system

D7550   Sequestrectomy for osteomyelitis

D7560   Maxillary sinusotomy for removal of tooth fragment or foreign body

TREATMENT OF FRACTURES - SIMPLE

D7610   Maxilla; open reduction (teeth immobilized, if present)

D7620   closed reduction (teeth immobilized, if present)

D7630   Mandible; open reduction (teeth immobilized, if present)

D7640   closed reduction (teeth immobilized, if present)

D7650   Malar and/or zygomatic arch; open reduction

D7660   closed reduction

D7670   Alveolus - stabilization of teeth, closed reduction splinting

D7680   Facial bones - complicated reduction with fixation and multiple surgical approaches

TREATMENT OF FRACTURES - COMPOUND

D7710   Maxilla; open reduction

D7720   closed reduction

D7730   Mandible; open reduction

D7740   closed reduction

D7750   Malar and/or zygomatic arch; open reduction

D7760   closed reduction

D7770   Alveolus - stabilization of teeth, open reduction splinting

D7780   Facial bones - complicated reduction with fixation and multiple surgical approaches

REDUCTION OF DISLOCATION AND MANAGEMENT OF OTHER TEMPOROMANDIBULAR JOINT DYSFUNCTIONS

D7810   Open reduction of dislocation

D7820   Closed reduction of dislocation

D7830   Manipulation under anesthesia

D7840   Condylectomy

D7850   Surgical discectomy, with/without implant

D7852   Disc repair

D7854   Synovectomy

D7856   Myotomy

D7858   Joint reconstruction

Not valid for Medicare	Non-covered by Medicare	Special coverage instructions	Carrier discretion

D7860	Arthrotomy
D7865	Arthroplasty
D7870	Arthrocentesis
D7871	Non-arthroscopic lysis and lavage
D7872	Arthroscopy - diagnosis, with or without biopsy
D7873	Arthroscopy - surgical; lavage and lysis of adhesions
D7874	disc repositioning and stabilization
D7875	synovectomy
D7876	discectomy
D7877	debridement
D7880	Occlusal orthotic device, by report
D7899	Unspecified TMD therapy, by report

REPAIR OF TRAUMATIC WOUNDS

D7910	Suture of recent small wounds up to 5 cm

COMPLICATED SUTURING (RECONSTRUCTION REQUIRING DELICATE HANDLING OF TISSUES AND WIDE UNDERMINING FOR METICULOUS CLOSURE)

D7911	Complicated suture; up to 5 cm
D7912	greater than 5 cm

OTHER REPAIR PROCEDURES

D7920	Skin graft (identify defect covered, location, and type of graft)
D7940	Osteoplasty - for orthognathic deformities
D7941	Osteotomy; mandibular rami
(D7942)	Code deleted 2000

● New code   ▲ Revised code   ( ) Deleted code

D7943 Osteotomy; mandibular rami with bone graft; includes obtaining the graft

D7944 segmented or subapical - per sextant or quadrant

D7945 body of mandible

D7946 LeFort I (maxilla - total)

D7947 LeFort I (maxilla - segmented)

D7948 LeFort II or LeFort III (osteoplasty of facial bones for midface hypoplasia or retrusion); without bone graft

D7949 LeFort II or LeFort III; with bone graft

D7950 Osseous, osteoperiosteal, or cartilage graft of the mandible or facial bones - autogeneous or nonautogeneous, by report

D7955 Repair of maxillofacial soft and hard tissue defect

D7960 Frenulectomy (frenectomy or frenotomy) - separate procedure

D7970 Excision of hyperplastic tissue - per arch

D7971 Excision of pericoronal gingiva

D7980 Sialolithotomy

D7981 Excision of salivary gland, by report

D7982 Sialodochoplasty

D7983 Closure of salivary fistula

D7990 Emergency tracheotomy

D7991 Coronoidectomy

D7995 Synthetic graft - mandible or facial bones, by report

D7996 Implant-mandible for augmentation purposes (excluding alveolar ridge), by report

Not valid for Medicare   Non-covered by Medicare   Special coverage instructions   Carrier discretion

D7997	Appliance removal (not by dentist who placed appliance), includes removal of archbar

D7999	Unspecified oral surgery procedure, by report

XI. ORTHODONTICS (D8000-D8999)

LIMITED ORTHODONTIC TREATMENT

D8010	Limited orthodontic treatment; of the primary dentition
D8020	of the transitional dentition
D8030	of the adolescent dentition
D8040	of the adult dentition

INTERCEPTIVE ORTHODONTIC TREATMENT

D8050	Interceptive orthodontic treatment; of the primary dentition
D8060	of the transitional dentition

COMPREHENSIVE ORTHODONTIC TREATMENT

D8070	Comprehensive orthodontic treatment; of the transitional dentition
D8080	of the adolescent dentition
D8090	of the adult dentition

MINOR TREATMENT TO CONTROL HARMFUL HABITS

D8210	Removable appliance therapy
D8220	Fixed appliance therapy

OTHER ORTHODONTIC SERVICES

D8660	Pre-orthodontic visit
D8670	Periodic orthodontic treatment visit (as part of contract)
D8680	Orthodontic retention (removal of appliances, construction and placement of retainer(s))

D8690 Orthodontic treatment (alternative billing to a contract fee)

D8691 Repair of orthodontic appliance

D8692 Replacement of lost or broken retainer

D8999 Unspecified orthodontic procedure, by report

XII. ADJUNCTIVE GENERAL SERVICES (D9000-D9999)

UNCLASSIFIED TREATMENT

D9110 Palliative (emergency) treatment of dental pain - minor procedures

ANESTHESIA

D9210 Local anesthesia not in conjunction with operative or surgical procedures

D9211 Regional block anesthesia

D9212 Trigeminal division block anesthesia

D9215 Local anesthesia

D9220 General anesthesia; first 30 minutes

D9221   each additional 15 minutes

D9230 Analgesia, anxiolysis, inhalation of nitrous oxide

(D9240) Code deleted 2000

D9241 Intravenous sedation/analgesia; first 30 minutes

D9242   each additional 15 minutes

D9248 Non-intravenous conscious sedation

PROFESSIONAL CONSULTATION

D9310 Consultation (diagnostic service provided by dentist or physician other than practitioner providing treatment)

PROFESSIONAL VISITS

D9410 House/extended care facility call

D9420 Hospital call

D9430 Office visit for observation (during regularly scheduled hours) - no other services performed

D9440 Office visit - after regularly scheduled hours

DRUGS

D9610 Therapeutic drug injection, by report

D9630 Other drugs and/or medicaments, by report

MISCELLANEOUS SERVICES

D9910 Application of desensitizing medicament

D9911 Application of desensitizing resin for cervical and/or root surface, per tooth

D9920 Behavior management, by report

D9930 Treatment of complications (post-surgical) - unusual circumstances, by report

D9940 Occlusal guard, by report

D9941 Fabrication of athletic mouthguards

D9950 Occlusion analysis; mounted case

D9951 Occlusal adjustment; limited

D9952   complete

D9970 Enamel microabrasion

D9971 Odontoplasty 1-2 teeth; includes removal of enamel projections

D9972 External bleaching; per arch

D9973   per tooth

D9974 Internal bleaching; per tooth

D9999 Unspecified adjunctive procedure, by report

NOTE: The Noble Metal Classification System has been adopted as a more precise method of reporting various alloys used in dentistry. The alloys are defined on the basis of the percentage of Noble Metal Content.

● New code ▲ Revised code ( ) Deleted code

DURABLE MEDICAL EQUIPMENT

Guidelines

In addition to the information presented in the INTRODUCTION, several other items unique to this section are defined or identified here:

1. **DEFINITION OF DURABLE MEDICAL EQUIPMENT:** Durable medical equipment (DME) can withstand repeated use and is used primarily to serve a medical purpose. It generally is not useful in the absence of an illness or injury, and is appropriate for use in the home. Expendable medical supplies, such as incontinent pads, lamb's wool pads, catheters, ace bandages, elastic stockings, surgical face masks, irrigating kits, sheets and bags, are not considered to be DME.

2. **REASONABLE AND NECESSARY:** DME may not be covered in every instance. The equipment must be reasonable and necessary for the illness or injury being treated or for improving the functioning of a malformed body part. A physician's prescription is normally sufficient to establish that the equipment is necessary. To determine reasonableness, the following conditions must be met: the expense must be proportionate to the therapeutic benefits of using the equipment; the cost must not substantially exceed a medically appropriate care plan; and, the item must not serve the same purpose as equipment already available to the patient. Claims for items that are not reasonable will be denied except when it is determined that no alternative plan of care is available for which payment could be made.

3. **SUBSECTION INFORMATION:** Some of the listed subheadings or subsections have special needs or instructions unique to that section. Where these are indicated, special "notes" will be presented preceding or following the listings. Those subsections within the DURABLE MEDICAL EQUIPMENT section that have "notes" are as follows:

Subsection	Code Numbers
Artificial kidney machines and accessories	E1510-E1699

4. **UNLISTED SERVICE OR PROCEDURE:** A service or procedure may be provided that is not listed in this edition of HCPCS. When reporting such a service, the appropriate "unlisted procedure" code may be used to indicate the service, identifying it by "special report"

E CODES

as defined below. HCPCS terminology is inconsistent in defining unlisted procedures. The procedure definition may include the term(s) "unlisted", "not otherwise classified", "unspecified", "unclassified", "other" and "miscellaneous". Prior to using these codes, try to determine if a Local Level III code or CPT code is available. The "unlisted procedures" and accompanying codes for DURABLE MEDICAL EQUIPMENT are as follows:

E1399   Durable medical equipment, miscellaneous
E1699   Dialysis equipment, not otherwise specified

5. **SPECIAL REPORT**: A service, material or supply that is rarely provided, unusual, variable or new may require a special report in determining medical appropriateness for reimbursement purposes. Pertinent information should include an adequate definition or description of the nature, extent, and need for the service, material or supply.

6. **MODIFIERS:** Listed services may be modified under certain circumstances. When appropriate, the modifying circumstance is identified by adding a modifier to the basic procedure code. CPT and HCPCS National Level II modifiers may be used with CPT and HCPCS National Level II procedure codes. Modifiers commonly used with DURABLE MEDICAL EQUIPMENT are as follows:

-CC   Procedure code change (use "CC" when the procedure code submitted was changed either for administrative reasons or because an incorrect code was filed)

-LL   Lease/rental (used the "LL" modifier when DME rental is to be applied against the purchase price)

-LT   Left side (used to identify procedures performed on the left sideof the body)

-MS   Six-month maintenance and servicing fee for reasonable and necessary parts and labor which are not covered under any manufacturer or supplier warranty

-NR   New when rented (use the "NR" modifier when DME which was new at the time of rental is subsequently purchased)

-NU   New equipment

-QE   Prescribed amount of oxygen less than 1 liter per minute (LPM)

-QF   Prescribed amount of oxygen exceeds 4 liters per minute (LPM) and portable oxygen is prescribed

-QG   Prescribed amount of oxygen is greater than 4 liters per minute (LPM)

-QH   Oxygen conserving device is being used with an oxygen delivery system

-QT   Recording and storage on tape by an analog tape recorder

-RP   Replacement and repair (may be used to indicate replacement of DME, orthotic and prosthetic devices which have been in use for some time. The claim shows the code for the part, followed by the "RP" modifier and the charge for the part.)

-RR   Rental (used when DME is to be rented)

-RT   Right side (used to identify procedures performed on the right side of the body)

-TC   Technical component. Under certain circumstances, a charge may be made for the technical component alone. Under those circumstances, the technical component charge is identified by adding modifier -TC to the usual procedure code. Technical component charges are institutional charges and are not billed separately by physicians. However, portable x-ray suppliers bill only for technical component and should utilize modifier -TC. The charge data from portable x-ray suppliers will then be used to build customary and prevailing profiles.

-UE   Used durable medical equipment

7. **CPT CODE CROSS-REFERENCE:** Unless otherwise specified, the equivalent CPT code for all listings in this section is 99070.

8. **DURABLE MEDICAL EQUIPMENT REGIONAL CARRIERS (DMERCS):** Effective October 1, 1993 claims for durable medical equipment (DME) must be billed to one of four regional carriers depending upon the residence of the beneficiary. The transition dates for DMERC claims is from November 1, 1993 to March 1, 1994 depending upon the state you practice in. See the Introduction for a complete discussion of DMERCs.

DURABLE MEDICAL EQUIPMENT

CANES

E0100 Cane, includes canes of all materials, adjustable or fixed, with tip

E0105 Cane, quad or three prong, includes canes of all materials, adjustable or fixed, with tips

CRUTCHES

E0110 Crutches, forearm, includes crutches of various materials, adjustable or fixed; pair, complete with tips and handgrip

E0111   each, with tip and handgrip

E0112 Crutches, underarm, wood, adjustable or fixed; pair, with pads, tips and handgrip

E0113   each, with pad, tip and handgrip

E0114 Crutches, underarm, other than wood, adjustable or fixed; pair, with pads, tips and handgrips

E0116 Crutches, underarm, other than wood, adjustable or fixed; each, with pad, tip and handgrips

WALKERS

E0130 Walker, rigid (pickup), adjustable or fixed height

E0135 Walker, folding (pickup), adjustable or fixed height

E0141 Rigid walker, wheeled, without seat

E0142 Rigid walker, wheeled, with seat

E0143 Folding walker, wheeled, without seat

E0144 Enclosed, framed folding walker, wheeled, with posterior seat

E0145 Walker, wheeled, with seat and crutch attachments

E0146 Folding walker, wheeled, with seat

E0147 Heavy duty, multiple breaking system, variable wheel resistance walker

E0148 Walker, heavy duty, without wheels, rigid or folding, any type, each

E0149 Walker, heavy duty, wheeled, rigid or folding, any type, each

ATTACHMENTS

E0153 Platform attachment; forearm crutch, each

E0154 walker, each

E0155 Wheel attachment, rigid pick-up walker, per pair

E0156 Seat attachment, walker

E0157 Crutch attachment, walker, each

E0158 Leg extensions for a walker, per set of four (4)

E0159 Brake attachment for wheeled walker, replacement, each

COMMODES

E0160 Sitz type bath or equipment, portable, used with or without commode;

E0161 with faucet attachments

E0162 Sitz bath chair

E0163 Commode chair; stationary, with fixed arms

E0164 mobile, with fixed arms

E0165 stationary, with detachable arms

E0166 mobile, with detachable arms

E0167 Pail or pan for use with commode chair

E0168 Commode chair, extra wide and/or heavy duty, stationary or mobile, with or without arms, any type, each

● **E0169** Commode chair with seat lift mechanism

E0175 Foot rest, for use with commode chair, each

E0176 Air pressure pad or cushion, nonpositioning

E0177 Water pressure pad or cushion, nonpositioning

E0178 Gel or gel-like pressure pad or cushion, nonpositioning

E0179 Dry pressure pad or cushion, nonpositioning

DECUBITUS CARE EQUIPMENT

E0180 Pressure pad, alternating with pump;

E0181   heavy duty

E0182 Pump for alternating pressure pad

E0184 Dry pressure mattress

E0185 Gel or gel-like pressure pad for mattress, standard mattress length and width

E0186 Air pressure mattress

E0187 Water pressure mattress

E0188 Synthetic sheepskin pad

E0189 Lambswool sheepskin pad, any size

E0191 Heel or elbow protector, each

E0192 Low pressure and positioning equalization pad, for wheelchair

E0193 Powered air floatation bed (low air loss therapy)

E0194 Air fluidized bed

E0196 Gel pressure mattress

E0197 Air pressure pad for mattress, standard mattress length and width

E0198 Water pressure pad for mattress, standard mattress length and width

E0199 Dry pressure pad for mattress, standard mattress length and width

HEAT/COLD APPLICATION

E0200 Heat lamp, without stand (table model), includes bulb, or infrared element

E0202 Phototherapy (bilirubin) light with photometer

E0205 Heat lamp, with stand, includes bulb, or infrared element

E0210 Electric heat pad; standard

E0215   moist

E0217 Water circulating heat pad with pump

E0218 Water circulating cold pad with pump

E0220 Hot water bottle

● **E0221** Infrared heating pad system

E0225 Hydrocollator unit, includes pads

E0230 Ice cap or collar

● **E0231** Non-contact wound warming device (temperature control unit, AC adapter and power cord) for use with warming card and wound cover

● **E0232** Warming card for use with the non-contact wound warming device and non-contact wound warming wound cover

E0235 Paraffin bath unit, portable (see medical supply code A4265 for paraffin)

E0236 Pump for water circulating pad

E0238 Non-electric heat pad, moist

E0239 Hydrocollator unit, portable

BATH AND TOILET AIDS

E0241   Bath tub wall rail, each

E0242   Bath tub rail, floor base

E0243   Toilet rail, each

E0244   Raised toilet seat

E0245   Tub stool or bench

E0246   Transfer tub rail attachment

E0249   Pad for water circulating heat unit

HOSPITAL BEDS AND ACCESSORIES

E0250   Hospital bed, fixed height, with any type side rails; with mattress

E0251   without mattress

E0255   Hospital bed, variable height, hi-lo, with any type side rails; with mattress

E0256   without mattress

E0260   Hospital bed, semi-electric (head and foot adjustment), with any type side rails; with mattress

E0261   without mattress

E0265   Hospital bed, total electric (head, foot and height adjustments), with any type side rails; with mattress

E0266   without mattress

E0270   Hospital bed, institutional type includes: oscillating, circulating and stryker frame, with mattress

E0271   Mattress; innerspring

E0272   foam rubber

E0273   Bed board

E0274 Over-bed table

E0275 Bed pan; standard, metal or plastic

E0276 fracture, metal or plastic

E0277 Powered pressure-reducing air mattress

E0280 Bed cradle, any type

E0290 Hospital bed; fixed-height, without side rails; with mattress

E0291 without mattress

E0292 Hospital variable height, hi-lo, without side rails; with mattress

E0293 without mattress

E0294 Hospital bed, semi-electric (head and foot adjustment), without side rails; with mattress

E0295 without mattress

E0296 Hospital bed, total electric (head, foot and height adjustments), without side rails; with mattress

E0297 without mattress

(E0298) Code deleted 2002; use K0549

HOSPITAL BED ACCESSORIES

E0305 Bed side rails; half length

E0310 full length

E0315 Bed accessory: board, table, or support device, any type

● **E0316** Safety enclosure frame/canopy for use with hospital bed, any type

E0325 Urinal; male, jug/type, any material

E0326 female, jug/type, any material

E0350 Control unit for electronic bowel irrigation/evacuation system

E0352 Disposable pack (water reservoir bag, speculum, valving mechanism and collection bag/box) for use with the electronic bowel irrigation/evacuation system

E0370 Air pressure elevator for heel

E0371 Nonpowered advanced pressure reducing overlay for mattress, standard mattress length and width

E0372 Powered air overlay for mattress, standard mattress length and width

E0373 Nonpowered advanced pressure reducing mattress

OXYGEN AND RELATED RESPIRATORY EQUIPMENT

E0424 Stationary compressed gaseous oxygen system, rental; includes container, contents, regulator, flowmeter, humidifier, nebulizer, cannula or mask, and tubing

E0425 Stationary compressed gas system, purchase; includes regulator, flowmeter, humidifier, nebulizer, cannula or mask, and tubing

E0430 Portable gaseous oxygen system, purchase; includes regulator flowmeter, humidifier, cannula or mask, and tubing

E0431 Portable gaseous oxygen system, rental; includes portable container, regulator, flowmeter, humidifier, cannula or mask, and tubing

E0434 Portable liquid oxygen system, rental; includes portable container, supply reservoir, humidifier, flowmeter, refill adaptor, contents gauge, cannula or mask, and tubing

E0435 Portable liquid oxygen system, purchase; includes portable container, supply reservoir, flowmeter, humidifier, contents gauge, cannula or masks, tubing and refill adaptor

E0439 Stationary liquid oxygen system; rental, includes container, contents, regulator, flowmeter, humidifier, nebulizer, cannula or mask, and tubing

E0440 purchase, includes use of reservoir, contents indicator, regulator, flowmeter, humidifier, nebulizer, cannula or mask, and tubing

E0441 Oxygen contents, gaseous (for use with owned gaseous stationary systems or when both a stationary and portable gaseous system are owned)

E0442 Oxygen contents, liquid (for use with owned liquid stationary systems or when both a stationary and portable liquid system are owned)

E0443 Portable oxygen contents, gaseous (for use only with portable gaseous systems when no stationary gas or liquid system is used)

E0444 Portable oxygen contents, liquid (for use only with portable liquid systems when no stationary gas or liquid system is used)

E0450 Volume ventilator, stationary or portable, with backup rate feature, used with invasive interface (e.g., tracheostomy tube)

(E0452) Code deleted 2000

(E0453) Code deleted 2000

E0455 Oxygen tent, excluding croup or pediatric tents

E0457 Chest shell (cuirass)

E0459 Chest wrap

E0460 Negative pressure ventilator, portable or stationary

E0462 Rocking bed with or without side rails

E0480 Percussor, electric or pneumatic, home model

● **E0481** Intrapulmonary percussive ventilation system and related accessories

● **E0482** Cough stimulating device, alternating positive and negative airway pressure

| | Not valid for Medicare | | Non-covered by Medicare | | Special coverage instructions | | Carrier discretion |

IPPB MACHINES

E0500 IPPB machine, all types, with built-in nebulization; manual or automatic valves; internal or external power source

HUMIDIFIERS/NEBULIZERS FOR USE WITH OXYGEN IPPB EQUIPMENT

COMPRESSORS

E0550 Humidifier, durable for extensive supplemental humidification during IPPB treatments or oxygen delivery

E0555 Humidifier, durable, glass or autoclavable plastic bottle type, for use with regulator or flowmeter

E0560 Humidifier, durable for supplemental humidification during IPPB treatment or oxygen delivery

E0565 Compressor, air power source for equipment which is not self-contained or cylinder driven

E0570 Nebulizer; with compressor

E0571 Aerosol compressor, battery powered, for use with small volume nebulizer

E0572 Aerosol compressor, adjustable pressure, light duty for intermittent use

E0574 Ultrasonic generator with small volume ultrasonic nebulizer

E0575 Nebulizer, ultrasonic, large volume

E0580 Nebulizer, with compressor, durable, glass or autoclavable plastic, bottle type, for use with regulator or flowmeter

E0585 Nebulizer with compressor and heater

E0590 Dispensing fee covered drug administered through DME nebulizer

---

SUCTION PUMP/ROOM VAPORIZERS

▲ **E0600** Respiratory suction pump, home model, portable or stationary, electric

E0601 Continuous airway pressure (CPAP) device

▲ **E0602** Breast pump, manual, any type

● **E0603** Breast pump, electric (AC and/or DC), any type

● **E0604** Breast pump, heavy duty, hospital grade, piston operated, pulsatile vacuum suction/release cycles, vacuum regulator, supplies, transformer, electric (AC and/or DC)

E0605 Vaporizer, room type

E0606 Postural drainage board

MONITORING EQUIPMENT

E0607 Home blood glucose monitor

E0608 Apnea monitor

(E0609) Code deleted 2002

PACEMAKER MONITOR

E0610 Pacemaker monitor, self-contained; (checks battery depletion, included audible and visible check systems)

E0615 (checks battery depletion and other pacemaker components, includes digital/visible check systems)

E0616 Implantable cardiac event recorder with memory, activator and programmer

E0617 External defibrillator with integrated electrocardiogram analysis

● **E0620** Skin piercing device for collection of capillary blood, laser, each

---

Not valid for Medicare | Non-covered by Medicare | Special coverage instructions | Carrier discretion **121**

PATIENT LIFTS

E0621 Sling or seat, patient lift, canvas or nylon

E0625 Patient lift, kartop, bathroom or toilet

E0627 Seat lift mechanism incorporated into a combination lift-chair mechanism

E0628 Separate seat life mechanism for use with patient owned furniture; electric

E0629 non-electric

E0630 Patient lift; hydraulic, with seat or sling

E0635 electric, with seat or sling

PNEUMATIC COMPRESSOR AND APPLIANCES (LYMPHEDEMA PUMP)

E0650 Pneumatic compressor; non-segmental home model

E0651 segmental home model without calibrated gradient pressure

E0652 segmental home model with calibrated gradient pressure

E0655 Non-segmental pneumatic appliance for use with pneumatic compressor; half arm

E0660 full leg

E0665 full arm

E0666 half leg

E0667 Segmental pneumatic appliance for use with pneumatic compressor; full leg

E0668 full arm

E0669 half leg

E0671 Segmental gradient pressure pneumatic appliance, full leg

E0672 full arm

E0673   half leg

ULTRAVIOLET CABINET

E0690   Ultraviolet cabinet, appropriate for home use

SAFETY EQUIPMENT

E0700   Safety equipment (e.g., belt, harness or vest)

RESTRAINTS

E0710   Restraints, any type (body, chest, wrist or ankle)

TRANSCUTANEOUS AND/OR NEUROMUSCULAR ELECTRICAL NERVE STIMULATORS-TENS

E0720   TENS; two lead, localized stimulation

E0730   four lead, larger area/multiple nerve stimulation

E0731   Form fitting conductive garment for delivery of TENS or NMES (with conductive fibers separated from the patient's skin by layers of fabric)

E0740   Incontinence treatment system, pelvic floor stimulator, monitor, sensor and/or trainer

E0744   Neuromuscular stimulator for scoliosis

E0745   Neuromuscular stimulator, electronic shock unit

E0746   Electromyography (EMG), biofeedback device

E0747   Osteogenesis stimulator; electrical, non-invasive, other than spinal applications

E0748   Osteogenisis stimulator; electrical, noninvasive, spinal applications

E0749   Osteogenisis stimulator, electrical, surgically implanted

(E0751)   Code deleted 2001

● **E0752**   Implantable neurostimulator electrode, each

(E0753)   Code deleted 2002

| | Not valid for Medicare | | Non-covered by Medicare | | Special coverage instructions | | Carrier discretion | **123** |

● **E0754** Patient programmer (external) for use with implantable programmable neurostimulator pulse generator

E0755 Electronic salivary reflex stimulator (intra-oral/non-invasive)

E0756 Implantable neurostimulator pulse generator

E0757 Implantable neurostimulator radiofrequency receiver

E0758 Radiofrequency transmitter (external) for use with implantable neurostimulator radiofrequency receiver

● **E0759** Radiofrequency transmitter (external) for use with implantable sacral root neurostimulator receiver for bowel and bladder management, replacement

E0760 Ostogenesis stimulator, low intensity ultrasound, non-invasive

E0765 FDA approved nerve stimulator with replaceable batteries for treatment of nausea and vomiting

E0776 IV pole

E0779 Ambulatory infusion pump, mechanical, reusable, for infusion 8 hours or greater

E0780 Ambulatory infusion pump, mechanical, reusable, for infusion less than 8 hours

E0781 Ambulatory infusion pump, single or multiple channels, electric or battery operated, with administrative equipment, worn by patient

E0782 Infusion pump, implantable, non-programmable

E0783 Infusion pump system, implantable, programmable (includes all components, e.g., pump, catheter, connectors, etc.)

E0784 External ambulatory infusion pump, insulin

E0785 Implantable intraspinal (epidural/intrathecal) catheter used with implantable infusion pump, replacement

E0786 Implantable programmable infusion pump, replacement (excludes implantable intraspinal catheter)

E0791 Parenteral infusion pump, stationary, single or multi-channel

TRACTION EQUIPMENT

TRACTION-CERVICAL

E0830 Ambulatory traction device, all types, each

E0840 Traction frame, attached to headboard, cervical traction

E0850 Traction stand, free standing, cervical traction

E0855 Cervical traction equipment not requiring additional stand or frame

TRACTION-OVERDOOR

E0860 Traction equipment, overdoor, cervical

TRACTION-EXTREMITY

E0870 Traction frame, attached to footboard, extremity traction, (e.g., Buck's)

E0880 Traction stand, free standing, extremity traction, (e.g., Buck's)

TRACTION-PELVIC

E0890 Traction frame, attached to footboard, pelvic traction

E0900 Traction stand, free standing, pelvic traction (e.g., Buck's)

TRAPEZE EQUIPMENT, FRACTURE FRAME AND OTHER ORTHOPEDIC DEVICES

E0910 Trapeze bars, A/K/A patient helper, attached to bed, with grab bar

E0920 Fracture frame; attached to bed, includes weights

E0930 free standing, includes weights

| | Not valid for Medicare | | Non-covered by Medicare | | Special coverage instructions | | Carrier discretion | **125** |

E0935 Passive motion exercise device

E0940 Trapeze bar, free standing, complete with grab bar

E0941 Gravity assisted traction device, any type

E0942 Cervical head harness/halter

E0943 Cervical pillow

E0944 Pelvic belt/harness/boot

E0945 Extremity belt/harness

E0946 Fracture frame; dual with cross bars, attached to bed, (e.g., Balken, 4 poster)

E0947 attachments for complex pelvic traction

E0948 attachments for complex cervical traction

WHEELCHAIRS

E0950 Tray

E0951 Loop heel, each

E0952 Loop toe, each

E0953 Pneumatic tire, each

E0954 Semi-pneumatic caster, each

WHEELCHAIR ACCESSORIES

E0958 Wheelchair attachment to convert any wheelchair to one arm drive

E0959 Amputee adapter (device used to compensate for transfer of weight due to lost limbs to maintain proper balance)

E0961 Brake extension, for wheelchair

E0962 1" cushion, for wheelchair

E0963 2" cushion, for wheelchair

E0964	3" cushion, for wheelchair
E0965	4" cushion, for wheelchair
E0966	Hook on head rest extension
E0967	Wheelchair hand rims with 8 vertical rubber tipped projections, pair
E0968	Commode seat, wheelchair
E0969	Narrowing device, wheelchair
E0970	No. 2 Footplates, except for elevating leg rest
E0971	Anti-tipping device wheelchair
E0972	Transfer board or device
E0973	Adjustable height detachable arms, desk or full length, wheelchair
E0974	'Grade-Aid' (device to prevent rolling back on an incline) for wheelchair
E0975	Reinforced seat upholstery, wheelchair
E0976	Reinforced back upholstery, wheelchair
E0977	Wedge cushion, wheelchair
E0978	Belt; safety with airplane buckle, wheelchair
E0979	safety with velcro closure, wheelchair
E0980	Safety vest, wheelchair
E0990	Elevating leg rest, each
E0991	Upholstery seat
E0992	Solid seat insert
E0993	Back, upholstery
E0994	Arm rest, each

Not valid for Medicare　　Non-covered by Medicare　　Special coverage instructions　　Carrier discretion

E0995   Calf rest, each

E0996   Tire, solid, each

E0997   Caster with a fork

E0998   Caster without fork

E0999   Pneumatic tire with wheel

E1000   Tire, pneumatic caster

E1001   Wheel, single

WHEELCHAIR-ECONOMY

ROLLABOUT CHAIR

E1031   Rollabout chair, any and all types with castors 5 inches or greater

E1035   Multi-positional patient transfer system, with integrated seat, operated by care giver

WHEELCHAIR-FULLY-RECLINING

E1050   Fully-reclining wheelchair; fixed full length arms, swing away detachable elevating leg rests

E1060   Fully-reclining wheelchair; detachable arms, desk or full length, swing away detachable elevating leg rests

E1065   Power attachment (to convert any wheelchair to motorized wheelchair, e.g., Solo)

E1066   Battery charger

E1069   Deep cycle battery

E1070   Fully-reclining wheelchair, detachable arms (desk or full length) swing away detachable footrest

E1083   Hemi-wheelchair; fixed full length arms, swing away detachable elevating leg rest

E1084   detachable arms desk or full length arms, swing away detachable elevating leg rests

E1085 fixed full length arms, swing away detachable footrests

E1086 detachable arms desk or full length, swing away detachable footrests

E1087 High strength lightweight wheelchair; fixed full length arms, swing away detachable elevating leg rests

E1088 detachable arms desk or full length, swing away detachable elevating leg rests

E1089 fixed length arms, swing away detachable footrest

E1090 detachable arms desk or full length, swing away detachable footrests

E1091 Youth wheelchair, any type

E1092 Wide heavy duty wheelchair, detachable arms (desk or full length); swing away detachable elevating leg rests

E1093 swing away detachable footrests

WHEELCHAIR-SEMI-RECLINING

E1100 Semi-reclining wheelchair; fixed full length arms, swing away detachable elevating leg rests

E1110 detachable arms (desk or full length), elevating leg rest

WHEELCHAIR-STANDARD

E1130 Standard wheelchair, fixed full length arms, fixed or swing away detachable footrests

E1140 Wheelchair, detachable arms, desk or full length; swing away detachable footrests

E1150 swing away detachable elevating leg rests

E1160 Wheelchair, fixed full length arms, swing away detachable elevating leg rests

WHEELCHAIR-AMPUTEE

E1170 Amputee wheelchair; fixed full length arms, swing away detachable elevating leg rests

| | Not valid for Medicare | | Non-covered by Medicare | | Special coverage instructions | | Carrier discretion | **129** |

E1171	fixed full length arms, without foot rests or leg rest
E1172	detachable arms (desk or full length), without foot rests or leg rest
E1180	detachable arms (desk or full length), swing away detachable foot rests
E1190	detachable arms (desk or full length), swing away detachable elevating leg rests
E1195	Heavy duty wheelchair, fixed full length arms, swing away detachable elevating leg rests
E1200	Amputee wheelchair, fixed full length arms, swing away detachable foot rest

WHEELCHAIR-POWER

E1210	Motorized wheelchair; fixed full length arms, swing away detachable elevating leg rests
E1211	detachable arms, desk or full length, swing away detachable elevating leg rests
E1212	fixed full length arms, swing away detachable foot rests
E1213	detachable arms desk or full length, swing away detachable foot rests

WHEELCHAIR-SPECIAL SIZE

E1220	Wheelchair specially sized or constructed (indicate brand name, model number, if any, and justification)
E1221	Wheelchair with fixed arm; footrests
E1222	elevating leg rests
E1223	Wheelchair with detachable arms; foot rests
E1224	elevating leg rests
E1225	Semi-reclining back for customized wheelchair
E1226	Full reclining back for customized wheelchair

E1227 Special height arms for wheelchair

E1228 Special back height for wheelchair

POWER OPERATED VEHICLE

E1230 Power operated vehicle (3 or 4 wheel non-highway) specify brand name and model number

WHEELCHAIR-LIGHTWEIGHT

E1240 Lightweight wheelchair; detachable arms, (desk or full length) swing away detachable, elevating leg rest

E1250 fixed full length arms, swing away detachable footrest

E1260 detachable arms (desk or full length) swing away detachable footrest

E1270 fixed full length arms, swing away detachable elevating leg rests

WHEELCHAIR-HEAVY DUTY

E1280 Heavy duty wheelchair; detachable arms (desk or full length) elevating leg rests

E1285 fixed full length arms, swing away detachable foot rest

E1290 detachable arms (desk or full length) swing away detachable foot rest

E1295 fixed full length arms, elevating leg rest

E1296 Special wheelchair; seat height from floor

E1297 seat depth, by upholstery

E1298 seat depth and/or width, by construction

WHIRLPOOL EQUIPMENT

E1300 Whirlpool; portable (overtub type)

E1310 non-portable (built-in type)

REPAIRS AND REPLACEMENT SUPPLIES

E1340   Repair or nonroutine service for DME requiring the skill of a technician, labor component, per 15 minutes

ADDITIONAL OXYGEN RELATED SUPPLIES AND EQUIPMENT

E1353   Regulator

E1355   Stand/Rack

E1372   Immersion external heater for nebulizer

(E1375)   Code deleted 2001; use E0570

(E1377)   Code deleted 2001

(E1378)   Code deleted 2001

(E1379)   Code deleted 2001

(E1380)   Code deleted 2001

(E1381)   Code deleted 2001

(E1382)   Code deleted 2001

(E1383)   Code deleted 2001

(E1384)   Code deleted 2001

(E1385)   Code deleted 2001

E1390   Oxygen concentrator, capable of delivering 85 percent or greater oxygen concentration at the prescribed flow rate

E1399   Durable medical equipment, miscellaneous

(E1400)   Code deleted 2000; use E1390

(E1401)   Code deleted 2000; use E1390

(E1402)   Code deleted 2000; use E1390

(E1403)   Code deleted 2000; use E1390

(E1404) Code deleted 2000; use E1390

E1405 Oxygen and water vapor enriching system; with heated delivery

E1406 without heated delivery

ARTIFICIAL KIDNEY MACHINES AND ACCESSORIES

NOTE: For supplies for ESRD, see codes A4650-A4999.

● **E1500** Centrifuge, for dialysis

E1510 Kidney dialysate delivery system; kidney machine, pump recirculating, air removal system, flowrate meter, power off, heater and temp control with alarm, I.V. poles, pressure gauge, concentrate container

▲ **E1520** Heparin infusion pump for hemodialysis

▲ **E1530** Air bubble detector for hemodialysis, each, replacement

▲ **E1540** Pressure alarm for hemodialysis, each, replacement

▲ **E1550** Bath conductivity meter for hemodialysis, each

▲ **E1560** Blood leak detector for hemodialysis, each, replacement

E1570 Adjustable chair, for ESRD patients

▲ **E1575** Transducer protectors/fluid barriers, for hemodialysis, any size, per 10

▲ **E1580** Unipuncture control system for hemodialysis

E1590 Hemodialysis machine

E1592 Automatic intermittent peritoneal dialysis system

E1594 Cycler dialysis machine for peritoneal dialysis

▲ **E1600** Delivery and/or installation charges for hemodialysis equipment

▲ **E1610** Reverse osmosis water purification system, for hemodialysis

▲ **E1615** Deionizer water purification system, for hemodialysis

▲ **E1620** Blood pump for hemodialysis, replacement

▲ **E1625** Water softening system, for hemodialysis

E1630 Reciprocating peritoneal dialysis system

▲ **E1632** Wearable artificial kidney, each

E1635 Compact (portable) travel hemodialyzer system

▲ **E1636** Sorbent cartridges, for hemodialysis, per 10

● **E1637** Hemostats, for dialysis, each

● **E1638** Heating pad, for peritoneal dialysis, any size, each

● **E1639** Scale, for dialysis, each

(E1640) Code deleted 2002

▲ **E1699** Dialysis equipment, not otherwise specified

E1700 Jaw motion rehabilitation system

E1701 Replacement cushions for jaw motion rehabilitation system, pkg. of 6

E1702 Replacement measuring scales for jaw motion rehabilitation system, pkg. of 200

▲ **E1800** Dynamic adjustable elbow extension/flexion device, includes soft interface material

● **E1801** Bi-directional static progressive stretch elbow device with range of motion adjustment, includes cuffs

▲ **E1805** Dynamic adjustable wrist extension/flexion device, includes soft interface material

● **E1806** Bi-directional static progressive stretch wrist device with range of motion adjustment, includes cuffs

▲ **E1810** Dynamic adjustable knee extension/flexion device, includes soft interface material

● **E1811** Bi-directional static progressive stretch knee device with range of motion adjustment, includes cuffs

▲ **E1815** Dynamic adjustable ankle extension/flexion device, includes soft interface material

● **E1816** Bi-directional static progressive stretch ankle device with range of motion adjustment, includes cuffs

● **E1818** Bi-directional static progressive stretch forearm pronation/supination device with range of motion adjustment, includes cuffs

▲ **E1820** Replacement soft interface material, dynamic adjustable extension/flexion device

● **E1821** Replacement soft interface material/cuffs for bi-directional static progressive stretch device

▲ **E1825** Dynamic adjustable finger extension/flexion device, includes soft interface material

▲ **E1830** Dynamic adjustable toe extension/flexion device, includes soft interface material

● **E1840** Dynamic adjustable shoulder flexion/abduction/rotation device, includes soft interface material

(**E1900**) Code deleted 2002

● **E1902** Communication board, non-electronic augmentative or alternative communication device

● **E2000** Gastric suction pump, home model, portable or stationary, electric

● **E2100** Blood glucose monitor with integrated voice synthesizer

● **E2101** Blood glucose monitor with integrated lancing/blood sample

PROCEDURES & PROFESSIONAL SERVICES

Guidelines

In addition to the information presented in the INTRODUCTION, several other items unique to this section are defined or identified here:

1. **TEMPORARY CODES:** The codes listed in this section are assigned by HCFA on a temporary basis to identify procedures/professional services.

PROCEDURES/PROFESSIONAL SERVICES

G0001 Routine venipuncture for collection of specimen(s) *16.00*

G0002 Office procedure, insertion of temporary indwelling catheter, foley type (separate procedure)

G0004 Patient demand single or multiple event recording with pre-symptom memory loop and 24-hour attended monitoring, per 30-day period; includes transmission, physician review and interpretation.

G0005 Patient demand single or multiple event recording with pre-symptom memory loop and 24-hour attended monitoring, per 30-day period; recording (includes hook-up, recording and disconnection)

G0006 Patient demand single or multiple event recording with pre-symptom memory loop and 24-hour attended monitoring, per 30-day period; 24-hour attended monitoring, receipt of transmissions, and analysis

G0007 Patient demand single or multiple event recording with pre-symptom memory loop and 24-hour attended monitoring, per 30-day period; physician review and interpretation only

G0008 Administration of influenza virus vaccine

G0009 Administration of pneumococcal vaccine

G-H
CODES

Not valid for Medicare	Non-covered by Medicare	Special coverage instructions	Carrier discretion	**137**

G0010 Administration of hepatitis B vaccine

G0015 Post-symptom telephonic transmission of electrocardiogram rhythm strip(s) and 24-hour attended monitoring, per 30-day period; tracing only

(G0016) Code deleted 2002

G0025 Collagen skin test kit

G0026 Fecal leucocyte examination

G0027 Semen analysis; presence and/or motility of sperm excluding Huhner

G0030 PET myocardial perfusion imaging, (following previous PET, G0030-G0047); single study, rest or stress (exercise and/or pharmacologic)

G0031 multiple studies, rest or stress (exercise and/or pharmacologic)

G0032 PET myocardial perfusion imaging, (following rest SPECT, 78464); single study, rest or stress (exercise and/or pharmacologic)

G0033 multiple studies, rest or stress (exercise and/or pharmacologic)

G0034 PET myocardial perfusion imaging, (following stress SPECT, 78465); single study, rest or stress (exercise and/or pharmacologic)

G0035 multiple studies, rest or stress (exercise and/or pharmacologic)

G0036 PET myocardial perfusion imaging (following coronary angiography, 93510-93529); single study, rest or stress (exercise and/or pharmacologic)

G0037 multiple studies, rest or stress (exercise and/or pharmacologic)

G0038 PET myocardial perfusion imaging (following stress planar myocardial perfusion, 78460); single study, rest or stress (exercise and/or pharmacologic)

G0039   multiple studies, rest or stress (exercise and/or pharmacologic)

G0040   PET myocardial perfusion imaging (following stress echocardiogram, 93350); single study, rest or stress (exercise and/or pharmacologic)

G0041   multiple studies, rest or stress (exercise and/or pharmacologic)

G0042   PET myocardial perfusion imaging (following stress nuclear ventriculogram 78481 or 78483); single study, rest or stress (exercise and/or pharmacologic)

G0043   multiple studies, rest or stress (exercise and/or pharmacologic)

G0044   PET myocardial perfusion imaging (following rest ECG 93000); single study, rest or stress (exercise and/or pharmacologic)

G0045   multiple studies, rest or stress (exercise and/or pharmacologic)

G0046   PET myocardial perfusion imaging (following stress ECG 93015); single study, rest or stress (exercise and/or pharmacologic)

G0047   multiple studies, rest or stress (exercise and/or pharmacologic)

G0050   Measurement of post-voiding residual urine and/or bladder capacity by ultrasound

G0101   Cervical or vaginal cancer screening; pelvic and clinical breast examination

G0102   Prostate cancer screening; digital rectal examination

G0103   Prostate cancer screening; prostate specific antigen test (PSA), total

G0104   Colorectal cancer screening; flexible sigmoidoscopy

G0105   colonoscopy on individual at high risk

G0106   alternative to G0104, screening sigmoidoscopy, barium enema

Not valid for Medicare | Non-covered by Medicare | Special coverage instructions | Carrier discretion

G0107   fecal-occult blood test, 1-3 simultaneous determinations

G0108   Diabetes outpatient self-management training services, individual, per 30 minutes

G0109   Diabetes outpatient self-management training services, group session (2 or more), per 30 minutes

G0110   Nett pulm-rehab; education/skills training, individual

G0111   education/skills training, group

G0112   nutritional guidance, initial

G0113   nutritional guidance, subsequent

G0114   psychosocial consultation

G0115   psychological testing

G0116   psychosocial counseling

● **G0117**   Glaucoma screening for high risk patients furnished by an optometrist or ophthalmologist

● **G0118**   Glaucoma screening for high risk patient furnished under the direct supervision of an optometrist or ophthalmologist

G0120   Colorectal cancer screening; alternative to G0105, screening colonoscopy, barium enema

G0121   colonoscopy on individual not meeting criteria for high risk

G0122   barium enema

G0123   Screening cytopathology, cervical or vaginal (any reporting system), collected in preservative fluid, automated thin layer preparation; screening by cytotechnologist under physician supervision

G0124   requiring interpretation by physician

▲ **G0125**   PET imaging regional or whole body; single pulmonary nodule, full- and partial-ring PET scanners only

(G0126) Code deleted 2002

G0127 Trimming of dystrophic nails, any number

G0128 Direct (fact-to-face with patient) skilled nursing services of a registered nurse provided in a comprehensive outpatient rehabilitation facility, each 10 minutes beyond the first 5 minutes

G0129 Occupational therapy requiring the skills of a qualified occupational therapist, furnished as a component of a partial hospitalization treatment program, per day

G0130 Single energy X-ray absorptiometry (sexa) bone density study, one or more sites; appendicular skeleton (peripheral) (e.g., radius, wrist, heel)

G0131 Computerized tomography bone mineral density study, one or more sites; axial skeleton (e.g., hips, pelvis, spine)

G0132 appendicular skeleton (peripheral) (e.g., radius, wrist, heel)

(G0133) Code deleted 1999; use 76977

G0141 Screening cytopathology smears, cervical or vaginal, performed by automated system, with manual rescreening, requiring interpretation by physician

G0143 Screening cytopathology, cervical or vaginal (any reporting system), collected in preservative fluid, automated thin layer preparation; with manual screening and rescreening by cytotechnologist under physician supervision

G0144 with manual screening and computer-assisted rescreening by cytotechnologist under physician supervision

G0145 with manual screening and computer-assisted rescreening using cell selection and review under physician supervision

G0147 Screening cytopathology smears, cervical or vaginal; performed by automated system under physician supervision

G0148 performed by automated system with manual rescreening

G0151 Services of physical therapist in home or health setting, each 15 minutes

G0152 Services of occupational therapist in home health setting, each 15 minutes

G0153 Services of speech and language pathologist in home health setting, each 15 minutes

G0154 Services of skilled nurse in home health setting, each 15 minutes

G0155 Services of clinical social worker in home health setting, each 15 minutes

G0156 Services of home health aide in home health setting, each 15 minutes

(G0159) Code deleted 2001

(G0160) Code deleted 2001

(G0161) Code deleted 2001

(G0163) Code deleted 2001; use G0215

(G0164) Code deleted 2001

(G0165) Code deleted 2001

G0166 External counterpulsation, per treatment session

G0167 Hyperbaric oxygen treatment not requiring physician attendance, per treatment session

G0168 Wound closure utilizing tissue adhesive(s) only

(G0169) Code deleted 2001

(G0170) Code deleted 2001

(G0171) Code deleted 2001

(G0172) Code deleted 2001; use G0177

G0173 Sterotactic radiosurgery, complete course of therapy in one session

(G0174) Code deleted 2002

G0175 Scheduled interdisciplinary team conference (minimum of three exclusive of patient care nursing staff) with patient present

G0176 Activity therapy, such as music, dance, art or play therapies not for recreation, related to the care and treatment of patient's disabling mental health problems, per session (45 minutes or more)

G0177 Training and education services related to the care and treatment of patient's disabling mental health problems per session (45 minutes or more)

(G0178) Code deleted 2002

G0179 Physician recertification services for Medicare-covered services provided by a participating home health agency (patient not present) including review of subsequent reports of patient status, review of patient's responses to the Oasis assessment instrument, contact with the home health agency to ascertain the follow-up implementation plan of care, and documentation in the patient's office record, per certification period

G0180 Physician certification services for Medicare-covered services provided by a participating home health agency (patient not present), including review of initial or subsequent reports of patient status, review of patient's responses to the oasis assessment instrument, contact with the home health agency to ascertain the initial implementation plan of care, and documentation in the patient's office record, per certification period

G0181 Physician supervision of a patient receiving Medicare-covered services provided by a participating home health agency (patient not present), requiring complex and multidisciplinary care modalities involving regular physician development and/or revision of care plans, review of subsequent reports of patient status, review of laboratory and other studies, communication (including telephone calls) with other health care professionals involved in the patient's care, integration of new information into the medical treatment plan and/or adjustment of medical therapy, within a calendar month, 30 minutes or more

Not valid for Medicare   Non-covered by Medicare   Special coverage instructions   Carrier discretion

G0182 Physician supervision of a patient under a Medicare-approved hospice (patient not present) requiring complex and multidisciplinary care modalities involving regular physician development and/or revision of care plans, review of subsequent reports of patient status, review of laboratory and other studies, communication (including telephone calls) with other health care professionals involved in the patient's care, integration of new information into the medical treatment plan and/or adjustment of medical therapy, within a calendar month, 30 minutes or more

(G0184) Code deleted 2002

G0185 Destruction of localized lesion of choroid (for example, choroidal neovascularization); transpupillary thermotherapy (one or more sessions)

G0186 Destruction of localized lesion of choroid (for example, choroidal neovascularization); photocoagulation, feeder vessel technique (one or more sessions)

G0187 Destruction of macular drusen, photocoagulation (one or more sessions)

(G0188) Code deleted 2002

(G0190) Code deleted 2002

(G0191) Code deleted 2002

G0192 Intranasal or oral administration; one vaccine (single or combination vaccine/toxoid)

G0193 Endoscopic study of swallowing function (also fiberoptic endoscopic evaluation of swallowing (FEES)

G0194 Sensory testing during endoscopic study of swallowing (add on code) referred to as fiberoptic endoscopic evaluation of swallowing with sensory testing (FEEST)

G0195 Clinical evaluation of swallowing function (not involving interpretation of dynamic radiological studies or endoscopic study of swallowing)

G0196 Evaluation of swallowing involving swallowing of radio-opaque materials

G0197 Evaluation of patient for prescription of speech generating devices

G0198 Patient adaptation and training for use of speech generating devices

G0199 Re-evaluation of patient using speech generating devices

G0200 Evaluation of patient for prescription of voice prosthetic

G0201 Modification or training in use of voice prosthetic

● **G0202** Screening mammography, producing direct digital image, bilateral, all views

(**G0203**) Code deleted 2002

● **G0204** Diagnostic mammography, producing direct digital image, bilateral, all views

(**G0205**) Code deleted 2002

● **G0206** Diagnostic mammography, producing direct digital image, unilateral, all views

(**G0207**) Code deleted 2002

● **G0210** PET imaging whole body; full- and partial-ring PET scanners only, diagnosis, lung cancer, non-small cell

● **G0211** PET imaging whole body; full- and partial-ring PET scanners only, initial staging, lung cancer, non-small cell

● **G0212** PET imaging whole body, full- and partial-ring PET scanners only, restaging, lung cancer, non-small cell

● **G0213** PET imaging whole body; full- and partial-ring PET scanners only, diagnosis, colorectal cancer

● **G0214** PET imaging whole body; full- and partial-ring PET scanners only, initial staging, colorectal cancer

● **G0215** PET imaging whole body; full- and partial-ring PET scanners only, restaging, colorectal cancer (replaces G0163)

● **G0216** PET imaging whole body; full- and partial-ring PET scanners only, diagnosis, melanoma

● **G0217** PET imaging whole body; full- and partial-ring PET scanners only, initial staging, melanoma

● **G0218** PET imaging whole body; full- and partial-ring PET scanners only, restaging, melanoma (replaces G0165)

● **G0219** PET imaging whole body; full and partial ring PET scanners only, for non-covered indications

● **G0220** PET imaging whole body; full- and partial-ring PET scanners only, diagnosis, lymphoma

● **G0221** PET imaging whole body; full- and partial-ring PET scanners only, initial staging, lymphoma (replaces G0164)

● **G0222** PET imaging whole body; full- and partial-ring PET scanners only, restaging, lymphoma (replaces G0164)

● **G0223** PET imaging whole body or regional; full- and partial-ring PET scanners only, diagnosis, head and neck cancer, excluding thyroid and CNS cancers

● **G0224** PET imaging whole body or regional; full- and partial-ring PET scanners only, initial staging, head and neck cancer, excluding thyroid and CNS cancers

● **G0225** PET imaging whole body or regional; full- and partial-ring PET scanners only, restaging, head and neck cancer, excluding thyroid and CNS cancers

● **G0226** PET imaging whole body; full and partial ring PET scanners only, diagnosis, esophageal cancer

● **G0227** PET imaging whole body, full- and partial-ring PET scanners only, initial staging, esophageal cancer

● **G0228** PET imaging whole body, full- and partial-ring PET scanners only, restaging, esophageal cancer

● **G0229** PET imaging; metabolic brain imaging for pre-surgical evaluation of refractory seizures, full- and partial-ring PET scanners only

● **G0230** PET imaging; metabolic assessment for myocardial viability following inconclusive spect study, full- and partial-ring PET scanners only

● **G0231** PET, whole body, for recurrence of colorectal or colorectal metastatic cancer; gamma cameras only

● **G0232** PET, whole body, for staging and characterization of lymphoma; gamma cameras only

● **G0233** PET, whole body, for recurrence of melanoma or melanoma metastatic cancer; gamma cameras only

● **G0234** PET, regional or whole body, for solitary pulmonary nodule following CT or for initial staging of pathologically diagnosed nonsmall cell lung cancer; gamma cameras only

● **G0236** Digitization of film radiographic images with computer analysis for lesion detection and further physician review for interpretation, diagnostic mammography (list separately in addition to code for primary procedure)

● **G0237** Therapeutic procedures to increase strength or endurance of respiratory muscles, face to face, one on one, each 15 minutes (includes monitoring)

● **G0238** Therapeutic procedures to improve respiratory function, other than described by G0237, one on one, face to face, per 15 minutes (includes monitoring)

● **G0239** Therapeutic procedures to improve respiratory function, other than services described by G0237, two or more (includes monitoring)

● **G0240** Critical care service delivered by a physician, face to face, during interfacility transport of a critically ill or critically injured patient; first 30-74 minutes of active transport

● **G0241** each additional 30 minutes (list separately in addition to G0240)

● **G0242** Multi-source photon stereotactic radiosurgery (cobalt 60 multi-source converging beams) plan, including dose volume histograms for target and critical structure

| | Not valid for Medicare | | Non-covered by Medicare | | Special coverage instructions | | Carrier discretion |

tolerances, plan optimization performed for highly conformal distributions, plan positional accuracy and dose verification, all lesions treated, per course of treatment

● **G0243** Multi-source photon stereotactic radiosurgery, delivery including collimator changes and custom plugging, complete course of treatment, all lesions

● **G0244** Observation care provided by a facility to a patient with CHF, chest pain, or asthma, minimum eight hours, maximum forty-eight hours

G9001 Coordinated care fee; initial rate

G9002 maintenance rate

G9003 risk adjusted high, initial

G9004 risk adjusted low, initial

G9005 risk adjusted maintenance

G9006 home monitoring

G9007 scheduled team conference

G9008 physician coordinated care oversight services

● **G9009** risk adjusted maintenance, level 3

● **G9010** risk adjusted maintenance, level 4

● **G9011** risk adjusted maintenance, level 5

● **G9012** Other specified case management service not elsewhere classified

G9016 Smoking cessation counseling, individual, in the absence of or in addition to any other evaluation and management service, per session (6-10 minutes) [DEMO PROJECT CODE ONLY]

REHABILITATIVE SERVICES

Rehabilitative Services

H0001   Alcohol and/or drug assessment

H0002   Alcohol and/or drug screening to determine eligibility for admission to treatment program

H0003   Alcohol and/or drug screening; laboratory analysis of specimens for presence of alcohol and/or drugs

H0004   Alcohol and/or drug services; individual counseling by a clinician

H0005   Alcohol and/or drug services; group counseling by a clinician

H0006   Alcohol and/or drug services; case management

H0007   Alcohol and/or drug services; crisis intervention (outpatient)

H0008   Alcohol and/or drug services; sub-acute detoxification (hospital inpatient)

H0009   Alcohol and/or drug services; acute detoxification (hospital inpatient)

H0010   Alcohol and/or drug services; sub-acute detoxification (residential addiction program inpatient)

H0011   Alcohol and/or drug services; acute detoxification (residential addiction program inpatient)

H0012   Alcohol and/or drug services; sub-acute detoxification (residential addiction program outpatient)

H0013   Alcohol and/or drug services; acute detoxification (residential addiction program outpatient)

H0014   Alcohol and/or drug services; ambulatory detoxification

Not valid for Medicare   Non-covered by Medicare   Special coverage instructions   Carrier discretion

H0015 Alcohol and/or drug services; intensive outpatient (treatment program that operates at least 3 hours/day and at least 3 days/week and is based on an individualized treatment plan), including assessment, counseling, crisis intervention, and activity therapies or education

H0016 Alcohol and/or drug services; medical/somatic (medical intervention in ambulatory setting)

H0017 Alcohol and/or drug services; residential (hospital residential treatment program)

H0018 Alcohol and/or drug services; short-term residential (non-hospital residential treatment program)

H0019 Alcohol and/or drug services; long-term residential (non-medical, non-acute care in residential treatment program where stay is typically longer than 30 days)

H0020 Alcohol and/or drug services; methadone administration and/or service (provision of the drug by a licensed program)

H0021 Alcohol and/or drug training service (for staff and personnel not employed by providers)

H0022 Alcohol and/or drug intervention service (planned facilitation)

H0023 Alcohol and/or drug outreach service (planned approach to reach a target population)

H0024 Alcohol and/or drug prevention information dissemination service (one-way direct or non-direct contact with service audiences to affect knowledge or attitude)

H0025 Alcohol and/or drug prevention education service (delivery of services with target population to affect knowledge, attitude and/or behavior)

H0026 Alcohol and/or drug prevention process services, community-based (delivery of services to develop skills of impactors)

H0027 Alcohol and/or drug prevention environmental services (broad range of external activities geared toward modifying systems in order to mainstream prevention through policy and law)

H0028 Alcohol and/or drug prevention problem identification and referral service (e.g., student assistance and employee assistance programs), does not include assessment

H0029 Alcohol and/or drug prevention alternatives service (services for populations that exclude alcohol and other drug use, e.g. alcohol-free social events)

H0030 Alcohol and/or drug hotline service

● **H1000** Prenatal care, at-risk assessment

● **H1001** Prenatal care, at-risk enhanced service; antepartum management

● **H1002** Prenatal care, at-risk enhanced service; care coordination

● **H1003** Prenatal care, at-risk enhanced service; education

● **H1004** Prenatal care, at-risk enhanced service; follow-up home visit

● **H1005** Prenatal care, at-risk enhanced service package (includes H1001-H1004)

● New code   ▲ Revised code   ( ) Deleted code

DRUGS ADMINISTERED OTHER THAN ORAL METHOD

(EXCEPTION: ORAL IMMUNOSUPPRESSIVE DRUGS)

Guidelines

In addition to the information presented in the INTRODUCTION, several other items unique to this section are defined or identified here:

1. **EXCEPTION:** Oral immunosuppressive drugs are not included in this section.

2. **ROUTE OF ADMINISTRATION:** Unless otherwise specified, the drugs listed in this section may be injected either subcutaneously, intramuscularly or intravenously.

3. **SUBSECTION INFORMATION:** Some of the listed subheadings or subsections have special needs or instructions unique to that section. Where these are indicated, special "notes" will be presented preceding or following the listings. Those subsections within the DRUGS ADMINISTERED OTHER THAN ORAL METHOD section that have "notes" are as follows:

Subsection	Code Numbers
Drugs administered other than oral method	J0000-J8999
Immunosuppressive drugs	J7500-J7506
Chemotherapy drugs	J9000-J9999

4. **UNLISTED SERVICE OR PROCEDURE:** A service or procedure may be provided that is not listed in this edition of HCPCS. When reporting such a service, the appropriate "unlisted procedure" code may be used to indicate the service, identifying it by "special report" as defined below. HCPCS terminology is inconsistent in defining unlisted procedures. The procedure definition may include the term(s) "unlisted", "not otherwise classified", "unspecified", "unclassified", "other" and "miscellaneous". Prior to using these codes, try to determine if a Local Level III code or CPT code is available. The "unlisted procedures" and accompanying codes for DRUGS ADMINISTERED OTHER THAN ORAL METHOD are as follows:

J CODES

Not valid for Medicare   Non-covered by Medicare   Special coverage instructions   Carrier discretion

> J3490   Unclassified drugs
> J9999   Not otherwise classified, antineoplastic drugs

5. **SPECIAL REPORT:** A service, material or supply that is rarely provided, unusual, variable or new may require a special report in determining medical appropriateness for reimbursement purposes. Pertinent information should include an adequate definition or description of the nature, extent, and need for the service, material or supply.

6. **MODIFIERS:** Listed services may be modified under certain circumstances. When appropriate, the modifying circumstance is identified by adding a modifier to the basic procedure code. CPT and HCPCS National Level II modifiers may be used with CPT and HCPCS National Level II procedure codes. Modifiers commonly used with DRUGS ADMINISTERED OTHER THAN ORAL METHOD are as follows:

-AA   Anesthesia services performed personally by anesthesiologist

-AD   Medical supervision by a physician: more than four concurrent anesthesia procedures.

-CC   Procedure code change (use "CC" when the procedure code submitted was changed either for administrative reasons or because an incorrect code was filed)

-G8   Monitored anesthesia care (MAC) for deep complex, complicated, or markedly invasive surgical procedure

-G9   Monitored anesthesia care (MAC) for patient who has history of severe cardio-pulmonary condition

-TC   Technical component. Under certain circumstances, a charge may be made for the technical component alone. Under those circumstances, the technical component charge is identified by adding modifier -TC to the usual procedure code. Technical component charges are institutional charges and are not billed separately by physicians. However, portable x-ray suppliers bill only for the technical component and should use modifier -TC. The charge data from portable x-ray suppliers will then be used to build customary and prevailing profiles.

7. **CPT CODE CROSS-REFERENCE:** Unless otherwise specified, the equivalent CPT codes for all listings in this section fall within the range 90701-90799.

Drugs Administered Other Than Oral Method

The following list of drugs can be injected either subcutaneous, intramuscular, or intravenous. The brand name(s) of the drugs has been included as bold-type in brackets [ ] in some cases.

NOTE: Third party payers may wish to determine a threshold and pay up to a certain dollar limit before developing for the drug. Use procedure code J0110 for processing these cases.

J0120 Injection, tetracycline, up to 250 mg

J0130 Injection abciximab, 10 mg

J0150 Injection, adenosine, 6 mg (not to be used to report any adenosine phosphate compounds, instead use A9270)

J0151 Injection, adenosine, 90 mg (not to be used to report any adenosine phosphate compounds, instead use A9270)

J0170 Injection, adrenalin, epinephrine, up to 1 ml ampul

J0190 Injection, biperiden lactate, per 5 mg

J0200 Injection, alatrofloxacin mesylate, 100 mg

J0205 Injection, alglucerase, per 10 units

J0207 Injection, amifostine, 500 mg

J0210 Injection, methyldopate HCl, [Aldomet], up to 250 mg

J0256 Injection, alpha 1—proteinase inhibitor—human, 10 mg

J0270 Injection, alprostadil, 1.25 mcg (code may be used for Medicare when drug administered under the direct supervision of a physician, not for use when drug is self administered)

J0275 Alprostadil urethral suppository (code may be used for Medicare when drug administered under the direct supervision of a physician, not for use when drug is self administered)

J0280 Injection, aminophylline, up to 250 mg

J0282   Injection, amiodarone hydrochloride, 30 mg

J0285   Injection, amphotericin B, 50 mg

J0286   Injection, amphotericin B, any lipid formulation, 50 mg

J0290   Injection, ampicillin sodium, 500 mg

J0295   Injection, ampicillin sodium/sulbactam sodium, per 1.5 gram

J0300   Injection, amobarbital, up to 125 mg

J0330   Injection, succinylcholine chloride, [Anectine], up to 20 mg

(J0340)   Code deleted 2002

J0350   Injection, anistreplase, per 30 units

J0360   Injection, hydralazine HCl, [Apresoline], up to 20 mg

J0380   Injection, metaraminol bitartrate, per 10 mg

J0390   Injection, chloroquine HCl, [Aralen HCl], up to 250 mg

J0395   Injection, arbutamine HCl, 1 mg

(J0400)   Code deleted 2002

J0456   Injection, azithromycin, 500 mg

J0460   Injection, atropine sulfate, up to 0.3 mg

J0470   Injection, dimercaprol, per 100 mg

J0475   Injection, baclofen, 10 mg

J0476   Injection, baclofen, 50 mcg for intrathecal trial

J0500   Injection, dicyclomine HCl, [Bentyl, Spasmoject], up to 20 mg

(J0510)   Code deleted 2002

J0515   Injection, benztropine mesylate, [Cogentin], per 1 mg

J0520 Injection, bethanechol chloride, myotonachol or urecholine, up to 5 mg

J0530 Injection, penicillin G benzathine and penicillin G procaine, [Bicillin C-R]; up to 600,000 units

J0540 up to 1,200,000 units

J0550 up to 2,400,000 units

J0560 Injection, penicillin G benzathine, [Bicillin long-acting]; up to 600,000 units

J0570 up to 1,200,000 units

J0580 up to 2,400,000 units

J0585 Botulinum toxin type A, per unit

● **J0587** Botulinum toxin type B, per 100 units

(J0590) Code deleted 2002

J0600 Injection, edetate calcium disodium, [calcium disodium versenate], up to 1,000 mg

J0610 Injection, calcium gluconate, per 10 ml

J0620 Injection, calcium glycerophosphate and calcium lactate, per 10 ml

J0630 Injection, calcitonin salmon, up to 400 units

J0635 Injection, calcitriol, [Calcijex] 1 mcg amp.

J0640 Injection, leucovorin calcium, per 50 mg

J0670 Injection, mepivacaine HCl, [Carbocaine], per 10 ml

J0690 Injection, cefazolin sodium, 500 mg

● **J0692** Injection, cefepime hydrochloride, 500 mg

J0694 Injection, cefoxitin sodium, [Mefoxin], 1 gram

(J0695) Code deleted 2002

J0696   Injection, ceftriaxone sodium, [Rocephin], per 250 mg

J0697   Injection sterile cefuroxime sodium, [Ceftin, Kefurox, Zihacef injection], per 750 mg

J0698   Injection, cefotaxime sodium, [Claforan], per gram

J0702   Injection, betamethasone acetate and betamethasone sodium phosphate, per 3 mg

J0704   Injection, betamethasone sodium phosphate, per 4 mg

● **J0706**   Injection, caffeine citrate, 5 mg

J0710   Injection, cephapirin sodium, [Cefadyl], up to 1 gram

J0713   Injection, ceftazidime, per 500 mg

J0715   Injection, ceftizoxime sodium, per 500 mg

J0720   Injection, chloramphenicol sodium succinate, [Chloromycetin Sodium Succinate], up to 1 gram

J0725   Injection, chorionic gonadotropin, per 1,000 USP units

(J0730)   Code deleted 2002

J0735   Injection, clonidine hydrochloride, 1 mg

J0740   Injection, cidofovir, 375 mg

J0743   Injection, cilastatin sodium/imipenem, [Primaxin], per 250 mg

● **J0744**   Injection, ciprofloxacin for intravenous infusion, 200 mg

J0745   Injection, codeine phosphate, per 30 mg

J0760   Injection, colchicine, per 1 mg

J0770   Injection, colistimethate sodium, [Coly-Mycin M], up to 150 mg

J0780   Injection, prochlorperazine, [Compazine], up to 10 mg

J0800   Injection, corticotropin, up to 40 units

(J0810) Code deleted 2002

J0835 Injection, cosyntropin, per 0.25 mg

J0850 Injection, cytomegalovirus immune globulin intravenous (human), per vial

J0895 Injection, deferoxamine mesylate, [Desferal] 500 mg

J0900 Injection, testosterone enanthate and estradiol valerate, up to 1 cc

J0945 Injection, brompheniramine maleate, per 10 mg

J0970 Injection, estradiol valerate, up to 40 mg

J1000 Injection, depo-estradiol cypionate, up to 5 mg

J1020 Injection, methylprednisolone acetate; 20 mg

J1030   40 mg

J1040   80 mg

J1050 Injection, medroxyprogesterone acetate, [Depo-Provera, Prempro], 100 mg

J1055 Injection, medroxyprogesterone acetate for contraceptive use, 150 mg

● **J1056** Injection, medroxyprogesterone acetate/estradiol cypionate, 5 mg/25 mg

J1060 Injection, testosterone cypionate and estradiol cypionate, up to 1 ml

J1070 Injection, testosterone cypionate, up to 100 mg

J1080 Injection, testosterone cypionate, 1 cc, 200 mg

(J1090) Code deleted 2002

J1095 Injection, dexamethasone acetate, per 8 mg

J1100 Injection, dexamethasone sodium phosphate, 1mg

J1110 Injection, dihydroergotamine mesylate, per 1 mg

J1120   Injection, acetazolamide sodium, [Diamox Sodium], up to 500 mg

J1160   Injection, digoxin, up to 0.5 mg

J1165   Injection, phenytoin sodium, [Dilantin], per 50 mg

J1170   Injection, hydromorphone, up to 4 mg

J1180   Injection, dyphylline, [Dilor, Lufyllin], up to 500 mg

J1190   Injection, dexrazoxane hydrochloride, per 250 mg

J1200   Injection, diphenhydramine HCl, [Benadryl], up to 50 mg

J1205   Injection, chlorothiazide sodium [Diuril], per 500 mg

J1212   Injection, DMSO, dimethyl sulfoxide, 50%, 50 ml

J1230   Injection, methadone HCl, [Dolophine HCl], up to 10 mg

J1240   Injection, dimenhydrinate, [Dramamine], up to 50 mg

J1245   Injection, dipyridamole, per 10 mg

J1250   Injection, dobutamine hydrochloride, per 250 mg

J1260   Injection, dolasetron mesylate, 10 mg

● **J1270**   Injection, doxercalciferol, 1 mcg

J1320   Injection, amitriptyline HCl, [Elavil HCl], up to 20 mg

J1325   Injection, epoprostenol, 0.5 mg

J1327   Injection, eptifibatide, 5 mg

J1330   Injection, ergonovine maleate, up to 0.2 mg

(J1362)   Code deleted 2002

J1364   Injection, erythromycin lactobionate, per 500 mg

J1380   Injection, estradiol valerate, up to 10 mg

J1390   Injection, estradiol valerate, up to 20 mg

J1410 Injection, estrogen conjugated, per 25 mg

J1435 Injection, estrone, per 1 mg

J1436 Injection, etidronate disodium per 300 mg

J1438 Injection, etanercept, 25 mg (code may be used for Medicare when drug administered under the direct supervision of a physician, not for use when drug is self administered)

J1440 Injection, filgrastim (G-CSF); 300 mcg

J1441 480 mcg

J1450 Injection, fluconazole, 200 mg

J1452 Injection, fomivirsen sodium, intraocular, 1.65 mg

J1455 Injection, foscarnet sodium, [Foscavir], per 1000 mg

J1460 Injection, gamma globulin; intramuscular 1 cc

J1470 intramuscular 2 cc

J1480 intramuscular 3 cc

J1490 intramuscular 4 cc

J1500 intramuscular 5 cc

J1510 intramuscular 6 cc

J1520 intramuscular 7 cc

J1530 intramuscular 8 cc

J1540 intramuscular 9 cc

J1550 intramuscular 10 cc

J1560 intramuscular over 10 cc

J1561 Injection, immune globulin; intravenous, 500 mg

(J1562) Code deleted 2001

J1563   Injection, immune globulin, intravenous, 1 gram

J1565   Injection, respiratory syncytial virus immune globulin, intravenous, 50 mg

J1570   Injection, ganciclovir sodium, [Cytovene], 500 mg

J1580   Injection, garamycin, gentamicin, up to 80 mg

● **J1590**   Injection, gatifloxacin, 10 mg

J1600   Injection, gold sodium thiomalate, up to 50 mg

J1610   Injection, glucagon hydrochloride, per 1 mg

J1620   Injection, gonadorelin hydrochloride, per 100 mcg

J1626   Injection, granisetron hydrochloride, 100 mcg

J1630   Injection, haloperidol, up to 5 mg

J1631   Injection, haloperidol decanoate, per 50 mg

J1642   Injection, heparin sodium, (heparin lock flush), per 10 units

J1644   Injection, heparin sodium, per 1,000 units

J1645   Injection, dalteparin sodium, per 2500 IU

J1650   Injection, enoxaparin sodium, 10 mg

● **J1655**   Injection, tinzaparin sodium, 1000 IU

J1670   Injection, tetanus immune globulin, human, up to 250 units

(J1690)   Code deleted 2002

J1700   Injection, hydrocortisone acetate, [Analpram HC, Hydrocortone Acetate], up to 25 mg

J1710   Injection, hydrocortisone sodium phosphate, [Hydrocortone Phosphate], up to 50 mg

J1720   Injection, hydrocortisone sodium succinate, [Solu-Cortef], up to 100 mg

J1730 Injection, diazoxide, [Hyperstat], up to 300 mg

(J1739) Code deleted 2002

(J1741) Code deleted 2002

J1742 Injection, ibutilide fumarate, 1 mg

J1745 Injection, infliximab, 10 mg

J1750 Injection, iron dextran, 50 mg

● **J1755** Injection, iron sucrose, 20 mg

(J1760) Code deleted 2000; use J1750

(J1770) Code deleted 2000; use J1750

(J1780) Code deleted 2000; use J1750

J1785 Injection, imiglucerase, per unit

J1790 Injection, droperidol, [Inapsine], up to 5 mg

J1800 Injection, propranolol HCl, [Inderal], up to 1 mg

J1810 Injection, droperidol and fentanyl citrate, [Innovar], up to 2 ml ampule

J1820 Injection, insulin, up to 100 units

J1825 Injection, interferon beta-1a, 33 mcg (code may be used for Medicare when drug administered under the direct supervision of a physician, not for use when drug is self administered)

J1830 Injection, interferon beta-1b, 0.25 mg (code may be used for Medicare when drug administered under the direct supervision of a physician, not for use when drug is self administered)

● **J1835** Injection, itraconazole, 50 mg

J1840 Injection, kanamycin sulfate, [Kantrex], up to 500 mg

J1850 Injection, kanamycin sulfate, [Kantrex Pediatric], up to 75 mg

J1885 Injection, ketorolac tromethamine, [Toradol IM], per 15 mg

J1890 Injection, cephalothin sodium, [Keflin], up to 1 gram

J1910 Injection, kutapressin, up to 2 ml

(J1930) Code deleted 2002

J1940 Injection, furosemide, [Lasix], up to 20 mg

J1950 Injection, leuprolide acetate (for depot suspension), per 3.75 mg

J1955 Injection, levocarnitine, per 1 gram

J1956 Injection, levofloxacin, 250 mg

J1960 Injection, levorphanal tartrate, up to 2 mg

(J1970) Code deleted 2002

J1980 Injection, hyoscyamine sulfate, [Levsin], up to 0.25 mg

J1990 Injection, chlordiazepoxide HCl, [Librium], up to 100 mg

J2000 Injection, lidocaine HCl, 50 cc

J2010 Injection, lincomycin HCl, up to 300 mg

● **J2020** Injection, linezolid, 200 mg

J2060 Injection, lorazepam, [Ativan], 2 mg

J2150 Injection, mannitol, 25% in 50 ml

J2175 Injection, meperidine HCl, per 100 mg

J2180 Injection, meperidine and promethazine HCl, [Mepergan], up to 50 mg

J2210 Injection, methylergonovine maleate, [Methergine Maleate], up to 0.2 mg

(J2240) Code deleted 2002

J2250 Injection, midazolam hydrochloride, per 1 mg

J2260	Injection, milrinone lactate, 5 mg
J2270	Injection, morphine sulfate, up to 10 mg
J2271	Injection, morphine sulfate, 100 mg
J2275	Injection, morphine sulfate (preservative-free sterile solution), per 10 mg
J2300	Injection, nalbuphine HCl, per 10 mg
J2310	Injection, naloxone hydrochloride, per 1 mg
J2320	Injection, nandrolone deconoate; up to 50 mg
J2321	up to 100 mg
J2322	up to 200 mg
(J2330)	Code deleted 2002
(J2350)	Code deleted 2002
J2352	Injection, octreotide acetate, 1 mg
J2355	Injection, oprelvekin, 5 mg
J2360	Injection, orphenadrine citrate, [Norflex, Norgesic], up to 60 mg
J2370	Injection, phenylephrine HCl, [Neo-Synephrine], up to 1 ml
J2400	Injection, chloroprocaine HCl [Nesacaine and Nesacaine-MPF], per 30 ml
J2405	Injection, ondansetron hydrochloride, per 1 mg
J2410	Injection, oxymorphone HCl [Numorphan], up to 1 mg
J2430	Injection, pamidronate disodium, per 30 mg
J2440	Injection, papaverine HCl, up to 60 mg
J2460	Injection, oxytetracycline HCl, up to 50 mg
(J2480)	Code deleted 2002

J2500   Injection, paricalcitol, 5 mcg

J2510   Injection, penicillin g procaine, aqueous, up to 600,000 units

(J2512)   Code deleted 2002

J2515   Injection, pentobarbital sodium, per 50 mg

J2540   Injection, penicillin G potassium, [Pfizerpen], up to 600,000 units

J2543   Injection, piperacillin sodium/tazobactam sodium, 1gram/0.125 grams (1.125 grams)

J2545   Pentamidine isethionate, inhalation solution, per 300 mg, administered through a DME

J2550   Injection, promethazine HCl, [Phenergan], up to 50 mg

J2560   Injection, phenobarbital sodium, [Phenobarbital], up to 120 mg

J2590   Injection, oxytocin, [Pitocin], up to 10 units

J2597   Injection, desmopressin acetate, per 1 mcg

(J2640)   Code deleted 2002

J2650   Injection, prednisolone acetate, up to 1 ml

J2670   Injection, tolazoline HCl, [Priscoline HCl], up to 25 mg

(J2675)   Code deleted 2002

J2680   Injection, fluphenazine deconoate, [Prolixin Deconoate], up to 25 mg

J2690   Injection, procainamide HCl, [Proenstyl], up to 1 gram

J2700   Injection, oxacillin sodium, [Prostaphlin], up to 250 mg

J2710   Injection, neostigmine methylsulfate, [Prostigmin Methylsulfate], up to 0.5 mg

J2720   Injection, protamine sulfate, per 10 mg

J2725 Injection, protirelin, per 250 mcg

J2730 Injection, pralidoxime chloride, [Protopam Chloride], up to 1 gram

J2760 Injection, phentolamine mesylate, [Regitine], up to 5 mg

J2765 Injection, metoclopramide HCl [Reglan], up to 10 mg

J2770 Injection, quinupristin/dalfopristin, 500 mg (150/350)

J2780 Injection, ranitidine hydrochloride, 25 mg

J2790 Injection, RHo(D) immune globulin, human, [Rhogam], one dose package

J2792 Injection, RHo(D) immune globulin, intravenous, human, solvent detergent, 100 IU

J2795 Injection, ropivacaine hydrochloride, 1 mg

J2800 Injection, methocarbamol, [Robaxin], up to 10 ml

J2810 Injection, theophylline, per 40 mg

J2820 Injection, sargramostim (GM-CSF), 50 mcg

(J2860) Code deleted 2002

J2910 Injection, aurothioglucose, [Solganal], up to 50 mg

J2912 Injection, sodium chloride, 0.9%, per 2 ml

J2915 Injection, sodium ferric gluconate complex in sucrose injection, 62.5 mg

J2920 Injection, methylprednisolone sodium succinate, [Solu-Medrol], up to 40 mg

J2930 Injection, methylprednisolone sodium succinate, [Solu-Medrol], up to 125 mg

● **J2940** Injection, somatrem, 1 mg

● **J2941** Injection, somatropin, 1 mg

J2950 Injection, promazine HCl, [Prozine, Sparine], up to 25 mg

(J2970)	Code deleted 2002
▲ **J2993**	Injection, reteplase, 18.1 mg
(J2994)	Code deleted 2001
J2995	Injection, streptokinase, per 250,000 IU
(J2996)	Code deleted 2001
J2997	Injection, alteplase recombinant, 1 mg
J3000	Injection, streptomycin, up to 1 gram
J3010	Injection, fentanyl citrate, 0.1 mg
J3030	Injection, sumatriptan succinate, 6 mg (code may be used for Medicare when drug administered under the direct supervision of a physician, not for use when drug is self administered)
J3070	Injection, pentazocine HCl, [Talwin], up to 30 mg
(J3080)	Code deleted 2002
● **J3100**	Injection, tenecteplase, 50 mg
J3105	Terbutaline sulfate, up to 1 mg
J3120	Injection, testosterone enanthate; up to 100 mg
J3130	up to 200 mg
J3140	Injection, testosterone suspension, up to 50 mg
J3150	Injection, testosterone propionate, up to 100 mg
J3230	Injection, chlorpromazine HCl, [Thorazine], up to 50 mg
J3240	Injection, thyrotropin alfa, 0.9 mg
J3245	Injection, tirofiban hydrochloride, 12.5 mg
J3250	Injection, trimethobenzamide HCl, up to 200 mg
J3260	Injection, tobramycin sulfate, [Nebcin], up to 80 mg

J3265	Injection, torsemide, 10 mg/ml
(J3270)	Code deleted 2002
J3280	Injection, thiethylperazine maleate, up to 10 mg
J3301	Injection, triamcinolone acetonide, [Kenalog], per 10 mg
J3302	Injection, triamcinolone diacetate, [Aristocort], per 5 mg
J3303	Injection, triamcinolone hexacetonide, [Aristospan], per 5 mg
J3305	Injection, trimetrexate glucoronate, per 25 mg
J3310	Injection, perphenazine, [Trilafon], up to 5 mg
J3320	Injection, spectinomycin hydrochloride, [Trobicin], up to 2 gram
J3350	Injection, urea, [Ureaphil], up to 40 grams
J3360	Injection, diazepam, [Valium], up to 5 mg
J3364	Injection, urokinase, 5000 IU vial
J3365	Injection, IV, urokinase, 250,000 IU vial
J3370	Injection, vancomycin HCl, 500 mg
(J3390)	Code deleted 2002
●**J3395**	Injection, verteporfin, 15 mg
J3400	Injection, triflupromazine HCl, [Vesprin], up to 20 mg
J3410	Injection, hydroxyzine HCl, [Vistaril], up to 25 mg
J3420	Injection, vitamin B-12 cyanocobalamin, up to 1000 mcg
J3430	Injection, phytonadione (vitamin K), per 1 mg
(J3450)	Code deleted 2002
J3470	Injection, hyaluronidase, [Wydase], up to 150 units
J3475	Injection, magnesium sulfate, per 500 mg

J3480	Injection, potassium chloride, per 2 mEq
J3485	Injection, zidovudine, 10 mg
J3490	Unclassified drugs
J3520	Edetate disodium, per 150 mg
J3530	Nasal vaccine inhalation
J3535	Drug administered through a metered dose inhaler
J3570	Laetrile, amygdalin, vitamin B17

MISCELLANEOUS DRUGS AND SOLUTIONS

J7030	Infusion, normal saline solution, 1000 cc
J7040	Infusion, normal saline solution, sterile (500 ml = 1 unit)
J7042	5% dextrose/normal saline solution (500 ml = 1 unit)
J7050	Infusion, normal saline solution, 250 cc
J7051	Sterile saline or water, up to 5 cc
J7060	5% dextrose/water (500 ml = 1 unit)
J7070	Infusion, D5W, 1000 cc
J7100	Infusion, dextran 40, 500 ml
J7110	Infusion, dextran 75, 500 ml
J7120	Ringers lactate infusion, up to 1000 cc
J7130	Hypertonic saline solution, 50 or 100 mEq, 20 cc vial
J7190	Factor VIII (antihemophilic factor, human), per IU
J7191	Factor VIII (antihemophilic factor (porcine)), per IU
J7192	Factor VIII (antihemophilic factor, recombinant), per IU
● **J7193**	Factor IX (antihemophilic factor, purified, non-recombinant) per IU

J7194   Factor IX, complex, per IU

● **J7195**   Factor IX (antihemophilic factor, recombinant) per IU

(**J7196**)   Code deleted 2001

J7197   Antithrombin III (human), per IU

J7198   Anti-inhibitor, per IU

J7199   Hemophilia clotting factor, not otherwise classified

J7300   Intrauterine copper contraceptive

● **J7302**   Levonorgestrel-releasing intrauterine contraceptive system, 52 mg

● **J7308**   Aminolevulinic acid HCL for topical administration, 20%, single unit dosage form (354 mg)

J7310   Ganciclovir, 4.5 mg, long-acting implant

(**J7315**)   Code deleted 2002

● **J7316**   Sodium hyaluronate, 5 mg for intra-articular injection

J7320   Hylan G-F 20, 16 mg, for intra articular injection

J7330   Autologous cultured chondrocytes, implant

● **J7340**   Dermal and epidermal, tissue of human origin, with or without bioengineered or processed elements, with metabolically active elements, per square centimeter

IMMUNOSUPPRESSIVE DRUGS (INCLUDES NON-INJECTIBLES)

J7500   Azathioprine, oral, 50 mg

J7501   Azathioprine, parenteral, 100 mg

J7502   Cyclosporine, oral, 100 mg

(**J7503**)   Code deleted 2000; use J7516

▲ **J7504**   Lymphocyte immune globulin, antithymocyte globulin, equine, parenteral, 250 mg

| | Not valid for Medicare | | Non-covered by Medicare | | Special coverage instructions | | Carrier discretion | **171** |

J7505 muromonab-CD3, parenteral, 5 mg

J7506 Prednisone, oral, per 5 mg

J7507 Tacrolimus, oral; per 1 mg

J7508 per 5 mg

J7509 Methylprednisolone, oral, per 4 mg

J7510 Prednisolone, oral, per 5 mg

● **J7511** Lymphocyte immune globulin, antithymocyte globulin, rabbit, parenteral, 25 mg

J7513 Daclizumab, parenteral, 25 mg

J7515 Cyclosporine, oral, 25 mg

J7516 Cyclosporine, parenteral, 250 mg

J7517 Mycophenolate mofetil, oral, 250 mg

J7520 Sirolimus, oral, 1 mg

J7525 Tacrolimus, parenteral, 5 mg

J7599 Immunosuppressive drug, not otherwise classified

J7608 Acetylcysteine, inhalation solution administered through DME, unit dose form, per gram

(J7610) Code deleted 2001

(J7615) Code deleted 2001

▲ **J7618** Albuterol, all formulations inlcuding separated isomers, inhalation solution administered through DME, concentrated form, per 1 mg (albuterol) or per 0.5 mg (levalbuterol)

▲ **J7619** Albuterol, all formulations including separated isomers, inhalation solution administered through DME, unit dose, per 1 mg (albuterol) or per 0.5 mg (levalbuterol)

(J7620) Code deleted 2001

● **J7622** Beclomethasone, inhalation solution administered through DME, unit dose form, per milligram

● **J7624** Betamethasone, inhalation solution administered through DME, unit dose form, per milligram

(J7625) Code deleted 2001

● **J7626** Budesonide inhalation solution, administered through DME, unit dose form, 0.25 mg

(J7627) Code deleted 2001

J7628 Bitolterol mesylate, inhalation solution administered through DME, concentrated form, per mg

J7629 Bitolterol mesylate, inhalation solution administered through DME, unit dose form, per mg

(J7630) Code deleted 2001

J7631 Cromolyn sodium, inhalation solution administered through DME, unit dose form, per 10 mg

J7635 Atropine, inhalation solution administered through DME, concentrated form, per mg

J7636 Atropine, inhalation solution administered through DME, unit dose form, per mg

J7637 Dexamethasone, inhalation solution administered through DME, concentrated form, per mg

J7638 Dexamethasone, inhalation solution administered through DME, unit dose form, per mg

J7639 Dornase alpha, inhalation solution administered through DME, unit dose form, per mg

(J7640) Code deleted 2001

● **J7641** Flunisolide, inhalation solution administered through DME, unit dose, per milligram

J7642 Glycopyrrolate, inhalation solution administered through DME, concentrated form, per mg

Not valid for Medicare	Non-covered by Medicare	Special coverage instructions	Carrier discretion	**173**

J7643   Glycopyrrolate, inhalation solution administered through DME, unit dose form, per mg

J7644   Ipratropium bromide, inhalation solution administered through DME, unit dose form, per mg

(J7645)   Code deleted 2001

J7648   Isoetharine HCl, inhalation solution administered through DME, concentrated form, per mg

J7649   Isoetharine HCl, inhalation solution administered through DME, unit dose form, per mg

(J7650)   Code deleted 2001

(J7651)   Code deleted 2001

(J7652)   Code deleted 2001

(J7653)   Code deleted 2001

(J7654))   Code deleted 2001

(J7655)   Code deleted 2001

J7658   Isoproterenol HCl, inhalation solution administered through DME, concentrated form, per mg

J7659   Isoproterenol HCl, inhalation solution administered through DME, unit dose form, per mg

(J7660)   Code deleted 2001

(J7665)   Code deleted 2001

J7668   Metaproterenol sulfate, inhalation solution administered through DME, concentrated form, per 10 mg

J7669   Metaproterenol sulfate, inhalation solution administered through DME, unit dose form, per 10 mg

(J7670)   Code deleted 2001

(J7672)   Code deleted 2001

(J7675)   Code deleted 2001

J7680 Terbutaline sulfate, inhalation solution administered through DME, concentrated form, per mg

J7681 Terbutaline sulfate, inhalation solution administered through DME, unit dose form, per mg

J7682 Tobramycin, unit dose form, 300 mg, inhalation solution, administered through DME

J7683 Triamcinolone, inhalation solution administered through DME, concentrated form, per mg

J7684 Triamcinolone, inhalation solution administered through DME, unit dose form, per mg

J7699 NOC drugs, inhalation solution administered through DME

J7799 NOC drugs, other than inhalation drugs, administered through DME

J8499 Prescription drug, oral, non-chemotherapeutic, NOS

J8510 Busulfan, oral, 2 mg

J8520 Capecitabine, oral, 150 mg

J8521 Capecitabine, oral, 500 mg

J8530 Cyclophosphamide, oral, 25 mg

J8560 Etoposide, oral, 50 mg

J8600 Melphalan, oral, 2 mg

J8610 Methotrexate, oral, 2.5 mg

J8700 Temozolmide, oral, 5 mg

J8999 Prescription drug, oral, chemotherapeutic, NOS

● New code ▲ Revised code ( ) Deleted code

CHEMOTHERAPY DRUGS

Guidelines

In addition to the information presented in the INTRODUCTION, several other items unique to this section are defined or identified here:

1. **EXCEPTION:** Oral immunosuppressive drugs are not included in this section.

2. **ROUTE OF ADMINISTRATION:** Unless otherwise specified, the drugs listed in this section may be injected either subcutaneously, intramuscularly or intravenously.

3. **DRUG COST ONLY:** The codes listed in this section include the cost of the chemotherapy drug only and do not include the administration of the drug.

4. **SUBSECTION INFORMATION:** Some of the listed subheadings or subsections have special needs or instructions unique to that section. Where these are indicated, special "notes" will be presented preceding or following the listings. Those subsections within the CHEMOTHERAPY DRUGS section that have "notes" are as follows:

Subsection	Code Numbers
Chemotherapy drugs	J9000-J9999

5. **UNLISTED SERVICE OR PROCEDURE:** A service or procedure may be provided that is not listed in this edition of HCPCS. When reporting such a service, the appropriate "unlisted procedure" code may be used to indicate the service, identifying it by "special report" as defined below. HCPCS terminology is inconsistent in defining unlisted procedures. The procedure definition may include the term(s) "unlisted", "not otherwise classified", "unspecified", "unclassified", "other" and "miscellaneous". Prior to using these codes, try to determine if a Local Level III code or CPT code is available. The "unlisted procedures" and accompanying codes for CHEMOTHERAPY DRUGS are as follows:

J9999   Not otherwise classified, antineoplastic drugs

6. **SPECIAL REPORT:** A service, material or supply that is rarely provided, unusual, variable or new may require a special report in determining medical appropriateness for reimbursement purposes. Pertinent information should include an adequate definition or description of the nature, extent, and need for the service, material or supply.

7. **MODIFIERS:** Listed services may be modified under certain circumstances. When appropriate, the modifying circumstance is identified by adding a modifier to the basic procedure code. CPT and HCPCS National Level II modifiers may be used with CPT and HCPCS National Level II procedure codes. Modifiers commonly used with CHEMOTHERAPY DRUGS are as follows:

-CC Procedure code change (used when the procedure code submitted was changed either for administrative reasons or because an incorrect code was filed)

-QB Physician providing service in a rural HPSA

-QU Physician providing service in an urban HPSA

-TC Technical component. Under certain circumstances, a charge may be made for the technical component alone. Under these circumstances, the technical component charge is identified by adding the modifier -TC to the usual procedure code. Technical component charges are institutional charges and are not billed separately by physicians. Portable x-ray suppliers bill only for the technical component however, and should use modifier -TC.

8. **CPT CODE CROSS-REFERENCE:** Unless otherwise specified, the equivalent CPT code for all listings in this section is 96545.

Chemotherapy Drugs

J9000 Doxorubicin HCl, [Adriamycin], 10 mg

J9001 Doxorubicin HCl, all lipid formulations, 10 mg

J9015 Aldesleukin, per single use vial

● **J9017** Arsenic trioxide, 1 mg

J9020 Asparaginase, 10,000 units

J9031 BCG (intravesical), per installation

J9040 Bleomycin sulfate, [Blenoxane], 15 units

J9045 Carboplatin, [Paraplatin], 50 mg

J9050 Carmustine, [BiCNU], 100 mg

J9060 Cisplatin, [Platinol], powder or solution, per 10 mg

J9062 Cisplatin, 50 mg

J9065 Injection, cladribine, [Leustatin], per 1 mg

J9070 Cyclophosphamide, [Cytoxan]; 100 mg

J9080 200 mg

J9090 500 mg

J9091 1.0 gram

J9092 2.0 gram

J9093 Cyclophosphamide, lyophilized, [Lyophilized Cytoxan]; 100 mg

J9094 200 mg

J9095 500 mg

J9096 1.0 gram

J9097 2.0 gram

J9100 Cytarabine, [Cytarabine Hydrochloride]; 100 mg

J9110 500 mg

J9120 Dactinomycin, 0.5 mg

J9130 Dacarbazine, 100 mg

J9140 200 mg

J9150 Daunorubicin, 10 mg

Not valid for Medicare   Non-covered by Medicare   Special coverage instructions   Carrier discretion

J9151	Daunorubicin citrate, liposomal formulation, 10 mg
J9160	Denileukin diftitox, 300 mcg
J9165	Diethylstilbestrol diphosphate, [Stilphostrol], 250 mg
J9170	Docetaxel, 20 mg
J9180	Epirubicin hydrochloride, 50 mg
J9181	Etoposide, [VePesid]; 10 mg
J9182	100 mg
J9185	Fludarabine phosphate, 50 mg
J9190	Fluorouracil, 500 mg
J9200	Floxuridine, 500 mg
J9201	Gemcitabine HCl, 200 mg
J9202	Goserelin acetate implant, [Zoladex], per 3.6 mg
J9206	Irinotecan, 20 mg
J9208	Ifosfomide, 1 gram
J9209	Mesna, [Mesnex], 200 mg
J9211	Idarubicin hydrochloride, 5 mg
J9212	Injection, interferon alfacon-1, recombinant, 1 mcg
J9213	Interferon, alfa-2A, recombinant, 3 million units
J9214	Interferon, alfa-2B, recombinant, 1 million units
J9215	Interferon, alfa-N3, (human leukocyte derived), 250,000 IU
J9216	Interferon, gamma 1-B, 3 million units
J9217	Leuprolide acetate, [Lupron Depot], (for depot suspension), 7.5 mg
J9218	Leuprolide acetate, [Lupron], per 1 mg

J9219   Leuprolide acetate implant, 65 mg

J9230   Mechlorethamine HCl, (nitrogen mustard), [Mustargen], 10 mg

J9245   Injection, melphalan HCl, 50 mg

J9250   Methotrexate sodium; 5 mg

J9260   50 mg

J9265   Paclitaxel, 30 mg

J9266   Pegaspargase, per single dose vial

J9268   Pentostatin, per 10 mg

J9270   Plicamycin, [Mithracin], 2.5 mg

J9280   Mitomycin; 5 mg

J9290   20 mg

J9291   40 mg

J9293   Injection, mitoxantrone HCl, per 5 mg

● **J9300**   Gemtuzumab ozogamicin, 5 mg

J9310   Rituximab, 100 mg

J9320   Streptozocin, 1 gram

J9340   Thiotepa, 15 mg

J9350   Topotecan, 4 mg

J9355   Trastuzumab, 10 mg

J9357   Valrubicin, intravesical, 200 mg

J9360   Vinblastine sulfate, [Velban], 1 mg

J9370   Vincristine sulfate, [Oncovin]; 1 mg

J9375   2 mg

J9380   5 mg

J9390   Vinorelbine tartrate, per 10 mg

J9600   Porfimer sodium, [Photofrin], 75 mg

J9999   Not otherwise classified, antineoplastic drugs

K CODES: FOR DMERCS USE ONLY

Guidelines

In addition to the information presented in the INTRODUCTION, several other items unique to this section are defined or identified here:

1. **EXCLUSIVE USE BY DMERCS:** The codes listed in this section are assigned by HCFA on a temporary basis and are for the exclusive use of the Durable Medical Equipment Regional Carriers (DMERCs). These codes are not to be used by providers for reporting purposes unless specifically instructed to do so by the local carrier.

2. **UNLISTED SERVICE OR PROCEDURE:** A service or procedure may be provided that is not listed in this edition of HCPCS. When reporting such a service, the appropriate "unlisted procedure" code may be used to indicate the service, identifying it by "special report" as defined below. HCPCS terminology is inconsistent in defining unlisted procedures. The procedure definition may include the term(s) "unlisted", "not otherwise classified", "unspecified", "unclassified", "other" and "miscellaneous". Prior to using these codes, try to determine if a Local Level III code or CPT code is available.

3. **SPECIAL REPORT:** A service, material or supply that is rarely provided, unusual, variable or new may require a special report in determining medical appropriateness for reimbursement purposes. Pertinent information should include an adequate definition or description of the nature, extent, and need for the service, material or supply.

4. **CPT CODE CROSS-REFERENCE:** Unless otherwise specified, the equivalent CPT code for all listings in this section is 99070.

K CODES

Temporary Codes for DMERCS

WHEELCHAIRS

K0001 Standard wheelchair

K0002 Standard hemi (low seat) wheelchair

K0003 Lightweight wheelchair

K0004 High strength, lightweight wheelchair

K0005 Ultralightweight wheelchair

K0006 Heavy duty wheelchair

K0007 Extra heavy duty wheelchair

(K0008) Code deleted 2001

K0009 Other manual wheelchair/base

K0010 Standard - weight frame motorized/power wheelchair

K0011 Standard - weight frame motorized/power wheelchair with programmable control parameters for speed adjustment, tremor dampening, acceleration control and braking

K0012 Lightweight portable motorized/power wheelchair

(K0013) Code deleted 2001

K0014 Other motorized/power wheelchair base

K0015 Detachable, non-adjustable height armrest, each

K0016 Detachable, adjustable height armrest; complete assembly, each

K0017   base, each

K0018   upper portion each

K0019 Arm pad, each

K0020	Fixed, adjustable height armrest, pair
K0021	Anti-tipping device, each
K0022	Reinforced back upholstery
K0023	Solid back insert, planar back, single density foam; attached with straps
K0024	with adjustable hook-on hardware
K0025	Hook-on headrest extension
K0026	Back upholstery for ultralightweight or high strength lightweight wheelchair
K0027	Back upholstery for wheelchair type other than ultralightweight or high strength lightweight wheelchair
K0028	Manual, fully reclining back
K0029	Reinforced seat upholstery
K0030	Solid seat insert, planar seat, single density foam
K0031	Safety belt/pelvic strap, each
K0032	Seat upholstery for ultralightweight or high strength lightweight wheelchair
K0033	Seat upholstery for wheelchair type other than ultralightweight or high strength lightweight wheelchair
K0034	Heel loop, each
K0035	Heel loop with ankle strap, each
K0036	Toe loop, each
K0037	High mount flip-up foot rest, each
K0038	Leg strap, each
K0039	Leg strap, H style, each
K0040	Adjustable angle footplate, each

Not valid for Medicare	Non-covered by Medicare	Special coverage instructions	Carrier discretion

K0041	Large size footplate, each
K0042	Standard size footplate, each
K0043	Foot rest, lower extension tube, each
K0044	Foot rest, upper hanger bracket, each
K0045	Foot rest, complete assembly
K0046	Elevating leg rest; lower extension tube, each
K0047	upper hanger bracket, each
K0048	complete assembly
K0049	Calf pad, each
K0050	Ratchet assembly
K0051	Cam release assembly, foot rest or leg rest, each
K0052	Swingaway, detachable foot rests, each
K0053	Elevating foot rests, articulating (telescoping), each
K0054	Seat width of 10", 11", 12", 15", 17", or 20" for a high strength, lightweight or ultralightweight wheelchair
K0055	Seat depth of 15", 17", or 18" for a high strength, lightweight or ultralightweight wheelchair
K0056	Seat height less than 17" or equal to or greater than 21" for a high strength, lightweight, or ultralightweight wheelchair
K0057	Seat width 19" or 20" for heavy duty or extra heavy duty chair
K0058	Seat depth 17" or 18" for motorized/power wheelchair
K0059	Plastic coated handrim, each
K0060	Steel handrim, each
K0061	Aluminum handrim, each

K0062 Handrim with 8-10 Vertical or oblique projections, each

K0063 Handrim with 12-16 Vertical or oblique projections, each

K0064 Zero pressure tube (flat free inserts), any size, each

K0065 Spoke protectors, each

K0066 Solid tire, any size each

K0067 Pneumatic tire, any size, each

K0068 Pneumatic tire tube, each

K0069 Rear wheel assembly, complete; with solid tire, spokes or molded, each

K0070 with pneumatic tire, spokes or molded, each

K0071 Front caster assembly, complete; with pneumatic tire, each

K0072 with semi-pneumatic tire, each

K0073 Caster pin lock, each

K0074 Pneumatic caster tire, any size, each

K0075 Semi-pneumatic caster tire, any size, each

K0076 Solid caster tire, any size, each

K0077 Front caster assembly, complete, with solid tire, each

K0078 Pneumatic caster tire tube, each

K0079 Wheel lock extension, pair

K0080 Anti-rollback device, pair

K0081 Wheel lock assembly, complete, each

K0082 22 NF deep cycle lead acid battery, each

K0083 22 NF gel cell battery, each

K0084 Group 24 deep cycle lead acid battery, each

| | Not valid for Medicare | | Non-covered by Medicare | | Special coverage instructions | | Carrier discretion | **187** |

K0085	Group 24 gel cell battery, each
K0086	U-1 lead acid battery, each
K0087	U-1 gel cell battery, each
K0088	Battery charger; lead acid or gel cell
K0089	dual mode
K0090	Rear wheel tire for power wheelchair, any size, each
K0091	Rear wheel tire tube other than zero pressure for power wheelchair, any size, each
K0092	Rear wheel assembly for power wheelchair, complete each
K0093	Rear wheel, zero pressure tire tube (flat free insert) for power wheelchair, any size, each
K0094	Wheel tire for power base, any size, each
K0095	Wheel tire tube other than zero pressure for each base, any size, each
K0096	Wheel assembly for power base, complete, each
K0097	Wheel zero pressure tire tube (flat free insert) for power base, any size, each
K0098	Drive belt for power wheelchair
K0099	Front caster for power wheelchair, each
K0100	Wheelchair adapter for amputee, pair (device used to compensate for transfer of weight due to lost limbs to maintain proper balance)
K0101	One-arm drive attachment, each
K0102	Crutch and cane holder, each
K0103	Transfer board, less than 25"
K0104	Cylinder tank carrier, each
K0105	IV hanger, each

K0106 Arm trough, each

K0107 Wheelchair tray

K0108 Wheelchair component or accessory, not otherwise specified

(K0109) Code deleted 1999

SPINAL ORTHOTICS

K0112 Trunk support device, vest type; with inner frame, prefabricated

K0113 without inner frame, prefabricated

K0114 Back support system for use with a wheelchair, with inner frame, prefabricated

K0115 Seating system, back module, posteriorlateral control, with or without lateral supports, custom fabricated for attachment to wheelchair base

K0116 Seating system, combined back and seat module, custom fabricated for attachment to wheelchair base

IMMUNOSUPPRESSIVE DRUGS

(K0119) Code deleted 2000; use J7500

(K0120) Code deleted 2000; use J7501

(K0121) Code deleted 2000; use J7515

(K0122) Code deleted 2000; use J7516

(K0123) Code deleted 2000; use J7504

INCONTINENCE SUPPLIES AND APPLIANCES

(K0137) Code deleted 2000; use A4369

(K0138) Code deleted 2000; use A4370

(K0139) Code deleted 2000; use A4371

TRACHEOSTOMY CARE SUPPLIES

(K0168) Code deleted 2000; use A7003

(K0169) Code deleted 2000; use A7004

(K0170) Code deleted 2000; use A7005

(K0171) Code deleted 2000; use A7006

(K0172) Code deleted 2000; use A7007

(K0173) Code deleted 2000; use A7008

(K0174) Code deleted 2000; use A7009

(K0175) Code deleted 2000; use A7010

(K0176) Code deleted 2000; use A7011

(K0177) Code deleted 2000; use A7012

(K0178) Code deleted 2000; use A7013

(K0179) Code deleted 2000; use A7014

(K0180) Code deleted 2000; use A7015

(K0181) Code deleted 2000; use A7016

(K0182) Code deleted 2001; use A7018

K0183 Nasal application device used with positive airway pressure device

▲ **K0184** Nasal single piece interface, replacement for nasal application device, pair or single piece interface

K0185 Headgear used with positive airway pressure device

K0186 Chin strap used with positive airway pressure device

K0187 Tubing used with positive airway pressure device

K0188 Filter, disposable, used with positive airway pressure device

K0189   Filter, non-disposable, used with positive airway pressure device

(K0190)   Code deleted 2000; use A7000

(K0191)   Code deleted 2000; use A7001

(K0192)   Code deleted 2000; use A7002

(K0193)   Code deleted 1999

(K0194)   Code deleted 1999

K0195   Elevating leg rests, pair (for use with capped rental wheelchair base)

K0268   Humidifier, non-heated, used with positive airway pressure device

(K0269)   Code deleted 2001; use E0572

(K0270)   Code deleted 2001; use E0574

(K0277)   Code deleted 2000; use A4372

(K0278)   Code deleted 2000; use A4373

(K0279)   Code deleted 2000; use A4374

(K0280)   Code deleted 2001; use A4331

(K0281)   Code deleted 2001; use A4332

(K0283)   Code deleted 2001; use A7019

(K0284)   Code deleted 2000; use E0779

(K0400)   Code deleted 2000; use A4280

(K0401)   Code deleted 2000; use A5508

(K0407)   Code deleted 2001; use A4333

(K0408)   Code deleted 2001; use A4334

(K0409)   Code deleted 2001; use A4319

(K0410)   Code deleted 2001; use A4324

(K0411)   Code deleted 2001; use A4325

(K0412)   Code deleted 2000; use J7517

K0415   Prescription antiemetic drug, oral, per 1 mg, for use in conjunction with oral anti-cancer drug, not otherwise specified

K0416   Prescription antiemetic drug, rectal, per 1 mg, for use in conjunction with oral anti-cancer drug, not otherwise specified

(K0417)   Code deleted 2000; use E0780

(K0418)   Code deleted 2000; use J7502

(K0419)   Code deleted 2000; use A4375

(K0420)   Code deleted 2000; use A4376

(K0421)   Code deleted 2000; use A4377

(K0422)   Code deleted 2000; use A4378

(K0423)   Code deleted 2000; use A4379

(K0424)   Code deleted 2000; use A4380

(K0425)   Code deleted 2000; use A4381

(K0426)   Code deleted 2000; use A4382

(K0427)   Code deleted 2000; use A4383

(K0428)   Code deleted 2000; use A4384

(K0429)   Code deleted 2000; use A4385

(K0430)   Code deleted 2000; use A4386

(K0431)   Code deleted 2000; use A4387

(K0432)   Code deleted 2000; use A4388

(K0433)   Code deleted 2000; use A4389

(K0434)   Code deleted 2000; use A4390

(K0435)   Code deleted 2000; use A4391

(K0436)   Code deleted 2000; use A4392

(K0437)   Code deleted 2000; use A4393

(K0438)   Code deleted 2000; use A4394

(K0439)   Code deleted 2000; use A4395

(K0440)   Code deleted 2001; use L8040

(K0441)   Code deleted 2001; use L8041

(K0442)   Code deleted 2001; use L8042

(K0443)   Code deleted 2001; use L8043

(K0444)   Code deleted 2001; use L8044

(K0445)   Code deleted 2001; use L8045

(K0446)   Code deleted 2001; use L8046

(K0447)   Code deleted 2001; use L8047

(K0448)   Code deleted 2001; use L8048

(K0449)   Code deleted 2001; use L8049

(K0450)   Code deleted 2001; use A4364

(K0451)   Code deleted 2001; use A4365

K0452   Wheelchair bearings, any type

(K0453)   Code deleted 1999; use J0285

K0455   Infusion pump used for uninterrupted administration of epoprostenol

(K0456)   Code deleted 2001; use E0298

(K0457)   Code deleted 2001; use E0168

(K0458) Code deleted 2001; use E0148

(K0459) Code deleted 2001; use E0149

K0460 Power add-on, to convert manual wheelchair to motorized wheelchair, joystick control

K0461 Power add-on, to convert manual wheelchair to power operated vehicle, tiller control

K0462 Temporary replacement for patient owned equipment being repaired, any type

(K0501) Code deleted 2001; use E0571

(K0503) Code deleted 2000; use J7608

(K0504) Code deleted 2000; use J7618

(K0505) Code deleted 2000; use J7619

(K0506) Code deleted 2000; use J7635

(K0507) Code deleted 2000; use J7636

(K0508) Code deleted 2000; use J7628

(K0509) Code deleted 2000; use J7629

(K0511) Code deleted 2000; use J7631

(K0512) Code deleted 2000; use J7637

(K0513) Code deleted 2000; use J7638

(K0514) Code deleted 2000; use J7639

(K0515) Code deleted 2000; use J7642

(K0516) Code deleted 2000; use J7643

(K0518) Code deleted 2000; use J7644

(K0519) Code deleted 2000; use J7648

(K0520) Code deleted 2000; use J7649

(K0521) Code deleted 2000; use J7658

(K0522) Code deleted 2000; use J7659

(K0523) Code deleted 2000; use J7668

(K0524) Code deleted 2000; use J7669

(K0525) Code deleted 2000; use J7680

(K0526) Code deleted 2000; use J7681

(K0527) Code deleted 2000; use J7683

(K0528) Code deleted 2000; use J7684

(K0529) Code deleted 2001; use A7020

(K0530) Code deleted 2000; use A7017

K0531 Humidifier, heated, used with positive airway pressure device

K0532 Respiratory assist device, bi-level pressure capability, without backup rate feature, used with noninvasive interface, e.g., nasal or facial mask (intermittent assist device with continuous positive airway pressure device)

K0533 Respiratory assist device, bi-level pressure capability, with backup rate feature, used with noninvasive interface, e.g., nasal or facial mask (intermittent assist device with continuous positive airway pressure device)

K0534 Respiratory assist device, bi-level pressure capability, with backup rate feature, used with invasive interface, e.g., tracheostomy tube (intermittent assist device with continuous positive airway pressure device)

(K0535) Code deleted 2001; use A6231

(K0536) Code deleted 2001; use A6232

(K0537) Code deleted 2001; use A6233

K0538 Negative pressure wound therapy electrical pump, stationary or portable

K0539 Dressing set for negative pressure wound therapy electrical pump, stationary or portable, each

K0540 Canister set for negative pressure wound therapy electrical pump, stationary or portable, each

▲**K0541** Speech generating device, digitized speech, using pre-recorded messages, less than or equal to 8 minutes recording time

K0542 Speech generating device, digitized speech using pre-recorded messages, greater than 8 minutes recording time

K0543 Speech generating device, synthesized speech, requiring message formulation by spelling and access by physical contact with the device

K0544 Speech generating device, synthesized speech, permitting multiple methods of message formulation and multiple methods of device access

K0545 Speech generating software program, for personal computer or personal digital assistant

K0546 Accessory for speech generating device, mounting system

K0547 Accessory for speech generating device, not otherwise classified

●**K0548** Injection, insulin lispro, up to 50 units

●**K0549** Hospital bed, heavy duty, extra wide, with weight capacity greater than 350 pounds but less than or equal to 600 pounds, with any type side rails, with mattress

●**K0550** Hospital bed, extra heavy duty, extra wide, with weight capacity greater than 600 pounds, with any type side rails, with mattress

●**K0551** Residual limb support system, solid base with adjustable drop hooks, mounts to wheelchair frame, each

ORTHOTIC PROCEDURES

Guidelines

In addition to the information presented in the INTRODUCTION, several other items unique to this section are defined or identified here:

1. **SUBSECTION INFORMATION:** Some of the listed subheadings or subsections have special needs or instructions unique to that section. Where these are indicated, special "notes" will be presented preceding or following the listings. Those subsections within the ORTHOTIC PROCEDURES section that have "notes" are as follows:

Subsection	Code Numbers
Scoliosis procedures	L1000-L1499
Orthotic devices-lower limb	L1600-L2999
Lower limb-hip-knee-angle-foot (or any combination)	L2000-L2199
Orthotic devices-upper limb	L3650-L3999

2. **UNLISTED SERVICE OR PROCEDURE:** A service or procedure may be provided that is not listed in this edition of HCPCS. When reporting such a service, the appropriate "unlisted procedure" code may be used to indicate the service, identifying it by "special report" as defined below. HCPCS terminology is inconsistent in defining unlisted procedures. The procedure definition may include the term(s) "unlisted", "not otherwise classified", "unspecified", "unclassified", "other" and "miscellaneous". Prior to using these codes, try to determine if a Local Level III code or CPT code is available. The "unlisted procedures" and accompanying codes for ORTHOTIC PROCEDURES are as follows:

L0999	Addition to spinal orthosis, not otherwise specified
L1499	Spinal orthosis, not otherwise specified
L2999	Lower extremity orthosis, not otherwise specified
L3649	Orthopedic shoe, modification, addition or transfer, not otherwise specified
L3999	Upper limb orthosis, not otherwise specified

3. **SPECIAL REPORT:** A service, material or supply that is rarely provided, unusual, variable or new may require a special report in determining medical appropriateness for reimbursement purposes.

Pertinent information should include an adequate definition or description of the nature, extent, and need for the service, material or supply.

4. **MODIFIERS:** Listed services may be modified under certain circumstances. When appropriate, the modifying circumstance is identified by adding a modifier to the basic procedure code. CPT and HCPCS National Level II modifiers may be used with CPT and HCPCS National Level II procedure codes. Modifiers commonly used with ORTHOTIC PROCEDURES are as follows:

-CC   Procedure code change (use "CC" when the procedure code submitted was changed either for administrative reasons or because an incorrect code was filed)

-LT   Left side (used to identify procedures performed on the left side of the body)

-RT   Right side (used to identify procedures performed on the right side of the body)

-TC   Technical component. Under certain circumstances, a charge may be made for the technical component alone. Under those circumstances, the technical component charge is identified by adding modifier -TC to the usual procedure number. Technical component charges are institutional charges and are not billed separately by physicians. However, portable x-ray suppliers bill only for the technical component and should use modifier -TC. The change data from portable x-ray suppliers will then be used to build customary and prevailing profiles.

5. **CPT CODE CROSS-REFERENCE:** Unless otherwise specified, the equivalent CPT code for all listings in this section is 99070.

6. **DURABLE MEDICAL EQUIPMENT REGIONAL CARRIERS (DMERCS):** Effective October 1, 1993, claims orthotics must be billed to one of four regional carriers depending upon the residence of the beneficiary. The transition dates for DMERC claims is from November 1, 1993 to March 1, 1994, depending upon the state you practice in. See the Introduction for a complete discussion of DMERCs.

Orthotic Procedures

ORTHOTIC DEVICES

SPINAL - CERVICAL

▲**L0100**   Cranial orthosis (helmet), with or without soft-interface, molded to patient model

▲**L0110**   Cranial orthosis (helmet), with or without soft-interface, non-molded

L0120   Cervical, flexible; non-adjustable (foam collar)

L0130   thermoplastic collar, molded to patient

L0140   Cervical, semi-rigid; adjustable (plastic collar)

L0150   adjustable molded chin cup (plastic collar with mandibular/occipital piece)

L0160   wire frame occipital/mandibular support

L0170   Cervical collar; molded to patient model

L0172   semi-rigid thermoplastic foam, two piece

L0174   semi-rigid, thermoplastic foam, two piece with thoracic extension

L0180   Cervical, multiple post collar, occipital/mandibular supports; adjustable

L0190   adjustable cervical bars (somi, guilford, taylor types)

L0200   adjustable cervical bars, and thoracic extension

SPINAL-THORACIC

L0210   Thoracic, rib belt;

L0220   custom fabricated

SPINAL-THORACIC-LUMBAR-SACRAL

FLEXIBLE

L0300 Thoracic-lumbar-sacral-orthosis (TLSO), flexible (dorso-lumbar surgical support);

L0310 custom fabricated

L0315 elastic type, with rigid posterior panel

L0317 hyperextension, elastic type, with rigid posterior panel

ANTERIOR-POSTERIOR CONTROL

L0320 TLSO, anterior-posterior control (Taylor type), with apron front

●**L0321** TLSO, anterior-posterior control, with rigid or semi-rigid posterior panel, prefabricated (includes fitting and adjustment)

L0330 TLSO, anterior-posterior-lateral control (Knight-Taylor type), with apron front

●**L0331** TLSO, anterior-posterior-lateral control, with rigid or semi-rigid posterior panel, prefabricated (includes fitting and adjustment)

ANTERIOR-POSTERIOR-LATERAL-ROTARY CONTROL

L0340 TLSO, anterior-posterior-lateral-rotary control; (Arnold, Magnuson, Steindler types), with apron front

L0350 flexion compression jacket, custom fitted

L0360 flexion compression jacket molded to patient model

L0370 hyperextension (Jewett, Lennox, Baker, Cash types)

L0380 with extensions

L0390 TLSO, anterior-posterior-lateral control; molded to patient model

● **L0391**   TLSO, anterior-posterior-lateral-rotary control, with rigid or semi-rigid posterior panel, prefabricated (includes fitting and adjustment)

L0400   TLSO, anterior-posterior-lateral control; molded to patient model, with interface material

L0410   two-piece construction, molded to patient model

L0420   two-piece construction, molded to patient model, with interface material

L0430   with interface material custom fitted

L0440   with overlapping front section, spring steel front, custom fitted

SPINAL — LUMBAR-SACRAL

FLEXIBLE

L0500   Lumbar-sacral-orthosis (LSO), flexible, (lumbo-sacral surgical support)

L0510   custom fabricated

▲ **L0515**   LSO, anterior-posterior control, with rigid or semi-rigid posterior panel, prefabricated

ANTERIOR-POSTERIOR-LATERAL CONTROL

L0520   LSO, anterior-posterior-lateral control (Knight, Wilcox types), with apron front

ANTERIOR-POSTERIOR CONTROL

L0530   LSO, anterior-posterior control (Macausland type), with apron front

LUMBAR FLEXION

L0540   LSO, lumbar flexion (Williams flexion type)

ANTERIOR-POSTERIOR-LATERAL CONTROL (BODY JACKET)

L0550 LSO, anterior-posterior-lateral control; molded to patient model

L0560 molded to patient model, with interface material

●**L0561** LSO, anterior-posterior-lateral control; with rigid or semi-rigid posterior panel, prefabricated

L0565 custom fitted

SPINAL-SACROILIAC

FLEXIBLE

L0600 Sacroiliac, flexible (sacroiliac surgical support);

L0610 custom fabricated

SEMI-RIGID

L0620 Sacroiliac, semi-rigid (Goldthwaite, Osgood types), with apron front

SPINAL-CERVICAL-THORACIC-LUMBER-SACRAL-HALO PROCEDURE

ANTERIOR-POSTERIOR-LATERAL CONTROL

L0700 Cervical-thoracic-lumber-sacral-orthoses (CTLSO), anterior-posterior-lateral control, molded to patient model; (Minerva type)

L0710 with interface material, (Minerva type)

HALO PROCEDURE

L0810 Halo procedure; cervical halo incorporated into jacket vest

L0820 cervical halo incorporated into plaster body jacket

L0830 cervical halo incorporated into Milwaukee type orthosis

SPINAL-TORSO SUPPORTS

PTOSIS SUPPORTS

L0860   Addition to halo procedures, magnetic resonance image compatible system

L0900   Torso support, ptosis support;

L0910   custom fabricated

PENDULOUS ABDOMEN SUPPORT

L0920   Torso support, pendulous abdomen support;

L0930   custom fabricated

POST SURGICAL SUPPORT

L0940   Torso support, post-surgical support;

L0950   custom fabricated

L0960   pads for post surgical support

ADDITIONS TO SPINAL ORTHOSES

L0970   TLSO, corset front

L0972   LSO, corset front

L0974   TLSO, full corset

L0976   LSO, full corset

L0978   Axillary crutch extension

L0980   Peroneal straps, pair

L0982   Stocking supporter grips, set of four (4)

L0984   Protective body sock, each

● **L0986**   Addition to spinal orthosis, rigid or semi-rigid abdominal panel, prefabricated

L0999   Addition to spinal orthosis, not otherwise specified

ORTHOTIC DEVICES-SCOLIOSIS PROCEDURES

NOTE: The orthotic care of scoliosis differs from other orthotic care in that the treatment is more dynamic in nature and utilizes ongoing, continual modification of the orthosis to the patient's changing condition. This coding structure uses the proper names or eponyms of the procedures because they have historic and universal acceptance in the profession. It should be recognized that variations to the basic procedures described by the founders/developers are accepted in various medical and orthotic practices throughout the country. All procedures include model of patient when indicated.

SCOLIOSIS-CERVICAL-THORACIC-LUMBAR-SACRAL (MILWAUKEE)

L1000   Cervical-thoracic-lumbar-sacral orthosis (CTLSO) (Milwaukee), inclusive of furnishing initial orthosis, including model

● **L1005**   Tension based scoliosis orthosis and accessory pads, includes fitting and adjustment

CORRECTION PADS

L1010   Additions to cervical-thoracic-lumber-sacral orthosis (CTLSO) or scoliosis orthosis; axilla sling

L1020   kyphosis pad

L1025   kyphosis pad, floating

L1030   lumbar bolster pad

L1040   lumbar or lumbar rib pad

L1050   sternal pad

L1060   thoracic pad

L1070   trapezius sling

L1080   outrigger

L1085 outrigger, bilateral with vertical extensions

L1090 lumbar sling

L1100 ring flange, plastic or leather

L1110 ring flange, plastic or leather, molded to patient model

L1120 covers for upright, each

SCOLIOSIS-THORACIC-LUMBAR-SACRAL (LOW PROFILE)

L1200 Thoracic-lumbar-sacral-orthosis (TLSO), inclusive of furnishing initial orthosis only

L1210 Addition to TLSO, (low profile); lateral thoracic extension

L1220 anterior thoracic extension

L1230 Milwaukee type superstructure

L1240 lumbar derotation pad

L1250 anterior asis pad

L1260 anterior thoracic derotation pad

L1270 abdominal pad

L1280 rib gusset (elastic), each

L1290 lateral trochanteric pad

OTHER SCOLIOSIS PROCEDURES

L1300 Other scoliosis procedure; body jacket molded to patient model

L1310 post-operative body jacket

L1499 Spinal orthosis, not otherwise specified

THORACIC-HIP-KNEE-ANKLE

L1500 Thoracic-hip-knee-ankle, orthosis (THKAO), mobility frame (Newington, Parapodium types)

▲**L1510** THKAO, standing frame, with or without tray and accessories

L1520 THKAO, swivel walker

ORTHOTIC DEVICES-LOWER LIMB

NOTE: The procedures L1600-L2999 are considered as "base" or the "basic procedures" and may be modified by listing other procedures from the "additions" (L2200-L2999) section and adding them to the base procedure.

LOWER LIMB-HIP

FLEXIBLE

L1600 Hip orthosis (HO), abduction control of hip joints, flexible, Frejka type with cover, prefabricated, includes fitting and adjustment

L1610 HO, abduction control of hip joints; flexible, (Frejka cover only), prefabricated, includes fitting and adjustment

L1620 HO, abduction control of hip joints; flexible, (Pavlik harness), prefabricated, includes fitting and adjustment

L1630 HO, abduction control of hip joints; semi-flexible (Von Rosen type), custom fabricated

L1640 HO, abduction control of hip joints; static, pelvic band or spreader bar, thigh cuffs, custom fabricated

L1650 HO, abduction control of hip joints; static, adjustable, (Ilfled type), prefabricated, includes fitting and adjustment

L1660 HO, abduction control of hip joints; static, plastic, prefabricated, includes fitting and adjustment

L1680 HO, abduction control of hip joints; dynamic, pelvic control, adjustable hip motion control, thigh cuffs (Rancho hip action type), custom fabricated

---

● New code   ▲ Revised code   ( ) Deleted code

L1685   HO, abduction control of hip joints; postoperative hip abduction type, custom fabricated

L1686   HO, abduction control of hip joints; postoperative hip abduction type, prefabricated, includes fitting and adjustment

L1690   Combination, bilateral, lumbo-sacral, hip, femur orthosis providing adduction and internal rotation control, prefabricated, includes fitting and adjustment

LOWER LIMB-LEGG PERTHES

L1700   Legg Perthes orthosis; (Toronto type), custom fabricated

L1710   (Newington type), custom fabricated

L1720   trilateral, (Tachidijan type), custom fabricated

L1730   (Scottish Rite type), custom fabricated

L1750   Legg Perthes sling (Sam Brown type), prefabricated, includes fitting and adjustment

L1755   (Patten Bottom type), custom fabricated

LOWER LIMB-KNEE

L1800   Knee orthosis (KO); elastic with stays, prefabricated, includes fitting and adjustment

L1810   elastic with joints, prefabricated, includes fitting and adjustment

L1815   elastic or other elastic type material with condylar pad(s), prefabricated, includes fitting and adjustment

L1820   elastic with condylar pads and joints, prefabricated, includes fitting and adjustment

L1825   elastic knee cap, prefabricated, includes fitting and adjustment

L1830   immobilizer, canvas longitudinal, prefabricated, includes fitting and adjustment

L1832 adjustable knee joints, positional orthosis, rigid support, prefabricated, includes fitting and adjustment

L1834 without knee joint, rigid, custom fabricated

L1840 derotation, medial-lateral, anterior cruciate ligament, custom fabricated

L1843 single upright, thigh and calf, with adjustable flexion and extension joint, medial-lateral and rotation control, pre-fabricated, includes fitting and adjustment

L1844 single upright, thigh and calf, with adjustable flexion and extension joint, medial-lateral and rotation control, custom fabricated

L1845 double upright, thigh and calf, with adjustable flexion and extension joint, medial-lateral and rotation control, pre-fabricated, includes fitting and adjustment

L1846 double upright, thigh and calf, with adjustable flexion and extension joint, medial-lateral and rotation control, custom fabricated

L1847 double upright with adjustable joint, with inflatable air support chamber(s), pre-fabricated, includes fitting and adjustment

L1850 Swedish type, pre-fabricated, includes fitting and adjustment

L1855 molded plastic, thigh and calf sections, with double upright knee joints, custom fabricated

L1858 molded plastic, polycentric knee joints, pneumatic knee pads (CTI), custom fabricated

L1860 modification of supracondylar prosthetic socket, custom fabricated (SK)

L1870 double upright, thigh and calf lacers with knee joint, custom fabricated

L1880 double upright, non-molded thigh and calf cuffs/lacers with knee joints, custom fabricated

---

L1885 single or double upright, thigh and calf, with functional active resistance control, pre-fabricated, includes fitting and adjustment

LOWER LIMB-ANKLE-FOOT

L1900 Ankle-foot orthosis (AFO); spring wire, dorsiflexion assist calf band, custom fabricated

L1902 ankle gauntlet, prefabricated, includes fitting and adjustment

L1904 molded ankle gauntlet, custom fabricated

L1906 multiligamentus ankle support, prefabricated, includes fitting and adjustment

L1910 posterior, single bar, clasp attachment to shoe counter, prefabricated, includes fitting and adjustment

L1920 single upright with static or adjustable stop (Phelps or Perlstein type), custom fabricated

▲**L1930** Ankle foot orthosis; plastic or other material, prefabricated, includes fitting and adjustment

▲**L1940** Ankle foot orthosis; plastic or other material, custom-fabricated

L1945 plastic, rigid anterior tibial section (floor reaction), custom fabricated

L1950 spiral, (IRM type), plastic, custom fabricated

L1960 posterior solid ankle, plastic, custom fabricated

L1970 plastic with ankle joint, custom fabricated

L1980 single upright free plantar dorsiflexion, solid stirrup, calf band/cuff (single bar "BK" orthosis), custom fabricated

L1990 double upright free plantar dorsiflexion, solid stirrup, calf band/cuff (double bar "BK" orthosis), custom fabricated

LOWER LIMB-HIP-KNEE-ANKLE-FOOT (OR ANY COMBINATION)

NOTE: L2000, L2020, and L2036 are base procedures to be used with any knee joint. L2010 and L2030 are to used only with no knee joint.

L2000   Knee-ankle-foot-orthosis (KAFO); single upright, free knee, free ankle, solid stirrup, thigh and calf bands/cuffs (single bar "AK" orthosis), custom fabricated

L2010   single upright, free ankle, solid stirrup, thigh and calf bands/cuffs (single bar "AK" orthosis), without knee joint, custom fabricated

L2020   double upright, free ankle, solid stirrup, thigh and calf bands/cuffs (double bar "AK" orthosis), custom fabricated

L2030   double upright, free ankle, solid stirrup, thigh and calf bands/cuffs, (double bar "AK" orthosis), without knee joint, custom fabricated

L2035   full plastic, static (pediatric size), prefabricated, includes fitting and adjustment

L2036   full plastic, double upright, free knee, custom fabricated

L2037   full plastic, single upright, free knee, custom fabricated

L2038   full plastic, with knee joint, multi-axis ankle, (Lively orthosis or equal), custom fabricated

L2039   full plastic, single upright, poly-axial hinge, medial lateral rotation control, cutom fabricated

TORSION CONTROL

L2040   Hip-knee-ankle-foot orthosis (HKAFO); torsion control, bilateral rotation straps, pelvic band/belt, custom fabricated

L2050   torsion control, bilateral torsion cables, hip joint, pelvic band/belt, custom fabricated

L2060   torsion control, bilateral torsion cables, ball bearing hip joint, pelvic band/belt, custom fabricated

L2070	torsion control, unilateral rotation straps, pelvic band/belt, custom fabricated
L2080	torsion control, unilateral torsion cable, hip joint, pelvic band/belt, custom fabricated
L2090	torsion control, unilateral torsion cable, ball bearing hip joint, pelvic band/belt, custom fabricated

FRACTURE ORTHOSES

L2102	Ankle-foot-orthosis (AFO), fracture orthosis, tibial fracture cast orthosis; plaster type casting material, custom fabricated
L2104	synthetic type casting material, custom fabricated
L2106	thermoplastic type casting material, custom fabricated
L2108	custom fabricated
L2112	soft, pre-fabricated, includes fitting and adjustment
L2114	semi-rigid, pre-fabricated, includes fitting and adjustment
L2116	rigid, pre-fabricated, includes fitting and adjustment
L2122	Knee-ankle-foot-orthosis (KAFO), fracture orthosis, femoral fracture cast orthosis; plaster type casting material, custom fabricated
L2124	synthetic type casting material, custom fabricated
L2126	thermoplastic type casting material, custom fabricated
L2128	custom fabricated
L2132	soft, prefabricated, includes fitting and adjustment
L2134	semi-rigid, prefabricated, includes fitting and adjustment
L2136	rigid, prefabricated, includes fitting and adjustment

ADDITIONS TO FRACTURE ORTHOSIS

L2180 Addition to lower extremity fracture orthosis; plastic shoe insert with ankle joints

L2182 drop lock knee joint

L2184 limited motion knee joint

L2186 adjustable motion knee joint, Lerman type

L2188 quadrilateral brim

L2190 waist belt

L2192 hip joint, pelvic band, thigh flange, and pelvic belt

ADDITIONS TO LOWER EXTREMITY ORTHOSIS

ADDITIONS-SHOE-ANKLE-SHIN-KNEE

L2200 Addition to lower extremity; limited ankle motion, each joint

L2210 dorsiflexion assist (plantar flexion resist), each joint

L2220 dorsiflexion and plantar flexion assist/resist, each joint

L2230 split flat caliper stirrups and plate attachment

L2240 round caliper and plate attachment

L2250 foot plate, molded to patient model, stirrup attachment

L2260 reinforced solid stirrup (Scott-Craig type)

L2265 long tongue stirrup

L2270 varus/valgus correction ("T") strap, padded/lined or malleolus pad

L2275 varus/valgus correction, plastic modification, padded/lined

L2280 molded inner boot

● New code   ▲ Revised code   ( ) Deleted code

L2300	abduction bar (bilateral hip involvement), jointed, adjustable
L2310	abduction bar-straight
L2320	non-molded lacer
L2330	lacer molded to patient model
L2335	anterior swing band
L2340	pre-tibial shell, molded to patient model
L2350	prosthetic type, (BK) socket, molded to patient model, (used for "PTB" "AFO" orthoses)
L2360	extended steel shank
L2370	patten bottom
L2375	torsion control, ankle joint and half solid stirrup
L2380	torsion control, straight knee joint, each joint
L2385	straight knee joint, heavy duty, each joint
L2390	offset knee joint, each joint
L2395	offset knee joint, heavy duty, each joint
L2397	Addition to lower extremity orthosis, suspension sleeve

ADDITIONS TO STRAIGHT OR OFFSET KNEE JOINTS

L2405	Addition to knee joint; drop lock, each joint
▲L2415	Addition to knee lock with integrated release mechanism (bail, cable, or equal), any material, each joint
L2425	Addition to knee joint; disc or dial lock for adjustable knee flexion, each joint
L2430	ratchet lock for active and progressive knee extension, each joint
L2435	polycentric joint, each joint

L2492   lift loop for drop lock ring

ADDITIONS-THIGH/WEIGHT BEARING

GLUTEAL/ISCHIAL WEIGHT

L2500   Addition to lower extremity, thigh/weight bearing; gluteal/ischial weight bearing, ring

L2510   quadrilateral brim, molded to patient model

L2520   quadrilateral brim, custom fitting

L2525   ischial containment/narrow M-L brim molded to patient model

L2526   ischial containment/narrow M-L brim, custom fitted

L2530   lacer, non-molded

L2540   lacer, molded to patient model

L2550   high roll cuff

ADDITIONS-PELVIC AND THORACIC CONTROL

L2570   Addition to lower extremity, pelvic control; hip joint, Clevis type two position joint; each

L2580   pelvic sling

L2600   hip joint, Clevis type, or thrust bearing, free, each

L2610   hip joint, Clevis or thrust bearing, lock, each

L2620   Addition to lower extremity, pelvic control, hip joint; heavy duty, each

L2622   adjustable flexion, each

L2624   adjustable flexion, extension, abduction control, each

L2627   Addition to lower extremity, pelvic control; plastic, molded to patient model, reciprocating hip joint and cables

L2628   metal frame, reciprocating hip joint and cables

L2630	band and belt, unilateral
L2640	band and belt, bilateral
L2650	Addition to lower extremity, pelvic and thoracic control, gluteal pad, each
L2660	Addition to lower extremity, thoracic control; thoracic band
L2670	paraspinal uprights
L2680	lateral support uprights

ADDITIONS-GENERAL

L2750	Addition to lower extremity orthosis; plating chrome or nickel, per bar
▲**L2755**	high strength, lightweight material, all hybrid lamination/prepreg composite, per segment
L2760	extension, per extension, per bar (for lineal adjustment for growth)
●**L2768**	orthotic side bar disconnect device, per bar
L2770	any material, per bar or joint
L2780	non-corrosive finish, per bar
L2785	drop lock retainer, each
L2795	knee control, full kneecap
L2800	knee control, knee cap, medial or lateral pull
L2810	knee control, condylar pad
L2820	soft interface for molded plastic, below knee section
L2830	soft interface for molded plastic, above knee section
L2840	tibial length sock, fracture or equal, each
L2850	femoral length sock, fracture or equal, each

L2860 Addition to lower extremity joint, knee or ankle, concentric adjustable torsion style mechanism, each

L2999 Lower extremity orthosis, not otherwise specified

FOOT ORTHOPEDIC SHOES, SHOE MODIFICATIONS, TRANSFERS

FOOT, INSERT, REMOVABLE, MOLDED TO PATIENT MODEL

L3000 Foot, insert, removable, molded to patient model; "UCB" type, Berkeley Shell, each

L3001 Spenco, each

L3002 plastazote or equal, each

L3003 silicone gel, each

L3010 longitudinal arch support, each

L3020 longitudinal/metatarsal support, each

L3030 Foot, insert, removable, formed to patient foot, each

FOOT, ARCH SUPPORT, REMOVABLE, PREMOLDED

L3040 Foot, arch support, removable, premolded; longitudinal, each

L3050 metatarsal, each

L3060 longitudinal/metatarsal, each

FOOT, ARCH SUPPORT, NONREMOVABLE, ATTACHED TO SHOE

L3070 Foot, arch support, non-removable attached to shoe; longitudinal, each

L3080 metatarsal, each

L3090 longitudinal/metatarsal, each

L3100 Hallus-valgus night dynamic splint

ABDUCTION AND ROTATION BARS

L3140   Foot, abduction rotation bar, including shoes

L3150   Foot, abduction rotation bars, without shoes

L3160   Foot, adjustable shoe-styled positioning device

L3170   Foot, plastic heel stabilizer

ORTHOPEDIC FOOTWEAR

L3201   Orthopedic shoe, oxford with supinator or pronator; infant

L3202   child

L3203   junior

L3204   Orthopedic shoe, hightop with supinator or pronator; infant

L3206   child

L3207   junior

L3208   Surgical boot, each; infant

L3209   child

L3211   junior

L3212   Benesch boot, pair; infant

L3213   child

L3214   junior

L3215   Orthopedic footwear, ladies shoes; oxford

L3216   depth inlay

L3217   hightop, depth inlay

L3218   Orthopedic footwear, ladies surgical boot; each

L3219   Orthopedic footwear, mens shoes; oxford

| | Not valid for Medicare | | Non-covered by Medicare | | Special coverage instructions | | Carrier discretion | **217** |

L3221   depth inlay

L3222   shoes, hightop, depth inlay

L3223   Orthopedic footwear, mens surgical boot, each

L3224   Orthopedic footwear, woman's shoe, oxford, used as an integral part of a brace (orthosis)

L3225   Orthopedic footwear, man's shoe, oxford, used as an integral part of a brace (orthosis)

L3230   Orthopedic footwear, custom shoes, depth inlay

L3250   Orthopedic footwear, custom molded shoe, removable inner mold, prosthetic shoe, each

L3251   Foot, shoe molded to patient model; silicone shoe, each

L3252   plastazote (or similar), custom fabricated, each

L3253   Foot, molded shoe plastazote (or similar) custom fitted, each

L3254   Non-standard size or width

L3255   Non-standard size or length

L3257   Orthopedic footwear, additional charge for split size

L3260   Ambulatory surgical boot, each

L3265   Plastazote sandal, each

SHOE MODIFICATION

LIFTS

L3300   Lift, elevation; heel, tapered to metatarsal, per inch

L3310   heel and sole, neoprene, per inch

L3320   heel and sole, cork, per inch

L3330   metal extension (skate)

L3332   inside shoe, tapered, up to one-half inch

L3334   heel, per inch

WEDGES

L3340   Heel wedge, SACH

L3350   Heel wedge

L3360   Sole wedge; outside sole

L3370   between sole

L3380   Clubfoot wedge

L3390   Outflare wedge

L3400   Metatarsal bar wedge; rocker

L3410   between sole

L3420   Full sole and heel wedge, between sole

HEELS

L3430   Heel; counter, plastic reinforced

L3440   counter, leather reinforced

L3450   SACH cushion type

L3455   new leather, standard

L3460   new rubber, standard

L3465   Thomas with wedge

L3470   Thomas extended to ball

L3480   pad and depression for spur

L3485   pad, removable for spur

ORTHOPEDIC SHOE ADDITIONS

L3500   Orthopedic shoe addition; insole, leather

L3510	insole, rubber
L3520	insole, felt covered with leather
L3530	sole, half
L3540	sole, full
L3550	toe tap, standard
L3560	toe tap, horseshoe
L3570	special extension to instep (leather with eyelets)
L3580	convert instep to velcro closure
L3590	convert firm shoe counter to soft counter
L3595	march bar

TRANSFER OR REPLACEMENT

L3600	Transfer of an orthosis from one shoe to another; caliper plate, existing
L3610	caliper plate, new
L3620	solid stirrup, existing
L3630	solid stirrup, new
L3640	Dennis Browne splint (Riveton), both shoes
L3649	Orthopedic shoe, modification, addition or transfer, not otherwise specified

ORTHOTIC DEVICES-UPPER LIMB

NOTE: The procedures in this section are considered as "base" or "basic" procedures and may be modified by listing other procedures from the "additions" section, and adding them to the base procedure.

UPPER LIMB-SHOULDER

L3650	Shoulder orthosis, (SO); figure of eight design abduction restrainer, prefabricated, includes fitting and adjusment

L3660   figure of eight design abduction restrainer, canvas and webbing, prefabricated, includes fitting and adjustment

L3670   acromio/clavicular (canvas and webbing type), prefabricated, includes fitting and adjustment

L3675   vest type abduction restrainer, canvas webbing type, or equal, prefabricated, includes fitting and adjustment

● **L3677**   hard plastic, shoulder stabilizer, pre-fabricated, includes fitting and adjustment

UPPER LIMB-ELBOW

L3700   Elbow orthosis (EO); elastic with stays, prefabricated, includes fitting and adjustment

L3710   elastic with metal joints, prefabricated, includes fitting and adjustment

L3720   double upright with forearm/arm cuffs, free motion, custom fabricated

L3730   double upright with forearm/arm cuffs, extension/flexion assist, custom fabricated

L3740   double upright with forearm/arm cuffs, adjustable position lock with active control, custom fabricated

L3760   with adjustable position locking joint(s), prefabricated, includes fitting and adjustment

UPPER LIMB — WRIST-HAND-FINGER

L3800   Wrist-hand-finger-orthoses (WHFO); short opponens, no attachments, custom fabricated

L3805   long opponens, no attachment, custom fabricated

L3807   without joint(s), prefabricated, inlcudes fitting and adjustment

ADDITIONS

L3810   Wrist-hand-finger-orthosis, addition to short and long opponens; thumb abduction ("C") bar

L3815   second M.P. abduction assist

L3820   I.P. extension assist, with M.P. extension stop

L3825   M.P. extension stop

L3830   M.P. extension assist

L3835   M.P. spring extension assist

L3840   spring swivel thumb

L3845   thumb I.P. extension assist, with M.P. stop

L3850   action wrist, with dorsiflexion assist

L3855   adjustable M.P. flexion control

L3860   adjustable M.P. flexion control and I.P.

L3890   Addition to upper extremity joint, wrist or elbow, concentric adjustable torsion style mechanism, each

DYNAMIC FLEXOR HINGE, RECIPROCAL WRIST EXTENSION/FLEXION, FINGER FLEXION/EXTENSION

L3900   Wrist-hand-finger-orthosis, dynamic flexor hinge, reciprocal wrist extension/flexion, finger flexion/ extension; wrist or finger driven, custom fabricated

L3901   cable driven, custom fabricated

EXTERNAL POWER

L3902   Wrist-hand-finger-orthosis, external powered; compressed gas, custom fabricated

L3904   electric, custom fabricated

OTHER WRIST-HAND-FINGER ORTHOSES-CUSTOM FITTED

L3906   Wrist-hand-orthosis, wrist gauntlet, custom fabricated

L3907   Wrist-hand-finger-orthosis, wrist guantlet with thumb spica, custom fabricated

---

L3908 Wrist-hand-orthosis (WHO), wrist extension control cock-up, prefabricated, includes fitting and adjustment

L3910 Wrist-hand-finger-orthosis (WHFO), Swanson design, prefabricated, includes fitting and adjustment

L3912 Hand-finger-orthosis, flexion glove with elastic finger control, prefabricated, includes fitting and adjustment

L3914 Wrist-hand-orthosis (WHO), wrist extension cock-up, prefabricated, includes fitting and adjustment

L3916 Wrist-hand-finger-orthosis, wrist extension cock-up with outrigger, prefabricated, includes fitting and adjustment

L3918 Hand-finger-orthosis (HFO); knuckle bender, prefabricated, inlcudes fitting and adjustment

L3920 knuckle bender with outrigger, prefabricated, includes fitting and adjustment

L3922 knuckle bender, two segment to flex joints, prefabricated, includes fitting and adjustment

L3923 Hand-finger-orthosis (HFO), without joint(s), prefabricated, includes fitting and adjustment, any type

L3924 Wrist-hand-finger orthosis (WHFO); Oppenheimer, prefabricated, includes fitting and adjustment

L3926 Thomas suspension, prefabricated, includes fitting and adjustment

L3928 Hand-finger orthosis (HFO), finger extension, with clock spring, prefabricated, includes fitting and adjustment

L3930 Wrist-hand-finger orthosis, finger extension, with wrist support, prefabricated, includes fitting and adjustment

L3932 Finger orthosis (FO); safety pin, spring wire, prefabricated, includes fitting and adjustment

L3934 safety pin, modified, prefabricated, includes fitting and adjustment

L3936 Wrist-hand-finger orthosis (WHFO); Palmer, prefabricated, includes fitting and adjustment

L3938   dorsal wrist, prefabricated, includes fitting and adjustment

L3940   dorsal wrist, with outrigger attachment, prefabricated, includes fitting and adjustment

L3942   Hand-finger orthosis (HFO); reverse knuckle bender, prefabricated, includes fitting and adjustment

L3944   reverse knuckle bender, with outrigger, prefabricated, includes fitting and adjustment

L3946   composite elastic, prefabricated, includes fitting and adjustment

L3948   Finger orthosis (FO), finger knuckle bender, prefabricated, includes fitting and adjustment

L3950   Wrist-hand-finger orthosis (WHFO); combination Oppenheimer, with knuckle bender and two attachments, prefabricated, includes fitting and adjustment

L3952   combination Oppenheimer, with reverse knuckle and two attachments, prefabricated, includes fitting and adjustment

L3954   Hand-finger orthosis (HFO), spreading hand, prefabricated, includes fitting and adjustment

L3956   Addition of joint to upper extremity orthosis, any material; per joint

UPPER LIMB — SHOULDER-ELBOW-WRIST-HAND

ABDUCTION POSITIONING — CUSTOM FITTED

L3960   Shoulder-elbow-wrist-hand orthoses, (SEWHO); abduction positioning, airplane design, prefabricated, includes fitting and adjustment

L3962   abduction positioning, Erbs palsey design, prefabricated, includes fitting and adjustment

L3963   molded shoulder, arm, forearm, and wrist, with articulating elbow joint, custom fabricated

L3964   Shoulder-elbow orthosis (SEO), mobile arm support attached to wheelchair, balanced; adjustable, prefabricated, includes fitting and adjustment

L3965   adjustable rancho type, prefabricated, includes fitting and adjustment

L3966   reclining, prefabricated, includes fitting and adjustment

L3968   friction arm support (friction dampening to proximal and distal joints), prefabricated, includes fitting and adjustment

L3969   Shoulder-elbow orthosis (SEO), mobile arm support, monosuspension arm and hand support, overhead elbow forearm hand sling support, yoke type suspension support, prefabricated, includes fitting and adjustment

ADDITIONS TO MOBILE ARM SUPPORTS

L3970   Shoulder-elbow orthosis (SEO), addition to mobile arm support; elevating proximal arm

L3972   offset or lateral rocker arm with elastic balance control

L3974   supinator

UPPER LIMB-FRACTURE ORTHOSES

L3980   Upper extremity fracture orthosis; humeral, prefabricated, includes fitting and adjustment

L3982   radius/ulnar, prefabricated, includes fitting and adjustment

L3984   wrist, prefabricated, includes fitting and adjustment

L3985   forearm, hand with wrist hinge, custom fabricated

L3986   combination of humeral, radius/ulnar, wrist, (example - Colles' fracture), custom fabricated

L3995   Addition to upper extremity orthosis, sock, fracture or equal, each

L3999   Upper limb orthosis, not otherwise specified

SPECIFIC REPAIR

▲L4000   Replace girdle for spinal orthosis (CTLSO or SO)

L4010   Replace trilateral socket brim

L4020   Replace quadrilateral socket brim; molded to patient model

L4030   custom fitted

L4040   Replace molded thigh lacer

L4045   Replace non-molded thigh lacer

L4050   Replace molded calf lacer

L4055   Replace non-molded calf lacer

L4060   Replace high roll cuff

L4070   Replace proximal and distal upright for KAFO

L4080   Replace metal bands KAFO, proximal thigh

L4090   Replace metal bands KAFO-AFO, calf or distal thigh

L4100   Replace leather cuff KAFO, proximal thigh

L4110   Replace leather cuff KAFO-AFO, calf or distal thigh

L4130   Replace pretibial shell

REPAIRS

L4205   Repair of orthotic device; labor component, per 15 minutes

L4210   repair or replace minor parts

ANCILLARY ORTHOTIC SERVICES

(L4310)   Code deleted 1999; use L4396

(L4320)   Code deleted 1999; use L4396

● New code   ▲ Revised code   ( ) Deleted code

L4350 Pneumatic ankle control splint (e.g., aircast), prefabricated, includes fitting and adjustment

L4360 Pneumatic walking splint (e.g., aircast), prefabricated, includes fitting and adjustment

L4370 Pneumatic full leg splint (e.g., aircast), prefabricated, includes fitting and adjustment

L4380 Pneumatic knee splint (e.g., aircast), prefabricated, includes fitting and adjustment

(L4390) Code deleted 1999; use L4392

L4392 Replacement, soft interface material; static AFO

L4394 foot drop splint

▲**L4396** Static ankle foot orthosis, including soft interface material, adjustable for fit, for positioning, pressure reduction, may be used for minimal ambulation, prefabricated, includes fitting and adjustment

L4398 Foot drop splint, recumbent positioning device, prefabricated, includes fitting and adjustment

● New code ▲ Revised code ( ) Deleted code

PROSTHETIC PROCEDURES

Guidelines

In addition to the information presented in the INTRODUCTION, several other items unique to this section are defined or identified here:

1. **PROSTHETIC DEVICES:** Prosthetic devices (other than dental) which replace all or part of an internal body organ (including contiguous tissue), or replace all or part of the function of a permanently inoperative or malfunctioning internal body organ, are covered when furnished upon a physician's order. This does not require a determination that there is no possibility that the patient's condition may improve in the future. If the medical record and the judgement of the attending physician indicate that the condition is of long and indefinite duration, the test of permanence is met. The device(s) may also be covered as a supply item when furnished incident to a physician's service.

2. **SUBSECTION INFORMATION:** Some of the listed subheadings or subsections have special needs or instructions unique to that section. Where these are indicated, special "notes" will be presented preceding or following the listings. Those subsections within the PROSTHETIC PROCEDURES section that have "notes" are as follows:

Subsection	Code Numbers
Prosthetic procedures-lower limb	L5000-L5999
Upper limb	L6000-L6590
Additions-upper limb	L6600-L6999

3. **UNLISTED SERVICE OR PROCEDURE:** A service or procedure may be provided that is not listed in this edition of HCPCS. When reporting such a service, the appropriate "unlisted procedure" code may be used to indicate the service, identifying it by "special report" as defined below. HCPCS terminology is inconsistent in defining unlisted procedures. The procedure definition may include the term(s) "unlisted", "not otherwise classified", "unspecified", "unclassified", "other" and "miscellaneous". Prior to using these codes, try to determine if a Local Level III code or CPT code is available. The "unlisted procedures" and accompanying codes for PROSTHETIC PROCEDURES are as follows:

L5999   Lower extremity prosthesis, not otherwise specified

L7499	Upper extremity prosthesis, not otherwise specified
L8039	Breast prosthesis, not otherwise specified
L8239	Gradient compression stocking, not otherwise specified
L8499	Unlisted procedure for miscellaneous prosthetic services
L8699	Prosthetic implant, not otherwise specified

4. **SPECIAL REPORT:** A service, material or supply that is rarely provided, unusual, variable or new may require a special report in determining medical appropriateness for reimbursement purposes. Pertinent information should include an adequate definition or description of the nature, extent, and need for the service, material or supply.

5. **MODIFIERS:** Listed services may be modified under certain circumstances. When appropriate, the modifying circumstance is identified by adding a modifier to the basic procedure code. CPT and HCPCS National Level II modifiers may be used with CPT and HCPCS National Level II procedure codes. Modifiers commonly used with PROSTHETIC PROCEDURES are as follows:

-CC Procedure code change (use "CC" when the procedure code submitted was changed either for administrative reasons or because an incorrect code was filed)

-LT Left side (used to identify procedures performed on the left side of the body)

-QB Physician providing service in a rural HMSA

-QU Physician providing service in an urban HMSA

-RT Right side (used to identify procedures performed on the right side of the body)

-TC Technical component. Under certain circumstances, a charge may be made for the technical component alone. Under those circumstances, the technical component charge is identified by adding modifier -TC to the usual procedure number. Technical component charges are institutional charges and are not billed separately by physicians. However, portable x-ray suppliers bill only for the technical component and should use modifier -TC. The charge data from portable x-ray suppliers will then be used to build customary and prevailing profiles.

6. **CPT CODE CROSS-REFERENCE:** Unless otherwise specified, the equivalent CPT code for all listings in this section is 99070.

7. **DURABLE MEDICAL EQUIPMENT REGIONAL CARRIERS (DMERCS):** Effective October 1, 1993 claims for prosthetics must be billed to one of four regional carriers depending upon the residence of the beneficiary. The transition dates for DMERC claims is from November 1, 1993 to March 1, 1994, depending upon the state you practice in. See the Introduction for a complete discussion of DMERCs.

Prosthetic Procedures

LOWER LIMB

> **NOTE:** The procedures in this section are considered as "base" or "basic" procedures, and they may be modified by listing items, procedures or special materials from the "additions" section, and adding them to the base procedure.

LOWER LIMB — PARTIAL FOOT

L5000 Partial foot; shoe insert with longitudinal arch, toe filler

L5010 molded socket, ankle height, with toe filler

L5020 molded socket, tibial tubercle height, with toe filler

LOWER LIMB-ANKLE

L5050 Ankle, symes; molded socket, SACH foot

L5060 metal frame, molded leather socket, articulated ankle/foot

LOWER LIMB-BELOW KNEE

L5100 Below knee; molded socket, shin, SACH foot

L5105 plastic socket, joints and thigh lacer, SACH foot

LOWER LIMB-KNEE DISARTICULATION

L5150 Knee disarticulation (or through knee), molded socket; external knee joints, shin, SACH foot

L5160 bent knee configuration, external knee joints, shin, SACH foot

| Not valid for Medicare | Non-covered by Medicare | Special coverage instructions | Carrier discretion | **231** |

LOWER LIMB-ABOVE KNEE

L5200 Above knee; molded socket, single axis constant friction knee, shin, SACH foot

L5210 short prosthesis, no knee joint ("stubbies"), with foot blocks, no ankle joints, each

L5220 short prosthesis, no knee joint ("stubbies"), with articulated ankle/foot, dynamically aligned, each

L5230 for proximal femoral focal deficiency, constant friction knee, shin, each foot

LOWER LIMB-HIP DISARTICULATION

L5250 Hip disarticulation; Canadian type, molded socket, hip joint, single axis constant friction knee, shin, SACH foot

L5270 tilt table type; molded socket, locking hip joint, single axis constant friction knee, shin, SACH foot

LOWER LIMB-HEMIPELVECTOMY

L5280 Hemipelvectomy, canadian type; molded socket, hip joint, single axis constant friction knee, shin, SACH foot

LOWER LIMB-ENDOSKELETAL-BELOW KNEE

(L5300) Code deleted 2002; use L5301

● **L5301** Below knee, molded socket, shin, each foot, endoskeletal system

LOWER LIMB-ENDOSKELETAL-KNEE DISARTICULATION

(L5310) Code deleted 2002; use L5311

● **L5311** Knee disarticulation (or through knee), molded socket, external knee joints, shin, sach foot, endoskeletal system

LOWER LIMB-ENDOSKELETAL-ABOVE KNEE

(L5320) Code deleted 2002; use L5321

● **L5321** Above knee, molded socket, open end, sach foot, endoskeletal system, single axis knee

LOWER LIMB-ENDOSKELETAL-HIP DISARTICULATION

(L5330) Code deleted 2002; use L5331

● **L5331** Hip disarticulation, Canadian type, molded socket, endoskeletal system, hip joint, single axis knee, sach foot

LOWER LIMB-ENDOSKELETAL-HEMIPELVECTOMY

(L5340) Code deleted 2002; use L5341

● **L5341** Hemipelvectomy, Canadian type, molded socket, endoskeletal system, hip joint, single axis knee, sach foot

IMMEDIATE-EARLY-INITIAL-PREPARATORY PROCEDURES

IMMEDIATE POST SURGICAL OR EARLY FITTING PROCEDURES

L5400 Immediate post surgical or early fitting; application of initial rigid dressing, including fitting, alignment, suspension, and one cast change, below knee

L5410 application of initial rigid dressing, including fitting, alignment and suspension, below knee, each additional cast change and realignment

L5420 application of initial rigid dressing, including fitting, alignment and suspension and one cast change "AK" or knee disarticulation

L5430 application of initial rigid dressing, including fitting, alignment and suspension, "AK" or knee disarticulation, each additional cast change and realignment

L5450 application of non-weight bearing rigid dressing, below knee

L5460 application of non-weight bearing rigid dressing, above knee

INITIAL PROSTHESIS

L5500 Initial, below knee "PTB" type socket, non-alignable system, pylon, no cover, SACH foot, plaster socket, direct formed

L5505 Initial, above knee - knee disarticulation, ischial level socket non-alignable system, pylon, no cover, SACH foot plaster socket, direct formed

PREPARATORY PROSTHESIS

L5510 Preparatory, below knee "PTB" type socket, non-alignable system, pylon, no cover, SACH foot; plaster socket, molded to model

L5520 thermoplastic or equal, direct formed

L5530 thermoplastic or equal, molded to model

L5535 Preparatory, below knee "PTB" type socket, non-alignable system, no cover, SACH foot, prefabricated, adjustable open end socket

L5540 Preparatory, below knee "PTB" type socket, non-alignable system, pylon, no cover, SACH foot, laminated socket, molded to model

L5560 Preparatory, above knee - knee disarticulation, ischial level socket, non-alignable system, pylon, no cover, SACH foot; plaster socket, molded to model

L5570 thermoplastic or equal, direct formed

L5580 thermoplastic or equal, molded to model

L5585 prefabricated adjustable open end socket

L5590 laminated socket, molded to model

L5595 Preparatory, hip disarticulation-hemipelvectomy, pylon, no cover, SACH foot; thermoplastic or equal, molded to patient model

L5600 laminated socket, molded to patient model

ADDITIONS TO LOWER EXTREMITY

L5610   Addition to lower extremity, endoskeletal system; above knee, hydracadence system

L5611   above knee - knee disarticulation, 4-bar linkage, with friction swing phase control

L5613   above knee-knee disarticulation, 4-bar linkage, with hydraulic swing phase control

L5614   above knee-knee disarticulation, 4-bar linkage, with pneumatic swing phase control

L5616   above knee, universal multiplex system, friction swing phase control

L5617   Addition to lower extremity, quick change self-aligning unit, above knee or below knee, each

ADDITIONS-TEST SOCKETS

L5618   Addition to lower extremity, test socket; Symes

L5620   below knee

L5622   knee disarticulation

L5624   above knee

L5626   hip disarticulation

L5628   hemipelvectomy

L5629   Addition to lower extremity, below knee, acrylic socket

ADDITIONS-SOCKET VARIATIONS

L5630   Addition to lower extremity, Symes type, expandable wall socket

L5631   Addition to lower extremity, above knee or knee disarticulation, acrylic socket

L5632   Addition to lower extremity, Symes type; "PTB" brim design socket

	Not valid for Medicare		Non-covered by Medicare		Special coverage instructions		Carrier discretion

L5634   posterior opening (Canadian) socket

L5636   medial opening socket

L5637   Addition to lower extremity, below knee; total contact

L5638   leather socket

L5639   wood socket

L5640   Addition to lower extremity, knee disarticulation, leather socket

L5642   Addition to lower extremity, above knee, leather socket

L5643   Addition to lower extremity, hip disarticulation, flexible inner socket, external frame

L5644   Addition to lower extremity, above knee, wood socket

L5645   Addition to lower extremity, below knee; flexible inner socket, external frame

L5646   air cushion socket

L5647   suction socket

L5648   Addition to lower extremity, above knee, air cushion socket

L5649   Addition to lower extremity, ischial containment/narrow M-L socket

L5650   Addition to lower extremity, total contact, above knee or knee disarticulation socket

L5651   Addition to lower extremity, above knee, flexible inner socket, external frame

L5652   Addition to lower extremity, suction suspension, above knee or knee disarticulation socket

L5653   Addition to lower extremity, knee disarticulation, expandable wall socket

ADDITIONS-SOCKET INSERT AND SUSPENSION

L5654   Addition to lower extremity, socket insert; Symes, (Kemblo, Pelite, Aliplast, Plastazote or equal)

L5655   below knee (Kemblo, Pelite, Aliplast, Plastazote or equal)

L5656   knee disarticulation, (Kemblo, Pelite, Aliplast, Plastazote or equal)

L5658   above knee (Kemblo, Pelite, Aliplast, Plastazote or equal)

L5660   Syme, silicone gel or equal

L5661   multi-durometer Symes

L5662   below knee, silicone gel or equal

L5663   knee disarticulation, silicone gel or equal

L5664   above knee, silicone gel or equal

L5665   multi-durometer, below knee

L5666   Addition to lower extremity; below knee, cuff suspension

(L5667)   Code deleted 2002

L5668   Addition to lower extremity; below knee, molded distal cushion

(L5669)   Code deleted 2002; use L5660, L5662, L5663, L5664

L5670   Addition to lower extremity; below knee, molded supracondylar suspension ("PTS" or similar)

● **L5671**   Addition to lower extremity; below knee/above knee suspension locking mechanism (shuttle, lanyard or equal), excludes socket insert

L5672   below knee, removable medial brim suspension

L5674   below knee, suspension sleeve, any material, each

L5675	below knee, suspension sleeve, heavy duty, any material, each
L5676	below knee, knee joints, single axis, pair
L5677	below knee, knee joints, polycentric, pair
L5678	below knee, joint covers, pair
L5680	below knee, thigh lacer, non-molded
L5682	below knee, thigh lacer, gluteal/ischial, molded
L5684	below knee, fork strap
L5686	below knee, back check (extension control)
L5688	below knee, waist belt, webbing
L5690	below knee, waist belt, padded and lined
L5692	Addition to lower extremity, above knee; pelvic control belt, light
L5694	pelvic control belt, padded and lined
L5695	pelvic control, sleeve suspension, neoprene or equal, each
L5696	Addition to lower extremity, above knee or knee disarticulation; pelvic joint
L5697	pelvic band
L5698	silesian bandage
L5699	All lower extremity protheses, shoulder harness
L5700	Replacement, socket; below knee, molded to patient model
L5701	above knee/knee disarticulation, including attachment plate, molded to patient model
L5702	hip disarticulation, including hip joint, molded to patient model
▲**L5704**	Custom shaped protective cover, below knee

▲**L5705**   Custom shaped protective cover, above knee

▲**L5706**   Custom shaped protective cover, knee disarticulation

▲**L5707**   Custom shaped protective cover, hip disarticulation

ADDITIONS-KNEE-SHIN SYSTEM

EXOSKELETAL

L5710   Addition, exoskeletal knee-shin system, single axis; manual lock

L5711   manual lock, ultra-light material

L5712   friction swing and stance phase control (safety knee)

L5714   variable friction swing phase control

L5716   Addition, exoskeletal knee-shin system, polycentric; mechanical stance phase lock

L5718   friction swing and stance phase control

L5722   Addition, exoskeletal knee-shin system, single axis; pneumatic swing, friction stance phase control

L5724   fluid swing phase control

L5726   external joints fluid swing phase control

L5728   fluid swing and stance phase control

L5780   pneumatic/hydrapneumatic swing phase control

L5785   Addition, exoskeletal system, below knee, ultra-light material (titanium, carbon fiber or equal)

L5790   Addition, exoskeletal system, above knee, ultra-light material (titanium, carbon fiber or equal)

L5795   Addition, exoskeletal system, hip disarticulation, ultra-light material (titanium, carbon fiber or equal)

ENDOSKELETAL

L5810 Addition, endoskeletal knee-shin system, single axis; manual lock

L5811 manual lock, ultra-light material

L5812 friction swing and stance phase control (safety knee)

L5814 Addition, endoskeletal knee-shin system, polycentric; hydraulic swing phase control, mechanical stance phase lock

L5816 mechanical stance phase lock

L5818 friction swing and stance phase control

L5822 Addition, endoskeletal knee-shin system, single axis; pneumatic swing, friction stance phase control

L5824 fluid swing phase control

L5826 hydraulic swing phase control, with miniature high activity frame

L5828 fluid swing and stance phase control

L5830 pneumatic swing phase control

L5840 Addition, endoskeletal knee-shin system, 4-bar linkage or multiaxial, pneumatic swing phase control

L5845 Addition, endoskeletal, knee-shin system; stance flexion feature, adjustable

L5846 microprocessor control feature, swing phase only

● **L5847** Addition, endoskeletal knee-shin system, microprocessor control feature, stance phase

L5850 Addition, endoskeletal system; above knee or hip disarticulation, knee extension assist

L5855 hip disarticulation, mechanical hip extension assist

L5910 below knee, alignable system

L5920   above knee or hip disarticulation, alignable system

L5925   above knee, knee disarticulation or hip disarticulation, manual lock

L5930   Addition, endoskeletal system; high activity knee control frame

L5940   below knee, ultra-light material (titanium, carbon fiber or equal)

L5950   above knee, ultra-light material (titanium, carbon fiber or equal)

L5960   hip disarticulation, ultra-light material (titanium, carbon fiber or equal)

L5962   below knee, flexible protective outer surface covering system

L5964   above knee, flexible protective outer surface covering system

L5966   hip disarticulation, flexible protective outer surface covering system

L5968   Addition to lower limb prosthesis, multiaxial ankle with swing phase active dorsiflexion feature

L5970   All lower extremity prostheses; foot, external keel, each foot

L5972   flexible keel foot (Safe, Sten, Bock Dynamic or equal)

L5974   foot, single axis ankle/foot

L5975   All lower extremity prosthesis; combination single axis ankle and flexible keel foot

L5976   energy storing foot (Seattle Carbon Copy II or equal)

L5978   foot, multiaxial ankle/foot

L5979   multiaxial ankle, dynamic response foot, one piece system

L5980   flex foot system

L5981   flex-walk system or equal

L5982   All exoskeletal lower extremity prostheses, axial rotation unit

L5984   All endoskeletal lower extremity prostheses, axial rotation unit

L5985   All endoskeletal lower extremity prostheses, dynamic prosthetic pylon

L5986   All lower extremity prostheses, multi-axial rotation unit ("MCP" or equal)

L5987   All lower extremity prosthesis, shank foot system with vertical loading pylon

L5988   Addition to lower limb prosthesis, vertical shock reducing pylon feature

● L5989   Addition to lower extremity prosthesis, endoskeletal system, pylon with integrated electronic force sensors

● L5990   Addition to lower extremity prothesis, user adjustable heel height

L5999   Lower extremity prosthesis, not otherwise specified

UPPER LIMB

NOTE: The procedures in L6000-L6599 are considered as "base" or "basic" procedures and may be modified by listing procedures from the "additions" sections. The base procedures include only standard friction wrist and control cable system unless otherwise specified.

UPPER LIMB-PARTIAL HAND

L6000   Partial hand, Robin-aids; thumb remaining (or equal)

L6010   little and/or ring ringer remaining (or equal)

L6020   no finger remaining (or equal)

UPPER LIMB-WRIST DISARTICULATION

L6050   Wrist disarticulation, molded socket, flexible elbow hinges, triceps pad

UPPER LIMB-BELOW ELBOW

L6055   Wrist disarticulation, molded socket with expandable interface, flexible elbow hinges, triceps pad

L6100   Below elbow, molded socket; flexible elbow hinge, triceps pad

L6110   (Muenster or Northwestern Suspension types)

L6120   Below elbow, molded double wall split socket; step-up hinges, half cuff

L6130   stump activated locking hinge, half cuff

UPPER LIMB-ELBOW DISARTICULATION

L6200   Elbow disarticulation, molded socket, outside locking hinge, forearm

UPPER LIMB-ABOVE ELBOW

L6205   Elbow disarticulation, molded socket with expandable interface, outside locking hinges, forearm

L6250   Above elbow, molded double wall socket, internal locking elbow, forearm

UPPER LIMB-SHOULDER DISARTICULATION

L6300   Shoulder disarticulation, molded socket, shoulder bulkhead, humeral section, internal locking elbow, forearm

L6310   Shoulder disarticulation, passive restoration; (complete prosthesis)

L6320   (shoulder cap only)

UPPER LIMB-INTERSCAPULAR THORACIC

L6350 Interscapular thoracic; molded socket, shoulder bulkhead, humeral section, internal locking elbow, forearm

L6360 passive restoration (complete prosthesis)

L6370 passive restoration (shoulder cap only)

UPPER LIMB-IMMEDIATE AND EARLY POST SURGICAL PROCEDURES

L6380 Immediate post surgical or early fitting, application of initial rigid dressing, including fitting alignment and suspension of components, and one cast change; wrist disarticulation or below elbow

L6382 elbow disarticulation or above elbow

L6384 shoulder disarticulation or interscapular thoracic

L6386 Immediate post surgical or early fitting; each additional cast change and realignment

L6388 application of rigid dressing only

UPPER LIMB-ENDOSKELETAL-BELOW ELBOW

L6400 Below elbow, molded socket endoskeletal system, including soft prosthetic tissue shaping

UPPER LIMB-ENDOSKELETAL-ELBOW DISARTICULATION

L6450 Elbow disarticulation, molded socket, endoskeletal system, including soft prosthetic tissue shaping

UPPER LIMB-ENDOSKELETAL-ABOVE ELBOW

L6500 Above elbow, molded socket, endoskeletal system, including soft prosthetic tissue shaping

UPPER LIMB-ENDOSKELETAL-SHOULDER DISARTICULATION

L6550 Shoulder disarticulation, molded socket, endoskeletal system, including soft prosthetic tissue shaping

UPPER LIMB-ENDOSKELETAL-INTERSCAPULAR THORACIC

L6570 Interscapular thoracic, molded socket, endoskeletal system, including soft prosthetic tissue shaping

L6580 Preparatory, wrist disarticulation or below elbow, single wall plastic socket, friction wrist, flexible elbow hinges, figure of eight harness, humeral cuff, Bowden cable control, USMC or equal pylon, no cover, molded to patient model

L6582 Preparatory, wrist disarticulation or below elbow, single wall socket, friction wrist, flexible elbow hinges, figure of eight harness, humeral cuff, bowden cable control, USMC or equal pylon, no cover, direct formed

L6584 Preparatory, elbow disarticulation or above elbow; single wall plastic socket, friction wrist, locking elbow, figure of eight harness, fair lead cable control, USMC or equal pylon, no cover, molded to patient model

L6586 single wall socket, friction wrist, locking elbow, figure of eight harness, fair lead cable control, USMC or equal pylon, no cover, direct formed

L6588 Preparatory shoulder disarticulation or interscapular thoracic; single wall plastic socket, shoulder joint, locking elbow, friction wrist, chest strap, fair lead cable control, USMC or equal pylon, no cover, molded to patient model

L6590 single wall socket, shoulder joint, locking elbow, friction wrist, chest strap, fair lead cable control, USMC or equal pylon, no cover, direct formed

ADDITIONS-UPPER LIMB

NOTE: The following procedures, modifications and/or components may be added to other base procedures. The items in this section should reflect the additional complexity of each modification procedure, in addition to base procedure, at the time of the original order.

L6600 Upper extremity additions; polycentric hinge, pair

L6605 single pivot hinge, pair

L6610	flexible metal hinge, pair
L6615	disconnect locking wrist unit
L6616	additional disconnect insert for locking wrist unit, each
L6620	flexion-friction wrist unit
L6623	spring assisted rotational wrist unit with latch release
L6625	rotation wrist unit with cable lock
L6628	quick disconnect hook adapter, Otto Bock or equal
L6629	quick disconnect lamination collar with coupling piece, Otto Bock or equal
L6630	stainless steel, any wrist
L6632	latex suspension sleeve, each
L6635	lift assist for elbow
L6637	nudge control elbow lock
L6640	shoulder abduction joint, pair
L6641	excursion amplifier, pulley type
L6642	excursion amplifier, lever type
L6645	shoulder flexion - abduction joint, each
L6650	shoulder universal joint, each
L6655	standard control cable, extra
L6660	heavy duty control cable
L6665	teflon, or equal, cable lining
L6670	hook to hand, cable adapter
L6672	harness, chest or shoulder, saddle type
L6675	harness, figure of ("8") eight type, for single control

L6676	harness, figure of ("8") eight type, for dual control
L6680	test socket, wrist disarticulation or below elbow
L6682	test socket, elbow disarticulation or above elbow
L6684	test socket, shoulder disarticulation or interscapular thoracic
L6686	suction socket
L6687	frame type socket, below elbow or wrist disarticulation
L6688	frame type socket, above elbow or elbow disarticulation
L6689	frame type socket, shoulder disarticulation
L6690	frame type socket, interscapular-thoracic
L6691	removable insert, each
L6692	silicone gel insert or equal, each
L6693	locking elbow, forearm counterbalance

TERMINAL DEVICES

HOOKS

L6700	Terminal device, hook, Dorrance, or equal; model #3
L6705	model #5
L6710	model #5X
L6715	model #5XA
L6720	model #6
L6725	model #7
L6730	model #7LO
L6735	model #8
L6740	model #8X

L6745   model #88X

L6750   model #10P

L6755   model #10X

L6765   model #12P

L6770   model #99X

L6775   model #555

L6780   model #SS555

L6790   Terminal device; hook-Accu hook, or equal

L6795   hook-2 load, or equal

L6800   hook-APRL VC, or equal

L6805   modifier wrist flexion unit

L6806   Terminal device, hook; TRS grip, grip III, VC or equal

L6807   grip I, grip II, VC or equal

L6808   TRS adept, infant or child, VC or equal

L6809   TRS Super sport, passive

L6810   Terminal device; pincher tool, Otto Bock or equal

HANDS

L6825   Terminal device, hand; Dorrance, VO

L6830   Aprl, VC

L6835   Sierra, VO

L6840   Becker imperial

L6845   Becker lock grip

L6850   Becker plylite

L6855   Robin-aids, VO

L6860   Robin-aids, VO soft

L6865   passive hand

L6867   Detroit infant hand (mechanical)

L6868   passive infant hand, (Steeper, Hosmer or equal)

L6870   child mitt

L6872   NYU child hand

L6873   mechanical infant hand, Steeper or equal

L6875   Bock, VC

L6880   Bock, VO

● **L6881**   Automatic grasp feature, addition to upper limb prosthetic terminal device

● **L6882**   Microprocessor control feature, addition to upper limb prosthetic terminal device

GLOVES FOR ABOVE HANDS

L6890   Terminal device, glove for above hands; production glove

L6895   custom glove

HAND RESTORATION

L6900   Hand restoration (casts, shading and measurements included), partial hand; with glove, thumb or one finger remaining

L6905   with glove, multiple fingers remaining

L6910   with glove, no fingers remaining

L6915   Hand restoration (shading, and measurements included), replacement glove for above

EXTERNAL POWER — BASE DEVICES

L6920 Wrist disarticulation, external power, self-suspended inner socket, removable forearm shell, Otto Bock or equal; switch, cables, two batteries and one charger, switch control of terminal device

L6925 electrodes, cables, two batteries and one charger, myoelectronic control of terminal device

L6930 Below elbow, external power, self-suspended inner socket, removable forearm shell; Otto Bock or equal switch, cables, two batteries and one charger, switch control of terminal device

L6935 Otto Bock or equal electrodes, cables, two batteries and one charger, myoelectronic control of terminal device

L6940 Elbow disarticulation, external power, molded inner socket, removable humeral shell, outside locking hinges, forearm; Otto Bock or equal switch, cables, two batteries and one charger, switch control of terminal device

L6945 Otto Bock or equal electrodes, cables, two batteries and one charger, myoelectronic control of terminal device

L6950 Above elbow, external power, molded inner socket, removable humeral shell, internal locking elbow, forearm; Otto Bock or equal switch, cables two batteries and one charger, switch control of terminal device

L6955 Otto Bock or equal electrodes, cables, two batteries and one charger, myoelectronic control of terminal device

L6960 Shoulder disarticulation, external power, molded inner socket, removable shoulder shell, shoulder bulkhead, humeral section, mechanical elbow, forearm; Otto Bock or equal switch, cables, two batteries and one charger, switch control of terminal device

L6965 Otto Bock or equal electrodes, cables, two batteries and one charger, myoelectronic control of terminal device

L6970 Interscapular-thoracic, external power, molded inner socket removable shoulder shell, shoulder bulkhead, humeral section, mechanical elbow, forearm; Otto Bock or equal switch, cables, two batteries and one charger, switch control of terminal device

L6975 Otto Bock or equal electrodes cables, two batteries and one charger, myoelectronic control of terminal device

EXTERNAL POWER-TERMINAL DEVICES

L7010 Electronic hand; Otto Bock, Steeper or equal, switch controlled

L7015 System Teknik, Variety Village or equal, switch controlled

L7020 Electronic Greifer, Otto Bock or equal, switch controlled

L7025 Electronic hand; Otto Bock or equal, myoelectronically controlled

L7030 System Teknik, Variety Village or equal, myoelectronically controlled

L7035 Electronic Greifer, Otto Bock or equal, myoelectronically controlled

L7040 Prehensile actuator, Hosmer or equal, switch controlled

L7045 Electronic hook, child, Michigan or equal, switch controlled

EXTERNAL POWER — ELBOW

L7170 Electronic elbow; hosmer or equal, switch controlled

L7180 Boston, Utah or equal, myoelectronically controlled

L7185 adolescent, Variety Village or equal, switch controlled

L7186 child, Variety Village or equal, switch controlled

L7190 adolescent, Variety Village or equal, myoelectronically controlled

L7191 child, Variety Village or equal, myoelectronically controlled

EXTERNAL POWER-CONTROL MODULES

L7260 Electronic wrist rotator; Otto Bock or equal

| Not valid for Medicare | Non-covered by Medicare | Special coverage instructions | Carrier discretion | **251** |

L7261	for Utah arm
L7266	Servo control, Steeper or equal
L7272	Analogue control, UNB or equal
L7274	Proportional control, 6-12 volt, Liberty, Utah or equal

EXTERNAL POWER-BATTERY COMPONENTS

L7360	Six volt battery, Otto Bock or equal, each
L7362	Battery charger, six volt, Otto Bock or equal
L7364	Twelve volt battery, Utah or equal, each
L7366	Battery charger, twelve volt, Utah or equal
L7499	Upper extremity prosthesis, not otherwise specified

REPAIRS

L7500	Repair of prosthetic device, hourly rate (excludes V5335 repair of oral or laryngeal prosthesis or artificial larynx)
L7510	Repair prosthetic device, repair or replace minor parts (excludes V5335 repair of oral or laryngeal prosthesis or artificial larynx)
L7520	Repair prosthetic device, labor component, per 15 minutes
L7900	Vacuum erection system

GENERAL-BREAST PROSTHESES

L8000	Breast prosthesis; mastectomy bra
● **L8001**	Breast prosthesis, mastectomy bra, with integrated breast prosthesis form, unilateral
● **L8002**	Breast prosthesis, mastectomy bra, with integrated breast prosthesis form, bilateral
L8010	mastectomy sleeve
L8015	External breast prosthesis garment, with mastectomy form, post mastectomy

L8020   Breast prosthesis; mastectomy form

L8030   silicone or equal

L8035   Custom breast prosthesis, post mastectomy, molded to patient model

L8039   Breast prosthesis, not otherwise specified

L8040   Nasal prosthesis, provided by a non-physician

L8041   Midfacial prosthesis, provided by a non-physician

L8042   Orbital prosthesis, provided by a non-physician

L8043   Upper facial prosthesis, provided by a non-physician

L8044   Hemi-facial prosthesis, provided by a non-physician

L8045   Auricular prosthesis, provided by a non-physician

L8046   Partial facial prosthesis, provided by a non-physician

L8047   Nasal septal prosthesis, provided by a non-physician

L8048   Unspecified maxillofacial prosthesis, by report, provided by a non-physician

L8049   Repair or modification of maxillofacial prosthesis, labor component, 15 minute increments, provided by a non-physician

GENERAL-ELASTIC SUPPORTS

L8100   Gradient compression stocking; below knee, 18-30 mmhg, each

L8110   below knee, 30-40 mmhg, each

L8120   below knee, 40-50 mmhg, each

L8130   thigh length, 18-30 mmhg, each

L8140   thigh length, 30-40 mmhg, each

L8150   thigh length, 40-50 mmhg, each

| Not valid for Medicare | Non-covered by Medicare | Special coverage instructions | Carrier discretion | **253** |

L8160   full length/chap style, 18-30 mmhg, each

L8170   full length/chap style, 30-40 mmhg, each

L8180   full length/chap style, 40-50 mmhg, each

L8190   waist length, 18-30 mmhg, each

L8195   waist length, 30-40 mmhg, each

L8200   waist length, 40-50 mmhg, each

L8210   custom made

L8220   lymphedema

L8230   garter belt

L8239   Gradient compression stocking, not otherwise specified

GENERAL-TRUSSES

L8300   Truss; single with standard pad

L8310   double with standard pads

L8320   addition to standard pad, water pad

L8330   addition to standard pad, scrotal pad

PROSTHETIC SOCKS

L8400   Prosthetic sheath; below knee, each

L8410   above knee, each

L8415   upper limb, each

L8417   Prosthetic sheath/sock, including a gel cushion layer, below knee or above knee, each

L8420   Prosthetic sock, multiple ply; below knee, each

L8430   above knee, each

L8435   upper limb, each

L8440 Prosthetic shrinker; below knee, each

L8460 above knee, each

L8465 upper limb, each

L8470 Prosthetic sock, single ply, fitting; below knee, each

L8480 above knee, each

L8485 upper limb, each

L8490 Addition to prosthetic sheath/sock, air seal suction retention system

L8499 Unlisted procedure for miscellaneous prosthetic services

PROSTHETIC IMPLANTS

L8500 Artificial larynx, any type

L8501 Tracheostomy speaking valve

● **L8505** Artificial larynx replacement battery/accessory, any type

● **L8507** Tracheo-esophageal voice prosthesis, patient inserted, any type, each

● **L8509** Tracheo-esophageal voice prosthesis, inserted by a licensed health care provider, any type

● **L8510** Voice amplifier

INTEGUMENTARY SYSTEM

L8600 Implantable breast prosthesis, silicone or equal

L8603 Injectable bulking agent, collagen implant, urinary tract, 2.5 ml syringe, includes shipping and necessary supplies

L8606 Injectable bulking agent, synthetic implant, urinary tract, 1 ml syringe, includes shipping and necessary supplies

HEAD (SKULL, FACIAL BONES AND TEMPOROMANDIBULAR JOINT)

L8610   Ocular implant

L8612   Aqueous shunt

L8613   Ossicula implant

L8614   Cochlear device/system

L8619   Cochlear implant external speech processor, replacement

UPPER EXTREMITY

L8630   Metacarpophalangeal joint implant

LOWER EXTREMITY (JOINT: KNEE, ANKLE, TOE)

L8641   Metatarsal joint implant

L8642   Hallux implant

MISCELLANEOUS MUSCULAR — SKELETAL

L8658   Interphalangeal joint implant

CARDIOVASCULAR SYSTEM

L8670   Vascular graft material, synthetic, implant

OTHER

L8699   Prosthetic implant, not otherwise specified

L9900   Orthotic and prosthetic supply, accessory, and/or service component of another HCPCS "L" code

MEDICAL SERVICES

Guidelines

In addition to the information presented in the INTRODUCTION, several other items unique to this section are defined or identified here:

1. **SUBSECTION INFORMATION:** Some of the listed subheadings or subsections have special needs or instructions unique to that section. Where these are indicated, special "notes" will be presented preceding or following the listings. Those subsections within the MEDICAL SERVICES section that have "notes" are as follows:

Subsection	Code Numbers
Office services	M0000-M0009
End-stage renal disease services	M0900-M0999

2. **SPECIAL REPORT:** A service, material or supply that is rarely provided, unusual, variable or new may require a special report in determining medical appropriateness for reimbursement purposes. Pertinent information should include an adequate definition or description of the nature, extent, and need for the service, material or supply.

3. **MODIFIERS:** Listed services may be modified under certain circumstances. When appropriate, the modifying circumstance is identified by adding a modifier to the basic procedure code. CPT and HCPCS National Level II modifiers may be used with CPT and HCPCS National Level II procedure codes. Modifiers commonly used with MEDICAL SERVICES are as follows:

    -AH   Clinical psychologist

    -AJ   Clinical social worker

    -CC   Procedure code change (use "CC" when the procedure code submitted was changed either for administrative reasons or because an incorrect code was filed)

    -EJ   Subsequent claims for a defined course of therapy (eg., EPO, sodium hyaluronate, infliximab)

    -EM   Emergency reserve supply (for ESRD benefit only)

-EP   Service provided as part of Medicaid early periodic screening diagnosis and treatment (EPSDT) program

-FP   Service provided as part of Medicaid family planning program

-Q5   Service furnished by a substitute physician under a reciprocal billing arrangement

-Q6   Service furnished by a locum tenens physician

-QB   Physician providing service in a rural HPSA

-QC   Single channel monitoring

-QD   Recording and storage in solid state memory by a digital recorder

-QT   Recording and storage on tape by an analog tape recorder

-QU   Physician providing service in an urban HPSA

-SF   Second opinion ordered by a professional review organization (PRO) per section 9401, P.L. 99-272 (100 percent reimbursement; no Medicare deductible or coinsurance)

-TC   Technical component. Under certain circumstances, a charge may be made for the technical component alone. Under those circumstances, the technical component charge is identified by adding modifier -TC to the usual procedure number. Technical component charges are institutional charges and are not billed separately by physicians. However, portable x-ray suppliers bill only for the technical component and should use modifier -TC. The charge data from portable x-ray suppliers will then be used to build customary and prevailing profiles.

4. **CPT CODE CROSS-REFERENCE:** See sections for equivalent CPT code(s) for listings in this section.

Medical Services

ASC SERVICES

M0064 Brief office visit for the sole purpose of monitoring or changing drug prescriptions used in the treatment of mental psychoneurotic and personality disorders

OTHER MEDICAL SERVICES

M0075 Cellular therapy

M0076 Prolotherapy

M0100 Intragastric hypothermia using gastric freezing (MNP)

(M0101) Code deleted 1999; use CPT

CARDIOVASCULAR SERVICES

M0300 IV chelation therapy (chemical endarterectomy)

M0301 Fabric wrapping of abdominal aneurysm (MNP)

(M0302) Code deleted 2002; use CPT

PHYSICAL MEDICINE SERVICES

OSTEOPATHIC MANIPULATION THERAPY (OMT)

NOTE: All OMT codes have been deleted; use CPT.

ESRD SERVICES

NOTE: For DME items for ESRD, see procedure codes E1500-E1699. For supplies for ESRD, see procedure codes A4650-A4999

Not valid for Medicare   Non-covered by Medicare   Special coverage instructions   Carrier discretion

● New code ▲ Revised code ( ) Deleted code

PATHOLOGY AND LABORATORY

Guidelines

In addition to the information presented in the INTRODUCTION, several other items unique to this section are defined or identified here:

1. **SPECIAL REPORT:** A service, material or supply that is rarely provided, unusual, variable or new may require a special report in determining medical appropriateness for reimbursement purposes. Pertinent information should include an adequate definition or description of the nature, extent, and need for the service, material or supply.

2. **MODIFIERS:** Listed services may be modified under certain circumstances. When appropriate, the modifying circumstance is identified by adding a modifier to the basic procedure code. CPT and HCPCS National Level II modifiers may be used with CPT and HCPCS National Level II procedure codes. Modifiers commonly used with PATHOLOGY AND LABORATORY SERVICES are as follows:

    -CC   Procedure code change (use "CC" when the procedure code submitted was changed either for administrative reasons or because an incorrect code was filed)

    -LR   Laboratory round trip

    -TC   Technical component. Under certain circumstances, a charge may be made for the technical component alone. Under these circumstances, the technical component charge is identified by adding the modifier -TC to the usual procedure code. Technical component charges are institutional charges and are not billed separately by physicians. Portable x-ray suppliers bill only for the technical component however, and should use modifier -TC. The charge data from portable x-ray suppliers will then be used to build customary and prevailing profiles.

3. **CPT CODE CROSS-REFERENCE:** See sections for equivalent CPT code(s) for all listings in this section.

Pathology And Laboratory

CHEMISTRY AND TOXICOLOGY TESTS

P2028   Cephalin flocculation, blood

P2029   Congo red, blood

P2031   Hair analysis (excluding arsenic)

P2033   Thymol turbidity, blood

P2038   Mucoprotein, blood (seromucoid) (medical necessity procedure)

PATHOLOGY SCREENING TESTS

P3000   Screening papanicolaou smear, cervical or vaginal, up to three smears; by technician under physician supervision

P3001   requiring interpretation by physician

MICROBIOLOGY TESTS

P7001   Culture, bacterial, urine; quantitative, sensitivity study

MISCELLANEOUS PATHOLOGY AND LABORATORY TESTS

P9010   Blood (whole), for transfusion, per unit

P9011   Blood (split unit), specify amount

P9012   Cryoprecipitate, each unit

(P9013)   Code deleted 2001

(P9014)   Code deleted 1999; use J1460

(P9015)   Code deleted 1999; use J1561

P9016   Red blood cells, leukocytes reduced, each unit

P9017   Fresh frozen plasma (single donor), each unit

(P9018)   Code deleted 2001

P9019 Platelets, each unit

P9020 Platelet rich plasma, each unit

P9021 Red blood cells, each unit

P9022 Red blood cells, washed, each unit

P9023 Plasma, pooled multiple donor, solvent/detergent treated, frozen, each unit

P9031 Platelets, leukocytes reduced, each unit

P9032 Platelets, irradiated, each unit

P9033 Platelets, leukocytes reduced, irradiated, each unit

P9034 Platelets, pheresis, each unit

P9035 Platelets, pheresis, leukocytes reduced, each unit

P9036 Platelets, pheresis, irradiated, each unit

P9037 Platelets, pheresis, leukocytes reduced, irradiated, each unit

P9038 Red blood cells, irradiated, each unit

P9039 Red blood cells, deglycerolized, each unit

P9040 Red blood cells, leukocytes reduced, irradiated, each unit

▲**P9041** Infusion, albumin (human), 5%, 50 ml

(P9042) Code deleted 2002; use P9046

▲**P9043** Infusion, plasma protein fraction (human), 5%, 50 ml

P9044 Plasma, cryoprecipitate reduced, each unit

●**P9045** Infusion, albumin (human), 5%, 250 ml

●**P9046** Infusion, albumin (human), 25%, 20 ml

●**P9047** Infusion, albumin (human), 25%, 50 ml

●**P9048** Infusion, plasma protein fraction (human), 5%, 250 ml

● **P9050**   Granulocytes, pheresis, each unit

P9603   Travel allowance one way in connection with medically necessary laboratory specimen collection drawn from home bound or nursing home bound patient; prorated miles actually travelled

P9604   prorated trip charge

(P9610)   Code deleted 1999; use P9612

P9612   Catheterization for collection of specimen; single patient, all places of service

P9615   multiple patients

TEMPORARY CODES

Guidelines

In addition to the information presented in the INTRODUCTION, several other items unique to this section are defined or identified here:

1. **SUBSECTION INFORMATION:** Some of the listed subheadings or subsections have special needs or instructions unique to that section. Where these are indicated, special "notes" will be presented preceding or following the listings. Those subsections within the TEMPORARY CODES section that have "notes" are as follows:

Subsection	Code Numbers
Temporary codes	Q0000-Q9999

2. **SPECIAL REPORT:** A service, material or supply that is rarely provided, unusual, variable or new may require a special report in determining medical appropriateness for reimbursement purposes. Pertinent information should include an adequate definition or description of the nature, extent, and need for the service, material or supply.

3. **MODIFIERS:** Listed services may be modified under certain circumstances. When appropriate, the modifying circumstance is identified by adding a modifier to the basic procedure code. CPT and HCPCS National Level II modifiers may be used with CPT and HCPCS National Level II procedure codes. Modifiers commonly used with TEMPORARY CODES are as follows:

   -CC Procedure code change (use "CC" when the procedure code submitted was changed either for administrative reasons or because an incorrect code was filed)

   -LL Lease/rental (used when DME equipment rental is to be applied against the purchase price)

   -LR Laboratory round trip

   -QC Single channel monitoring

   -QD Recording and storage in solid state memory by a digital recorder

-QE   Prescribed amount of oxygen is less than 1 liter per minute (LPM)

-QF   Prescribed amount of oxygen exceeds 4 liters per minute (LPM) and portable oxygen is prescribed

-QG   Prescribed amount of oxygen is greater than 4 liters per minute (LPM)

-QH   Oxygen conserving device is being used with an oxygen delivery system

-QT   Recording and storage on tape by an analog tape recorder

-RP   Replacement and repair (may be used to indicate replacement of DME, orthotic and prosthetic devices that have been in use for some time. The claim shows the code for the part, followed by the "RP" modifier and the charge for the part.)

-RR   Rental (used when DME is to be rented)

-TC   Technical component. Under certain circumstances, a charge may be made for the technical component alone. Under these circumstances, the technical component charge is identified by adding the modifier -TC to the usual procedure code. Technical component charges are institutional charges and are not billed separately by physicians. Portable x-ray suppliers bill only for the technical component however, and should use modifier -TC. The charge data from portable x-ray suppliers will then be used to build customary and prevailing profiles.

-UE   Used durable medical equipment

4. **CPT CODE CROSS-REFERENCE:** See sections for equivalent CPT code(s) for all listings in this section.

Temporary Codes

NOTE: Temporary codes are national codes given by HCFA on a temporary basis. The list contains current codes, as well as those which have been superseded by permanent alphanumeric codes as indicated by the cross-reference.

(Q0034) Code deleted 2001

Q0035 Cardiokymography

(Q0068) Code deleted 2000; use CPT Level I HCPCS code 36521

Q0081 Infusion therapy, using other than chemotherapeutic drugs, per visit

(Q0082) Code deleted 2001

Q0083 Chemotherapy administration by other than infusion technique only (e.g., subcutaneous, intramuscular, push), per visit

Q0084 Chemotherapy administration by infusion technique only, per visit

Q0085 Chemotherapy administration by both infusion technique and other technique(s) (e.g., subcutaneous, intramuscular, push), per visit

Q0086 Physical therapy evaluation/treatment, per visit

Q0091 Screening papanicolaou smear; obtaining, preparing and conveyance of cervical or vaginal smear to laboratory

Q0092 Set-up portable x-ray equipment

Q0111 Wet mounts, including preparations of vaginal, cervical or skin specimens

Q0112 All potassium hydroxide (koh) preparations

Q0113 Pinworm examinations

Q0114 Fern test

Q0115 Post-coital direct, qualitative examinations of vaginal or cervical mucous

(Q0132)   Code deleted 2000; use E0590

Q0136   Injection, epoetin alpha, (for non ESRD use), per 1,000 units

(Q0144)   Code deleted 2002

(Q0156)   Code deleted 2001

(Q0157)   Code deleted 2001

(Q0159)   Code deleted 1999; use J0151

(Q0160)   Code deleted 2002; use J7193

(Q0161)   Code deleted 2002; use J7195

(Q0162)   Code deleted 1999; use P9612

Q0163   Diphenhydramine HCl, 50 mg, oral, FDA approved prescription anti-emetic, for use as a complete therapeutic substitute for an IV anti-emetic at time of chemotherapy treatment not to exceed a 48 hour dosage regimen

Q0164   Prochlorperazine maleate, 5 mg, oral, FDA approved prescription anti-emetic, for use as a complete therapeutic substitute for an IV anti-emetic at the time of chemotherapy treatment, not to exceed a 48 hour dosage regimen

Q0165   Prochlorperazine maleate, 10 mg, oral, FDA approved prescription anti-emetic, for use as a complete therapeutic substitute for an IV anti-emetic at the time of chemotherapy treatment, not to exceed a 48 hour dosage regimen

Q0166   Granisetron HCl, 1 mg, oral, FDA approved prescription anti-emetic, for use as a complete therapeutic substitute for an IV anti-emetic at the time of chemotherapy treatment, not to exceed a 24 hour dosage regimen

Q0167   Dronabinol, 2.5 mg, oral, FDA approved prescription anti-emetic, for use as a complete therapeutic substitute for an IV anti-emetic at the time of chemotherapy treatment, not to exceed a 48 hour dosage regimen

Q0168   Dronabinol, 5 mg, oral, FDA approved prescription anti-emetic, for use as a complete therapeutic substitute for an IV anti-emetic at the time of chemotherapy treatment, not to exceed a 48 hour dosage regimen

Q0169   Promethazine HCl, 12.5 mg, oral, FDA approved prescription anti-emetic, for use as a complete therapeutic substitute for an IV anti-emetic at the time of chemotherapy treatment, not to exceed a 48 hour dosage regimen

Q0170   Promethazine HCl, 25 mg, oral, FDA approved prescription anti-emetic, for use as a complete therapeutic substitute for an IV anti-emetic at the time of chemotherapy treatment, not to exceed a 48 hour dosage regimen

Q0171   Chlorpromazine HCl, 10 mg, oral, FDA approved prescription anti-emetic, for use as a complete therapeutic substitute for an IV anti-emetic at the time of chemotherapy treatment, not to exceed a 48 hour dosage regimen

Q0172   Chlorpromazine HCl, 25 mg, oral, FDA approved prescription anti-emetic, for use as a complete therapeutic substitute for an IV anti-emetic at the time of chemotherapy treatment, not to exceed a 48 hour dosage regimen

Q0173   Trimethobenzamide HCl, 250 mg, oral, FDA approved prescription anti-emetic, for use as a complete therapeutic substitute for an IV anti-emetic at the time of chemotherapy treatment, not to exceed a 48 hour dosage regimen

Q0174   Thiethylperazine maleate, 10 mg, oral, FDA approved prescription anti-emetic, for use as a complete therapeutic substitute for an IV anti-emetic at the time of chemotherapy treatment, not to exceed a 48 hour dosage regimen

Q0175   Perphenzaine, 4 mg, oral, FDA approved prescription anti-emetic, for use as a complete therapeutic substitute for an IV anti-emetic at the time of chemotherapy treatment, not to exceed a 48 hour dosage regimen

Q0176 Perphenzaine, 8 mg, oral, FDA approved prescription anti-emetic, for use as a complete therapeutic substitute for an IV anti-emetic at the time of chemotherapy treatment, not to exceed a 48 hour dosage regimen

Q0177 Hydroxyzine pamoate, 25 mg, oral, FDA approved prescription anti-emetic, for use as a complete therapeutic substitute for an IV anti-emetic at the time of chemotherapy treatment, not to exceed a 48 hour dosage regimen

Q0178 Hydroxyzine pamoate, 50 mg, oral, FDA approved prescription anti-emetic, for use as a complete therapeutic substitute for an IV anti-emetic at the time of chemotherapy treatment, not to exceed a 48 hour dosage regimen

Q0179 Ondansetron HCl, 8 mg, oral, FDA approved prescription anti-emetic, for use as a complete therapeutic substitute for an IV anti-emetic at the time of chemotherapy treatment, not to exceed a 48 hour dosage regimen

Q0180 Dolasetron mesylate, 100 mg, oral, FDA approved prescription anti-emetic, for use as a complete therapeutic substitute for an IV anti-emetic at the time of chemotherapy treatment, not to exceed a 24 hour dosage regimen

Q0181 Unspecified oral dosage form, FDA approved prescription anti-emetic, for use as a complete therapeutic substitute for an IV anti-emetic at the time of chemotherapy treatment, not to exceed a 48 hour dosage regimen

(Q0182) Code deleted 1999; use J0275

Q0183 Dermal tissue, of human origin, with and without other bioengineered or processed elements; but without metabolically active elements, per square centimeter

Q0184 with metabolically active elements, per square centimeter

(Q0185) Code deleted 2002; use J7340

(Q0186) Code deleted 2001; use A0432

Q0187 Factor VIIa (coagulation factor, recombinant) per 1.2 mg

(Q0188) Code deleted 2001; use A9700

Q1001 New technology intraocular lense category 1 as defined in Federal Register notice, vol 65 (May 3, 2000)

Q1002 New technology intraocular lense category 2 as defined in Federal Register notice, vol 65 (May 3, 2000)

Q1003 New technology intraocular lense category 3 as defined in Federal Register notice

Q1004 New technology intraocular lense category 4 as defined in Federal Register notice

Q1005 New technology intraocular lense category 5 as defined in Federal Register notice

Q2001 Oral, cabergoline, 0.5 mg

Q2002 Injection, Elliotts b solution, per ml

Q2003 Injection, aprotinin, 10,000 KIU

Q2004 Irrigation solution for treatment of bladder calculi, for example Renacidin, per 500 ml

Q2005 Injection, corticorelin ovine triflutate, per dose

Q2006 Injection, digoxin immune fab (ovine), per vial

Q2007 Injection, ethanolamine oleate, 100 mg

Q2008 Injection, fomepizole, 1.5 mg

Q2009 Injection, fosphenytoin, 50 mg

Q2010 Injection, glatiramer acetate, per dose

Q2011 Injection, hemin, per 1 mg

Q2012 Injection, pegademase bovine, 25 IU

Q2013 Injection, pentastarch, 10 % solution, per 100 ml

Q2014 Injection, sermorelin acetate, 0.5 mg

(Q2015) Code deleted 2002

(Q2016) Code deleted 2002

Q2017   Injection, teniposide, 50 mg

Q2018   Injection, urofollitropin, 75 IU

Q2019   Injection, basiliximab, 20 mg

Q2020   Injection, histrelin acetate, 10 mg

Q2021   Injection, lepirudin, 50 mg

Q2022   Von Willebrand factor complex, human, per IU

Q3001   Radioelements for brachytherapy, any type, each

Q3002   Supply of radiopharmaceutical diagnostic imaging agent; gallium Ga 67, per mci

Q3003   technetium Tc99M bicisate, per unit dose

Q3004   xenon Xe 133, per 10 mci

Q3005   technetium Tc99M mertiatide, per mci

Q3006   technetium Tc99M glucepatate, per 5 mci

Q3007   sodium phosphate P32, per mci

Q3008   indium 111-In pentetreotide, per 3 mci

Q3009   technetium Tc99M oxidronate, per mci

Q3010   technetium Tc99M-labeled red blood cells, per mci

Q3011   chromic phosphate P32 suspension, per mci

Q3012   Supply of oral radiopharmaceutical diagnostic imaging agent, cyanocobalamin cobalt Co57, per 0.5 mci

(**Q3013**)   Code deleted 2002; use J3395

● **Q3014**   Telehealth originating site facility fee

● **Q3017**   Ambulance service, advanced life support (ALS) assessment, no other ALS services provided

● **Q4001**   Cast supplies, body cast adult, with or without head, plaster

● **Q4002**   Cast supplies, body cast adult, with or without head, fiberglass

● **Q4003**   Cast supplies, shoulder cast, adult (11 years +), plaster

● **Q4004**   Cast supplies, shoulder cast, adult (11 years +), fiberglass

● **Q4005**   Cast supplies, long arm cast, adult (11 years +), plaster

● **Q4006**   Cast supplies, long arm cast, adult (11 years +), fiberglass

● **Q4007**   Cast supplies, long arm cast, pediatric (0-10 years), plaster

● **Q4008**   Cast supplies, long arm cast, pediatric (0-10 years), fiberglass

● **Q4009**   Cast supplies, short arm cast, adult (11 years +), plaster

● **Q4010**   Cast supplies, short arm cast, adult (11 years +), fiberglass

● **Q4011**   Cast supplies, short arm cast, pediatric (0-10 years), plaster

● **Q4012**   Cast supplies, short arm cast, pediatric (0-10 years), fiberglass

● **Q4013**   Cast supplies, gauntlet cast (includes lower forearm and hand), adult (11 years +), plaster

● **Q4014**   Cast supplies, gauntlet cast (includes lower forearm and hand), adult (11 years +), fiberglass

● **Q4015**   Cast supplies, gauntlet cast (includes lower forearm and hand), pediatric (0-10 years), plaster

● **Q4016**   Cast supplies, gauntlet cast (includes lower forearm and hand), pediatric (0-10 years), fiberglass

● **Q4017**   Cast supplies, long arm splint, adult (11 years +), plaster

● **Q4018**   Cast supplies, long arm splint, adult (11 years +), fiberglass

● **Q4019**   Cast supplies, long arm splint, pediatric (0-10 years), plaster

● **Q4020**   Cast supplies, long arm splint, pediatric (0-10 years), fiberglass

● **Q4021**   Cast supplies, short arm splint, adult (11 years +), plaster

● **Q4022**   Cast supplies, short arm splint, adult (11 years +), fiberglass

● **Q4023**   Cast supplies, short arm splint, pediatric (0-10 years), plaster

● **Q4024**   Cast supplies, short arm splint, pediatric (0-10 years), fiberglass

● **Q4025**   Cast supplies, hip spica (one or both legs), adult (11 years +), plaster

● **Q4026**   Cast supplies, hip spica (one or both legs), adult (11 years +), fiberglass

● **Q4027**   Cast supplies, hip spica (one or both legs), pediatric (0-10 years), plaster

● **Q4028**   Cast supplies, hip spica (one or both legs), pediatric (0-10 years), fiberglass

● **Q4029**   Cast supplies, long leg cast, adult (11 years +), plaster

● **Q4030**   Cast supplies, long leg cast, adult (11 years +), fiberglass

● **Q4031**   Cast supplies, long leg cast, pediatric (0-10 years), plaster

● **Q4032**   Cast supplies, long leg cast, pediatric (0-10 years), fiberglass

● **Q4033**   Cast supplies, long leg cylinder cast, adult (11 years +), plaster

● **Q4034**   Cast supplies, long leg cylinder cast, adult (11 years +), fiberglass

● **Q4035**   Cast supplies, long leg cylinder cast, pediatric (0-10 years), plaster

● **Q4036**   Cast supplies, long leg cylinder cast, pediatric (0-10 years), fiberglass

● **Q4037**   Cast supplies, short leg cast, adult (11 years +), plaster

● **Q4038**   Cast supplies, short leg cast, adult (11 years +), fiberglass

● **Q4039**   Cast supplies, short leg cast, pediatric (0-10 years), plaster

● **Q4040**   Cast supplies, short leg cast, pediatric (0-10 years), fiberglass

● **Q4041**   Cast supplies, long leg splint, adult (11 years +), plaster

● **Q4042**   Cast supplies, long leg splint, adult (11 years +), fiberglass

● **Q4043**   Cast supplies, long leg splint, pediatric (0-10 years), plaster

● **Q4044**   Cast supplies, long leg splint, pediatric (0-10 years), fiberglass

● **Q4045**   Cast supplies, short leg splint, adult (11 years +), plaster

● **Q4046**   Cast supplies, short leg splint, adult (11 years +), fiberglass

● **Q4047**   Cast supplies, short leg splint, pediatric (0-10 years), plaster

● **Q4048**   Cast supplies, short leg splint, pediatric (0-10 years), fiberglass

● **Q4049**   Finger splint, static

● **Q4050**   Cast supplies, for unlisted types and materials of casts

● **Q4051**   Splint supplies, miscellaneous (includes thermoplastics, strapping, fasteners, padding and other supplies)

INJECTION CODES FOR EPO

Q9920   Injection of EPO, per 1000 units; at patient HCT of 20 or less

Q9921   at patient HCT of 21

Q9922   at patient HCT of 22

| | Not valid for Medicare | | Non-covered by Medicare | | Special coverage instructions | | Carrier discretion | **275** |

Q9923	at patient HCT of 23
Q9924	at patient HCT of 24
Q9925	at patient HCT of 25
Q9926	at patient HCT of 26
Q9927	at patient HCT of 27
Q9928	at patient HCT of 28
Q9929	at patient HCT of 29
Q9930	at patient HCT of 30
Q9931	at patient HCT of 31
Q9932	at patient HCT of 32
Q9933	at patient HCT of 33
Q9934	at patient HCT of 34
Q9935	at patient HCT of 35
Q9936	at patient HCT of 36
Q9937	at patient HCT of 37
Q9938	at patient HCT of 38
Q9939	at patient HCT of 39
Q9940	at patient HCT of 40 or above

DIAGNOSTIC RADIOLOGY SERVICES

Guidelines

In addition to the information presented in the INTRODUCTION, several other items unique to this section are defined or identified here:

1. **SPECIAL REPORT:** A service, material or supply that is rarely provided, unusual, variable or new may require a special report in determining medical appropriateness for reimbursement purposes. Pertinent information should include an adequate definition or description of the nature, extent, and need for the service, material or supply.

2. **MODIFIERS:** Listed services may be modified under certain circumstances. When appropriate, the modifying circumstance is identified by adding a modifier to the basic procedure code. CPT and HCPCS National Level II modifiers may be used with CPT and HCPCS National Level II procedure codes. Modifiers commonly used with DIAGNOSTIC RADIOLOGY SERVICES are as follows:

   -CC   Procedure code change (use "CC" when the procedure code submitted was changed either for administrative reasons or because an incorrect code was filed)

   -LT   Left side (used to identify procedures performed on the left side of the body)

   -RT   Right side (used to identify procedures performed on the right side of the body)

   -TC   Technical component. Under certain circumstances, a charge may be made for the technical component alone. Under those circumstances, the technical component charge is identified by adding modifier -TC to the usual procedure number. Technical component charges are institutional charges and are not billed separately by physicians. However, portable x-ray suppliers bill only for the technical component and should use modifier -TC. The charge data from portable x-ray suppliers will then be used to build customary and prevailing profiles.

3. **CPT CODE CROSS-REFERENCE:** There are no equivalent CPT codes for procedures listed in this section.

Diagnostic Radiology Services

R0070   Transportation of portable x-ray equipment and personnel to home or nursing home, per trip to facility or location; one patient seen

R0075   more than one patient seen, per patient

R0076   Transportation of portable EKG to facility or location, per patient

PRIVATE PAYER CODES

Guidelines

HCPCS "S" codes are temporary national codes established by the private payers for private payer use. Prior to using "S" codes on insurance claims to private payers, you should consult with the payer to confirm that the "S" codes are acceptable. "S" codes are not valid for Medicare use.

In addition to the information presented in the INTRODUCTION, several other items unique to this section are defined or identified here.

1. **SPECIAL REPORT:** A service, material or supply that is rarely provided, unusual, variable or new may require a special report in determining medical appropriateness for reimbursement purposes. Pertinent information should include an adequate definition or description of the nature, extent, and need for the service, material or supply.

2. **MODIFIERS:** Listed services may be modified under certain circumstances. When appropriate, the modifying circumstance is identified by adding a modifier to the basic procedure code. CPT and HCPCS National Level II modifiers may be used with CPT and HCPCS National Level II procedure codes.

Private Payer Codes

S0009   Injection, butorphanol tartrate, 1 mg

(S0010)   Code deleted 2001; use Q2015

(S0011)   Code deleted 2001; use Q2016

S0012   Butorphanol tartrate, nasal spray, 25 mg

S0014   Tacrine HCl, 10 mg

S0016   Injection, amikacin sulfate, 500 mg

S0017   Injection, aminocaproic acid, 5 g

S0020   Injection, bupivicaine HCl, 30 ml

S0021   Injection, ceftoperazone sodium, 1 g

Not valid   Non-covered   Special   Carrier   **279**
for Medicare   by Medicare   coverage   discretion
                              instructions

S0023	Injection, cimetidine HCl, 300 mg
(S0024)	Code deleted 2002
S0028	Injection, fanotidine, 20 mg
(S0029)	Code deleted 2002; use J1450
S0030	Injection, metronidazole, 500 mg
S0032	Injection, nafcillin sodium, 2 g
S0034	Injection, ofloxacin, 400 mg
S0039	Injection, sulfamethoxazole and trimethoprim, 10 ml
S0040	Injection, ticarcillin disodium and clavulanate potassium, 3.1 g
S0071	Injection, acyclovir sodium, 50 mg
S0072	Injection, amikacin sulfate, 100 mg
S0073	Injection, aztreonam, 500 mg
S0074	Injection, cefotetan disodium, 500 mg
S0077	Injection, clindamycin phosphate, 300 mg
S0078	Injection, fosphenytoin sodium, 750 mg
● S0079	Injection, octreotide acetate, 100 mcg (for doses over 1 mg use J2352 or C1207)
S0080	Injection, pentamidine isethionate, 300 mg
S0081	Injection, piperacillin sodium, 500 mg
S0085	Injection, gatifloxacin, 200 mg
(S0086)	Code deleted 2002; use J3395
● S0087	Injection, alemtuzumab, 30 mg
● S0088	Imatinib, 100 mg
S0090	Sildenafil citrate, 25 mg

● **S0091** Granisetron hydrochloride, 1mg (for circumstances falling under the medicare statute, use Q0166)

● **S0092** Injection, hydromorphone hydrochloride, 250 mg (loading dose for infusion pump)

● **S0093** Injection, morphine sulfate, 500 mg (loading dose for infusion pump)

(S0096) Code deleted 2002

(S0097) Code deleted 2001; use J1742

(S0098) Code deleted 2001

● **S0155** Sterile dilutant for epoprostenol, 50 ml

S0156 Exemestane, 25 mg

S0157 Becaplermin gel 0.01%, 0.5 gram

● **S0170** Anastrozole, oral, 1 mg

● **S0171** Injection, bumetanide, 0.5 mg

● **S0172** Chlorambucil, oral, 2 mg

● **S0173** Dexamethasone, oral, 4 mg

● **S0174** Dolasetron mesylate, oral 50 mg (for circumstances falling under the medicare statute, use Q0180)

● **S0175** Flutamide, oral, 125 mg

● **S0176** Hydroxyurea, oral, 500 mg

● **S0177** Levamisole hydrochloride, oral, 50 mg

● **S0178** Lomustine, oral, 10 mg

● **S0179** Megestrol acetate, oral, 20 mg

● **S0181** Ondansetron hydrochloride, oral, 4 mg (for circumstances falling under the medicare statute, use Q0179)

● **S0182** Procarbazine hydrochloride, oral, 50 mg

● **S0183**   Prochlorperazine maleate, oral, 5 mg (for circumstances falling under the medicare statute, use Q0164 - Q0165)

● **S0187**   Tamoxifen citrate, oral, 10 mg

● **S0189**   Testosterone pellet, 75 mg

● **S0190**   Mifepristone, oral, 200 mg

● **S0191**   Misoprostol, oral, 200 mcg

● **S0199**   Medically induced abortion by oral ingestion of medication including all associated services and supplies (e.g., patient counseling, office visits, confirmation of pregnancy by HCG, ultrasound to confirm duration of pregnancy, ultrasound to confirm completion of abortion) except drugs

● **S0206**   Procedure performed in surgery suite in physician's office (list separately in addition to code for primary procedure to denote use of facility and equipment)

● **S0208**   Paramedic intercept, hospital-based ALS service (non-voluntary), non-transport

● **S0209**   Wheelchair van, mileage, per mile

● **S0215**   Non-emergency transportation; mileage

   S0220   Medical conference by a physician with interdisciplinary team of health professionals or representatives of community agencies to coordinate activities of patient care (patient is present); approximately 30 minutes

   S0221   Medical conference by a physician with interdisciplinary team of health professionals or representatives of community agencies to coordinate activities of patient care (patient is present); approximately 60 minutes

● **S0250**   Comprehensive geriatric assessment and treatment planning performed by assessment team

● **S0255**   Hospice referral visit (advising patient and family of care options) performed by nurse, social worker, or other designated staff

● **S0260** History and physical (outpatient or office) related to surgical procedure (list separately in addition to code for appropriate evaluation and management service)

● **S0302** Completed early periodic screening diagnosis and treatment (EPSDT) service (list in addition to code for appropriate evaluation and management service)

● **S0310** Hospitalist services (list separately in addition to code for appropriate evaluation and management service)

● **S0340** Lifestyle modification program for management of coronary artery disease, including all supportive services; first quarter/stage

● **S0341** Lifestyle modification program for management of coronary artery disease, including all supportive services; second or third quarter/stage

● **S0342** Lifestyle modification program for management of coronary artery disease, including all supportive services; fourth quarter/stage

● **S0395** Impression casting of a foot performed by a practitioner other than the manufacturer of the orthotic

● **S0400** Global fee for extracorporeal shock wave lithotripsy treatment of kidney stone(s)

● **S0500** Disposable contact lens, per lens

● **S0504** Single vision prescription lens (safety, athletic or sunglass), per lens

● **S0506** Bifocal vision prescription lens (safety, athletic or sunglass), per lens

● **S0508** Trifocal vision prescription lens (safety, athletic or sunglass), per lens

● **S0510** Non-prescription lens (safety, athletic or sunglass), per lens

● **S0512** Daily wear specialty contact lens, per lens

● **S0514** Color contact lens, per lens

● **S0516** Safety eyeglass frames

	Not valid for Medicare		Non-covered by Medicare		Special coverage instructions		Carrier discretion

● **S0518**   Sunglasses frames

● **S0580**   Polycarbonate lens (List this code in addition to the basic code for the lens)

● **S0581**   Nonstandard lens (List this code in addition to the basic code for the lens)

● **S0590**   Integral lens service, miscellaneous services reported separately

● **S0592**   Comprehensive contact lens evaluation

S0601   Screening proctoscopy

S0605   Digital rectal examination, annual

S0610   Annual gynecological examination; new patient

S0612   established patient

S0620   Routine ophthalmological examination including refraction; new patient

S0621   established patient

● **S0622**   Physical exam for college, new or established patient (list separately in addition to appropriate evaluation and management code)

S0630   Removal of sutures by a physician other than the physician who originally closed the wound

S0800   Laser in situ keratomileusis (LASIK)

S0810   Photorefractive keratectomy (PRK)

● **S0812**   Phototherapeutic keratectomy (PTK)

S0820   Computerized corneal topography, unilateral

S0830   Ultrasound pachymetry to determine corneal thickness, with interpretation and report, unilateral

● **S1001**   Deluxe item, patient aware (List in addition to code for basic item)

● **S1002** Customized item (List in addition to code for basic item)

S1015 IV tubing extension set

S1016 Non-PVC (polyvinyl chloride) intravenous administration set, for use with drugs that are not stable in PVC, e.g., paclitaxel

● **S1025** Inhaled nitric oxide for the treatment of hypoxic respiratory failure in the neonate; per diem

● **S1030** Continuous noninvasive glucose monitoring device, purchase (for physician interpretation of data, use CPT code)

● **S1031** Continuous noninvasive glucose monitoring device, rental, including sensor, sensor replacement, and download to monitor (for physician interpretation of data, use CPT code)

(S2050) Code deleted 2001; use 44132

(S2052) Code deleted 2002

S2053 Transplantation of small intestine and liver allografts

S2054 Transplantation of multivisceral organs

S2055 Harvesting of donor multivisceral organs, with preparation and maintenance of allografts; from cadaver donor

S2060 Lobar lung transplantation

S2061 Donor lobectomy (lung) for transplantation, living donor

● **S2065** Simultaneous pancreas kidney transplantation

● **S2080** Laser-assisted uvulopalatoplasty (laup)

S2102 Islet cell tissue transplant from pancreas; allogenic

S2103 Adrenal tissue transplant to brain

(S2109) Code deleted 2001; use J7330

| | Not valid for Medicare | | Non-covered by Medicare | | Special coverage instructions | | Carrier discretion | **285** |

● S2112   Arthroscopy, knee, surgical for harvesting cartilage (chondrocyte cells)

● S2115   Osteotomy, periacetabular, with internal fixation

S2120   Low density lipoprotein (LDL) apheresis using heparin-induced extracorporeal LDL precipitation

S2140   Cord blood harvesting for transplantation, allogenic

S2142   Cord blood-derived stem cell transplantation, allogenic

● S2150   Bone marrow or blood-derived peripheral stem cell harvesting and transplantation, allogenic or autologous, including pheresis, high-dose chemotherapy, and 28 days of post-transplant care (including drugs, hospitalization, medical, surgical, diagnostic and emergency services)

S2180   Donor leukocyte infusion (e.g., DLI, donor lymphocyte infusion, donor buffy coat cell transfusion, donor peripheral blood monocyte transfusion)

(S2190)   Code deleted 2001; use 11980

S2202   Echosclerotherapy

(S2204)   Code deleted 2001; use 33140

S2205   Minimally invasive direct coronary artery bypass surgery involving mini-thoracotomy or mini-sternotomy surgery, performed under direct vision; using arterial graft(s), single coronary arterial graft

S2206   using arterial graft(s), two coronary arterial grafts

S2207   using venous graft only, single coronary venous graft

S2208   using single arterial and venous graft(s), single venous graft

S2209   using two arterial grafts and single venous graft

(S2210)   Code deleted 2002

(S2220)   Code deleted 2002

● S2250   Uterine artery embolization for uterine fibroids

● **S2260** Induced abortion, 17 to 24 weeks, any surgical method

S2300 Arthroscopy, shoulder, surgical; with thermally-induced capsulorrhaphy

S2340 Chemodenervation of abductor muscle(s) of vocal cord

● **S2341** Chemodenervation of adductor muscle(s) of vocal cord

● **S2342** Nasal endoscopy for post-operative debridement following functional endoscopic sinus surgery, nasal and/or sinus cavity(s), unilateral or bilateral

S2350 Diskectomy, anterior, with decompression of spinal cord and/or nerve root(s), including osteophytectomy; lumbar, single interspace

S2351 Diskectomy, anterior, with decompression of spinal cord and/or nerve root(s), including osteophytectomy; lumbar, each additional interspace (list separately in addition to code for primary procedure)

● **S2360** Percutaneous vertebroplasty, one vertebral body, unilateral or bilateral injection; cervical

● **S2361** Each additional cervical vertebral body (list separately in addition to code for primary procedure)

S2370 Intradiscal electrothermal therapy, single interspace

S2371 Each additional interspace (list separately in addition to code for primary procedure)

● **S2400** Repair, congenital hernia in the fetus, procedure performed in utero

● **S2401** Repair, urinary tract obstruction in the fetus, procedure performed in utero

● **S2402** Repair, congenital cystic adenomatoid malformation in the fetus, procedure performed in utero

● **S2403** Repair, extralobar pulmonary sequestration in the fetus, procedure performed in utero

● **S2404** Repair, myelomeningocele in the fetus, procedure performed in utero

● **S2409** Repair, congenital malformation of fetus, procedure performed in utero, not otherwise classified

● **S2411** Fetoscopic laser therapy for treatment of twin-to-twin transfusion syndrome

● **S3600** Stat laboratory request (situations other than S3601)

● **S3601** Emergency stat laboratory charge for patient who is homebound or residing in a nursing facility

S3620 Newborn metabolic screening panel, includes test kit, postage and the following tests: hemoglobin; electrophoresis; hydroxyprogesterone; 17-D; phenalanine (PKU); and thyroxine, total

● **S3630** Eosinophil count, blood, direct

S3645 HIV-1 antibody testing of oral mucosal transudate

S3650 Saliva test, hormone level; during menopause

S3652 to assess preterm labor risk

(S3700) Code deleted 2002

● **S3701** Immunoassay for nuclear matrix protein 22 (NMP-22), quantitative

S3708 Gastrointestinal fat absorption study

● **S3818** Complete gene sequence analysis; BRCA1 gene

● **S3819** Complete gene sequense analysis; BRCA2 gene

● **S3830** Complete mlh1 and mlh2 gene sequence analysis for hereditary nonpolyposis colorectal cancer (HNPCC) genetic testing

● **S3831** Single-mutation analysis (in individual with a known mlh1 and mlh2 mutation in the family) for hereditary nonpolyposis colorectal cancer (HNPCC) genetic testing

● **S3835** Complete gene sequence analysis for cystic fibrosis genetic testing

● **S3837** Complete gene sequence analysis for hemochromatosis genetic testing

● **S3900** Surface electromyography (EMG)

S3902 Ballistocardiogram

S3904 Masters two step

(S3906) Code deleted 2002

● **S4011** In vitro fertilization; including but not limited to identification and incubation of mature oocytes, fertilization with sperm, incubation of embryo(s), and subsequent visualization for determination of development

● **S4015** Complete in vitro fertilization cycle, case rate

● **S4016** Frozen in vitro fertilization cycle, case rate

● **S4018** Frozen embryo transfer procedure canceled before transfer, case rate

● **S4020** In vitro fertilization procedure canceled before aspiration, case rate

● **S4021** In vitro fertilization procedure canceled after aspiration, case rate

● **S4022** Assisted oocyte fertilization, case rate

● **S4025** Donor services for in vitro fertilization (sperm or embryo), case rate

● **S4026** Procurement of donor sperm from sperm bank

● **S4027** Storage of previously frozen embryos

● **S4028** Microsurgical epididymal sperm aspiration (mesa)

● **S4030** Sperm procurement and cryopreservation services; initial visit

● **S4031** Sperm procurement and cryopreservation services; subsequent visit

(S4980) Code deleted 2002

● **S4981**   Insertion of levonorgestrel-releasing intrauterine system

● **S4989**   Contraceptive intrauterine device (e.g., progestacert IUD), including implants and supplies

● **S4990**   Nicotine patches, legend

● **S4991**   Nicotine patches, non-legend

S5000   Prescription drug, generic

S5001   Prescription drug, brand name

(S5002)   Code deleted 2002

(S5003)   Code deleted 2002

▲ **S5010**   5% dextrose and 0.45% normal saline, 1000 ml

S5011   5% dextrose in lactated ringer's, 1000 ml

S5012   5% dextrose with potassium chloride, 1000 ml

▲ **S5013**   5% dextrose/0..45% normal saline with potassium chloride and magnesium sulfate, 1000 ml

▲ **S5014**   5% dextrose/0.45% normal saline with potassium chloride and magnesium sulfate, 1500 ml

(S5016)   Code deleted 2002

(S5017)   Code deleted 2002

(S5018)   Code deleted 2002

(S5019)   Code deleted 2002

(S5020)   Code deleted 2002

(S5021)   Code deleted 2002

(S5022)   Code deleted 2002

(S5025)   Code deleted 2002

● **S5035**   Home infusion therapy, routine service of infusion device (e.g., pump maintenance)

● **S5036** Home infusion therapy, repair of infusion device (e.g., pump repair)

● **S5497** Home infusion therapy, catheter care/maintenance, not otherwise classified; includes administrative services, professional pharmacy services, care coordination, and all necessary supplies and equipment (drugs and nursing visits coded separately), per diem

● **S5498** Home infusion therapy, catheter care/maintenance, simple (single lumen), includes administrative services, professional pharmacy services, care coordination and all necessary supplies and equipment, (drugs and nursing visits coded separately), per diem

● **S5501** Home infusion therapy, catheter care/maintenance, complex (more than one lumen), includes administrative services, professional pharmacy services, care coordination, and all necessary supplies and equipment (drugs and nursing visits coded separately), per diem

● **S5502** Home infusion therapy, catheter care/maintenance, implanted access device, includes administrative services, professional pharmacy services, care coordination and all necessary supplies and equipment, (drugs and nursing visits coded separately), per diem (use this code for interim maintenance of vascular access not currently in use)

(S5503) Code deleted 2002

● **S5517** Home infusion therapy, all supplies necessary for restoration of catheter patency or declotting

● **S5518** Home infusion therapy, all supplies necessary for catheter repair

● **S5520** Home infusion therapy, all supplies (including catheter) necessary for a peripherally inserted central venous catheter (PICC) line insertion

● **S5521** Home infusion therapy, all supplies (including catheter) necessary for a midline catheter insertion

● **S5522** Home infusion therapy, insertion of peripherally inserted central venous catheter (PICC), nursing services only (no supplies or catheter included)

● **S5523** Home infusion therapy, insertion of midline central venous catheter, nursing services only (no supplies or catheter included)

(S8001) Code deleted 2002

● **S8030** Scleral application of tantalum ring(s) for localization of lesions for proton beam therapy

S8035 Magnetic source imaging

● **S8037** Magnetic resonance cholangiopancreatography (MRCP)

S8040 Topographic brain mapping

(S8048) Code deleted 2001; use 36823

S8049 Intraoperative radiation therapy (single administration)

● **S8055** Ultrasound guidance for multifetal pregnancy reduction(s), technical component (only to be used when the physician doing the reduction procedure does not perform the ultrasound, guidance is included in the CPT code for multifetal pregnancy reduction - 59866)

(S8060) Code deleted 2001; use A9700

S8080 Scintimammography (radioimmunoscintigraphy of the breast), unilateral, including supply of radiopharmaceutical

S8085 Fluorine-18 fluorodeoxyglucose (F-18 FDG) imaging using dual-head coincidence detection system (non-dedicated PET scan)

S8092 Electron beam computed tomography (also known as ultrafast CT, cine CT)

▲ **S8095** Wig (for medically-induced or congenital hair loss)

S8096 Portable peak flow meter

● **S8097** Asthma kit (including but not limited to portable peak expiratory flow meter, instructional video, brochure, and/or spacer)

● **S8100** Holding chamber or spacer for use with an inhaler or nebulizer; without mask

● **S8101** Holding chamber or spacer for use with an inhaler or nebulizer; with mask

S8105 Oximeter for measuring blood oxygen levels noninvasively

S8110 Peak expiratory flow rate (physician services)

● **S8180** Tracheostomy shower protector

● **S8181** Tracheostomy tube holder

● **S8182** Humidifier, heated, used with ventilator, non-servo-controlled

● **S8183** Humidifier, heated, used with ventilator, dual servo-controlled with temperature monitoring

● **S8185** Flutter device

● **S8186** Swivel adaptor

● **S8189** Tracheostomy supply, not otherwise classified

● **S8190** Electronic spirometer (or microspirometer)

S8200 Chest compression vest

S8205 Chest compression system generator and hoses (for use with chest compression vest - S8200)

S8210 Mucus trap

S8260 Oral orthotic for treatment of sleep apnea, includes fitting, fabrication, and materials

(S8300) Code deleted 2001

(S8400) Code deleted 2002

● **S8401** Child-size incontinence garment, diaper, each

(S8402) Code deleted 2002

● **S8403** Adult-sized incontinence garment, disposable, pull-up brief, each

● **S8404**   Child-size incontinence garment, disposable, pull-up brief, each

▲ **S8405**   Disposable liner/shield for incontinence, each

● **S8415**   Supplies for home delivery of infant

● **S8420**   Gradient pressure aid (sleeve and glove combination), custom made

● **S8421**   Gradient pressure aid (sleeve and glove combination), ready made

● **S8422**   Gradient pressure aid (sleeve), custom made, medium weight

● **S8423**   Gradient pressure aid (sleeve), custom made, heavy weight

● **S8424**   Gradient pressure aid (sleeve), ready made

● **S8425**   Gradient pressure aid (glove), custom made, medium weight

● **S8426**   Gradient pressure aid (glove), custom made, heavy weight

● **S8427**   Gradient pressure aid (glove), ready made

● **S8428**   Gradient pressure aid (gauntlet), ready made

● **S8429**   Gradient pressure exterior wrap

● **S8430**   Padding for compression bandage, roll

● **S8431**   Compression bandage, roll

● **S8450**   Splint, prefabricated, digit (specify digit by use of modifier)

● **S8451**   Splint, prefabricated, wrist or ankle

● **S8452**   Splint, prefabricated, elbow

● **S8490**   Insulin syringes (100 syringes, any size)

S8950   Complex lymphedema therapy, each 15 min

S8999 Resuscitation bag (for use by patient on artificial respiration during power failure or other catastrophic event)

S9001 Home uterine monitor with or without associated nursing services

S9007 Ultrafiltration monitor

S9015 Automated EEG monitoring

S9022 Digital subraction angiography (use in addition to CPT code for the procedure for further identification)

(S9023) Code deleted 2002

S9024 Paranasal sinus ultrasound

S9025 Omnicardiogram/cardiointegram

(S9033) Code deleted 2001; use 95979, 95986

(S9035) Code deleted 2002

S9055 Procuren or other growth factor preparation to promote wound healing

S9056 Coma stimulation per diem

▲**S9061** Home administration of aerosolized drug therapy (e.g., pentamidine); administative services, professional pharmacy services, care coordination, all necesary supplies and equipment (drugs and nursing visits coded separately), per diem

S9075 Smoking cessation treatment

●**S9083** Global fee urgent care centers

(S9085) Code deleted 2002

▲**S9088** Services provided in an urgent care center (list in addition to code for service)

S9090 Vertebral axial decompression, per session

● **S9098**   Home visit, phototherapy services (e.g., Bili-lite), including equipment rental, nursing services, blood draw, supplies, and other services, per diem

● **S9109**   Congestive heart failure telemonitoring, equipment rental, including telescale, computer system and software, telephone connections, and maintenance, per month

● **S9117**   Back school, per visit

S9122   Home health aide or certified nurse assistant, providing care in the home; per hour

S9123   Nursing care, in the home; by registered nurse, per hour

S9124   by licensed practical nurse, per hour

S9125   Respite care, in the home, per diem

S9126   Hospice care, in the home, per diem

S9127   Social work visit, in the home, per diem

S9128   Speech therapy, in the home, per diem

S9129   Occupational therapy, in the home, per diem

● **S9131**   Physical therapy; in the home, per diem

S9140   Diabetic management program; follow-up visit to non-MD provider

S9141   follow-up visit to MD provider

(S9200)   Code deleted 2002

● **S9208**   Home management of pre-term labor, including administrative services, professional pharmacy services, care coordination, and all necessary supplies or equipment (drugs and nursing visits coded separately), per diem (do not use this code with any home infusion per diem code)

● **S9209**   Home management of pre-term premature rupture of membranes (PPROM), including administrative services, professional pharmacy services, care coordination, and all

---

necessary supplies or equipment (drugs and nursing visits coded separately), per diem (do not use this code with any home infusion per diem code)

(S9210) Code deleted 2002

● **S9211** Home management of gestational hypertension, includes administrative services, professional pharmacy services, care coordination and all necessary supplies and equipment (drugs and nursing visits coded separately); per diem (do not use this code with any home infusion per diem code)

● **S9212** Home management of postpartum hypertension, includes administrative services, professional pharmacy services, care coordination, and all necessary supplies and equipment (drugs and nursing visits coded separately), per diem (do not use this code with any home infusion per diem code)

● **S9213** Home management of preeclampsia, includes administrative services, professional pharmacy services, care coordination, and all necessary supplies and equipment (drugs and nursing services coded separately); per diem (do not use this code with any home infusion per diem code)

● **S9214** Home management of gestational diabetes, includes administrative services, professional pharmacy services, care coordination, and all necessary supplies and equipment (drugs and nursing visits coded separately); per diem (do not use this code with any home infusion per diem code)

● **S9216** Nursing services and all necessary equipment and supplies for gestational hypertension program (includes maternal assessment as needed, telephonic collection of blood pressure, urine protein, weight and fetal movement counting via a home data collection system, patient status reports, 24 hour/7 day a week nursing support, and all education to the patient and care giver); per diem

● **S9217** Nursing services and all necessary equipment and supplies for postpartum hypertension program (includes maternal assessment as needed, telephonic collection of blood pressure, urine protein, weight, compliance management support, patient status reports, 24 hour/7 day a week nursing support, and all education to the patient and care giver); per diem

● **S9218** Nursing services and all necessary equipment and supplies for preeclampsia program (includes maternal assessment as needed, telephonic collection of blood pressure, urine protein, weight and daily fetal movement counts via a home data collection system, compliance management support, patient status reports, 24 hour/7 day a week nursing support, and all education to the patient and care giver); per diem

(**S9220**) Code deleted 2002

(**S9225**) Code deleted 2002

(**S9230**) Code deleted 2002

(**S9300**) Code deleted 2002

(**S9308**) Code deleted 2002

(**S9310**) Code deleted 2002

● **S9325** Home infusion therapy, pain management infusion; administrative services, professional pharmacy services, care coordination, and all necessary supplies and equipment, (drugs and nursing visits coded separately), per diem (do not use this code with S9326, S9327 or S9328)

● **S9326** Home infusion therapy, continuous pain management infusion; administrative services, professional pharmacy services, care coordination and all necessary supplies and equipment (drugs and nursing visits coded separately), per diem

● **S9327** Home infusion therapy, intermittent pain management infusion; administrative services, professional pharmacy services, care coordination, and all necessary supplies and equipment (drugs and nursing visits coded separately), per diem

● **S9328** Home infusion therapy, implanted pump pain management infusion; administrative services, professional pharmacy services, care coordination, and all necessary supplies and equipment (drugs and nursing visits coded separately), per diem

● **S9329** Home infusion therapy, chemotherapy infusion; administrative services, professional pharmacy services, care coordination, and all necessary supplies and equipment (drugs and nursing visits coded separately), per diem (do not use this code with S9330 or S9331)

● **S9330** Home infusion therapy, continuous chemotherapy infusion; administrative services, professional pharmacy services, care coordination, and all necessary supplies and equipment (drugs and nursing visits coded separately), per diem

● **S9331** Home infusion therapy, intermittent chemotherapy infusion; administrative services, professional pharmacy services, care coordination, and all necessary supplies and equipment (drugs and nursing visits coded separately), per diem

● **S9336** Home infusion therapy, continuous anticoagulant infusion therapy (e.g., Heparin), administrative services, professional pharmacy services, care coordination and all necessary supplies and equipment (drugs and nursing visits coded separately), per diem

● **S9338** Home infusion therapy, immunotherapy therapy; administrative services, professional pharmacy services, care coordination, and all necessary supplies and equipment (drug and nursing visits coded separately), per diem

● **S9339** Home therapy; peritoneal dialysis, administrative services, professional pharmacy services, care coordination and all necessary supplies and equipment (drugs and nursing visits coded separately), per diem

● **S9340** Home therapy; enteral nutrition; administrative services, professional pharmacy services, care coordination, and all necessary supplies and equipment (enteral formula and nursing visits coded separately), per diem

Not valid for Medicare | Non-covered by Medicare | Special coverage instructions | Carrier discretion **299**

● **S9341** Home therapy; enteral nutrition via gravity; administrative services, professional pharmacy services, care coordination, and all necessary supplies and equipment (enteral formula and nursing visits coded separately), per diem

● **S9342** Home therapy; enteral nutrition via pump; administrative services, professional pharmacy services, care coordination, and all necessary supplies and equipment (enteral formula and nursing visits coded separately), per diem

● **S9343** Home therapy; enteral nutrition via bolus; administrative services, professional pharmacy services, care coordination, and all necessary supplies and equipment (enteral formula and nursing visits coded separately), per diem

● **S9345** Home infusion therapy, anti-hemophilic agent infusion therapy (e.g., Factor VIII); administrative services, professional pharmacy services, care coordination, and all necessary supplies and equipment (drugs and nursing visits coded separately), per diem

● **S9346** Home infusion therapy, alpha-1-proteinase inhibitor (e.g., Prolastin); administrative services, professional pharmacy services, care coordination, and all necessary supplies and equipment (drugs and nursing visits coded separately), per diem

● **S9347** Home infusion therapy, uninterrupted, long-term, controlled rate intravenous infusion therapy (e.g., Epoprostenol); administrative services, professional pharmacy services, care coordination, all necessary supplies and equipment (drugs and nursing visits coded separately), per diem

● **S9348** Home infusion therapy, sympathomimetic/inotropic agent infusion therapy (e.g., Dobutamine); administrative services, professional pharmacy services, care coordination, all necessary supplies and equipment (drugs and nursing visits coded separately), per diem

● **S9349** Home infusion therapy, tocolytic infusion therapy; administrative services, professional pharmacy services, care coordination, and all necessary supplies and equipment (drugs and nursing visits coded separately), per diem

● **S9351** Home infusion therapy, continuous anti-emetic infusion therapy; administrative services, professional pharmacy services, care coordination, all necessary supplies and equipment (drugs and nursing visits coded separately), per diem

● **S9353** Home infusion therapy, continuous insulin infusion therapy; administrative services, professional pharmacy services, care coordination, and all necessary supplies and equipment (drugs and nursing visits coded separately), per diem

● **S9355** Home infusion therapy, chelation therapy; administrative services, professional pharmacy services, care coordination, and all necessary supplies and equipment (drugs and nursing visits coded separately), per diem

● **S9357** Home infusion therapy, enzyme replacement intravenous therapy; (e.g., Imiglucerase); administrative services, professional pharmacy services, care coordination, and all necessary supplies and equipment (drugs and nursing visits coded separately), per diem

● **S9359** Home infusion therapy, anti-tumor necrosis factor intravenous therapy; (e.g., Infliximab); administrative services, professional pharmacy services, care coordination, and all necessary supplies and equipment (drugs and nursing visits coded separately), per diem

● **S9361** Home infusion therapy, diuretic intravenous therapy; administrative services, professional pharmacy services, care coordination, and all necessary supplies and equipment (drugs and nursing visits coded separately), per diem

● **S9363** Home infusion therapy, anti-spasmotic intravenous therapy; administrative services, professional pharmacy services, care coordination, and all necessary supplies and equipment (drugs and nursing visits coded separately), per diem

● **S9364** Home infusion therapy, total parenteral nutrition (TPN); administrative services, professional pharmacy services, care coordination, and all necessary supplies and equipment (includes standard TPN formula, lipids, specialty amino acid formulas, drugs, and nursing visits coded separately), per diem (do not use with home infusion codes S9365-S9368 using daily volume scales)

● **S9365**   Home infusion therapy, total parenteral nutrition (TPN); one liter per day, administrative services, professional pharmacy services, care coordination, and all necessary supplies and equipment (includes standard TPN formula, lipids, specialty amino acid formulas, drugs, and nursing visits coded separately), per diem

● **S9366**   Home infusion therapy, total parenteral nutrition (TPN); more than one liter but no more than two liters per day, administrative services, professional pharmacy services, care coordination, and all necessary supplies and equipment (includes standard TPN formula, lipids, specialty amino acid formulas, drugs, and nursing visits coded separately), per diem

● **S9367**   Home infusion therapy, total parenteral nutrition (TPN); more than two liters but no more than three liters per day, administrative services, professional pharmacy services, care coordination, and all necessary supplies and equipment (includes standard TPN formula, lipids, specialty amino acids, drugs, and nursing visits coded separately), per diem

● **S9368**   Home infusion therapy, total parenteral nutrition (TPN); more than three liters per day, administrative services, professional pharmacy services, care coordination, and all necessary supplies and equipment (includes standard TPN formula, lipids, specialty amino acid formulas, drugs, and nursing visits coded separately), per diem

● **S9370**   Home therapy, intermittent anti-emetic injection therapy; administrative services, professional pharmacy services, care coordination, and all necessary supplies and equipment (drugs and nursing visits coded separately), per diem

● **S9372**   Home therapy; intermittent anticoagulant injection therapy (e.g., heparin); administrative services, professional pharmacy services, care coordination, and all necessary supplies and equipment (drugs and nursing visits coded separately), per diem (do not use this code for flushing of infusion devices with heparin to maintain patency)

● **S9373**   Home infusion therapy, hydration therapy; administrative services, professional pharmacy services, care coordination, and all necessary supplies and equipment

---

   ●   New code   ▲   Revised code   ( )   Deleted code

(drugs and nursing visits coded separately), per diem (do not use with hydration therapy codes S9374-S9377 using daily volume scales)

● **S9374** Home infusion therapy, hydration therapy; one liter per day, administrative services, professional pharmacy services, care coordination, and all necessary supplies and equipment (drugs and nursing visits coded separately), per diem

● **S9375** Home infusion therapy, hydration therapy; more than one liter but no more than two liters per day, administrative services, professional pharmacy services, care coordination, and all necessary supplies and equipment (drugs and nursing visits coded separately), per diem

● **S9376** Home infusion therapy, hydration therapy; more than two liters but no more than three liters per day, administrative services, professional pharmacy services, care coordination, and all necessary supplies and equipment (drugs and nursing visits coded separately), per diem

● **S9377** Home infusion therapy, hydration therapy; more than three liters per day, administrative services, professional pharmacy services, care coordination, and all necessary supplies (drugs and nursing visits coded separately), per diem

● **S9379** Home infusion therapy, infusion therapy, not otherwise classified; administrative services, professional pharmacy services, care coordination, and all necessary supplies and equipment (drugs and nursing visits coded separately), per diem

● **S9381** Delivery or service to high risk areas requiring escort or extra protection, per visit

(S9395) Code deleted 2002

(S9420) Code deleted 2002

(S9423) Code deleted 2002

(S9425) Code deleted 2002

S9435 Medical foods for inborn errors of metabolism

● **S9441** Asthma education, non-physician provider, per session

● **S9442**   Birthing classes, non-physician provider, per session

● **S9443**   Lactation classes, non-physician provider, per session

● **S9445**   Patient education, not otherwise classified, non-physician provider, individual, per session

● **S9446**   Patient education, not otherwise classified, non-physician provider, group, per session

S9455   Diabetic management program; group session

S9460   nurse visit

S9465   dietician visit

S9470   Nutritional counseling, dietitian visit

S9472   Cardiac rehabilitation program, non-physician provider, per diem

S9473   Pulmonary rehabilitation program, non-physician provider, per diem

S9474   Enterostomal therapy by a registered nurse certified in enterostomal therapy, per diem

S9475   Ambulatory setting substance abuse treatment or detoxification services, per diem

S9480   Intensive outpatient psychiatric services, per diem

S9485   Crisis intervention mental health services, per diem

● **S9494**   Home infusion therapy, antibiotic, antiviral, or antifungal therapy; administrative services, professional pharmacy services, care coordination, and all necessary supplies and equipment (drug and nursing visits coded separately), per diem (do not use with home infusion codes for hourly dosing schedules S9497-S9504)

● **S9497**   Home infusion therapy, antibiotic, antiviral, or antifungal therapy; once every 3 hours; administrative services, professional pharmacy services, care coordination, and all necessary supplies and equipment (drugs and nursing visits coded separately), per diem

● **S9500** Home infusion therapy, antibiotic, antiviral, or antifungal therapy; once every 24 hours; administrative services, professional pharmacy services, care coordination, and all necessary supplies and equipment (drugs and nursing visits coded separately), per diem

● **S9501** Home infusion therapy, antibiotic, antiviral, or antifungal therapy; once every 12 hours; administrative services, professional pharmacy services, care coordination, and all necessary supplies and equipment (drugs and nursing visits coded separately), per diem

● **S9502** Home infusion therapy, antibiotic, antiviral, or antifungal therapy; once every 8 hours, administrative services, professional pharmacy services, care coordination, and all necessary supplies and equipment (drugs and nursing visits coded separately), per diem

● **S9503** Home infusion therapy, antibiotic, antiviral, or antifungal; once every 6 hours; administrative services, professional pharmacy services, care coordination, and all necessary supplies and equipment (drugs and nursing visits coded separately), per diem

● **S9504** Home infusion therapy, antibiotic, antiviral, or antifungal; once every 4 hours; administrative services, professional pharmacy services, care coordination, and all necessary supplies and equipment (drugs and nursing visits coded separately), per diem

S9524 Nursing services related to home IV therapy, per diem

(S9526) Code deleted 2002

(S9527) Code deleted 2002

(S9528) Code deleted 2002

● **S9529** Routine venipuncture for collection of specimen(s), single home bound, nursing home, or skilled nursing facility patient

(S9533) Code deleted 2002

(S9535) Code deleted 2002

● **S9537** Home therapy; hematopoietic hormone injection therapy (e.g., Crythropoietin, g-csf, gm-csf); administrative services, professional pharmacy services, care coordination, and all necessary supplies and equipment (drugs and nursing visits coded separately), per diem

● **S9538** Home transfusion of blood product(s); administrative services, professional pharmacy services, care coordination and all necessary supplies and equipment (blood products, drugs, and nursing visits coded separately), per diem

(**S9539**) Code deleted 2002

● **S9542** Home injectable therapy; not otherwise classified, including administrative services, professional pharmacy services, coordination of care, and all necessary supplies and equipment (drugs and nursing visits coded separately), per diem

S9543 Administration of medication, intramuscularly, epidurally, or subcutaneously, in the home setting, including all nursing care, equipment, and supplies; per diem

(**S9545**) Code deleted 2002

(**S9550**) Code deleted 2002

(**S9555**) Code deleted 2002

● **S9558** Home injectable therapy; growth hormone, including administrative services, professional pharmacy services, coordination of care, and all necessary supplies and equipment (drugs and nursing visits coded separately), per diem

● **S9559** Home injectable therapy; interferon, including administrative services, professional pharmacy services, coordination of care, and all necessary supplies and equipment (drugs and nursing visits coded separately), per diem

● **S9560** Home injectable therapy; hormonal therapy (e.g., leuprolide, goserelin), including administrative services, professional pharmacy services, care coordination, and all necessary supplies and equipment (drugs and nursing visits coded separately), per diem

---

● New code ▲ Revised code ( ) Deleted code

● **S9800**   Home therapy; provision of infusion, specialty drug administration, and/or associated nursing services and procedures, by highly technical RN, per hour (do not use this code with S9524)

● **S9810**   Home therapy; professional pharmacy services for provision of infusion, specialty drug administration, and/or disease state management, not otherwise classified, per hour (do not use this code with any per diem code)

● **S9981**   Medical records copying fee, administrative

● **S9982**   Medical records copying fee, per page

● **S9986**   Not medically necessary service (patient is aware that service not medically necessary)

● **S9989**   Services provided outside of the United States of America (list in addition to code(s) for services(s))

S9990   Services provided as part of a phase II clinical trial

S9991   Services provided as part of a phase III clinical trial

S9992   Transportation costs to and from trial location and local transportation costs (e.g., fares for taxicab or bus) for clinical trial participant and one caregiver/companion

S9994   Lodging costs (e.g., hotel charges) for clinical trial participant and one caregiver/companion

S9996   Meals for clinical trial participant and one caregiver/companion

S9999   Sales tax

STATE MEDICAID AGENCY CODES

Guidelines

For the year 2002, "T" codes have been added to HCPCS. These codes are exclusively for the use of state Medicaid agencies. Prior to using "T" codes on health insurance claims to your state Medicaid processor, you should verify that these codes are acceptable. "T" codes are not valid for Medicare use.

In addition to the information presented in the INTRODUCTION, several other items unique to this section are defined or identified here.

1. **SPECIAL REPORT:** A service, material or supply that is rarely provided, unusual, variable or new may require a special report in determining medical appropriateness for reimbursement purposes. Pertinent information should include an adequate definition or description of the nature, extent, and need for the service, material or supply.

2. **MODIFIERS:** Listed services may be modified under certain circumstances. When appropriate, the modifying circumstance is identified by adding a modifier to the basic procedure code. CPT and HCPCS National Level II modifiers may be used with CPT and HCPCS National Level II procedure codes.

State Medicaid Agency Codes

● **T1000** Private duty/independent nursing service(s), licensed, up to 15 minutes

● **T1001** Nursing assessment/evaluation

● **T1002** RN services, up to 15 minutes

● **T1003** LPN/LVN services, up to 15 minutes

● **T1004** Services of a qualified nursing aide, up to 15 minutes

● **T1005** Respite care services, up to 15 minutes

Not valid for Medicare   Non-covered by Medicare   Special coverage instructions   Carrier discretion

● **T1006** Alcohol and/or substance abuse services, family/couple counseling

● **T1007** Alcohol and/or substance abuse services, treatment plan development and/or modification

● **T1008** Day treatment for individual alcohol and/or substance abuse services

● **T1009** Child sitting services for children of the individual receiving alcohol and/or substance abuse services

● **T1010** Meals for individuals receiving alcohol and/or substance abuse services (when meals are not included in the program)

● **T1011** Alcohol and/or substance abuse services, not otherwise classified

● **T1012** Alcohol and/or substance abuse services, skills development

● **T1013** Sign language or oral interpreter services

● **T1014** Telehealth transmission, per minute, professional services bill separately

● **T1015** Clinic visit/encounter, all-inclusive

VISION SERVICES

Guidelines

In addition to the information presented in the INTRODUCTION, several other items unique to this section are defined or identified here:

1. **SUBSECTION INFORMATION:** Some of the listed subheadings or subsections have special needs or instructions unique to that section. Where these are indicated, special "notes" will be presented preceding or following the listings. Those subsections within the VISION SERVICES section that have "notes" are as follows:

Subsection	Code Numbers
Spectacle lenses	V2100-V2499
Contact lenses	V2500-V2599
Low vision aids	V2600-V2615

2. **UNLISTED SERVICE OR PROCEDURE:** A service or procedure may be provided that is not listed in this edition of HCPCS. When reporting such a service, the appropriate "unlisted procedure" code may be used to indicate the service, identifying it by "special report" as defined below. HCPCS terminology is inconsistent in defining unlisted procedures. The procedure definition may include the term(s) "unlisted", "not otherwise classified", "unspecified", "unclassified", "other" and "miscellaneous". Prior to using these codes, try to determine if a Local Level III code or CPT code is available. The "unlisted procedures" and accompanying codes for VISION SERVICES are as follows:

V2199	Not otherwise classified, single vision lens, bifocal, glass or plastic
V2499	Variable sphericity lens, other type
V2599	Not otherwise classified, contact lens
V2629	Prosthetic eye, other type
V2799	Vision service, miscellaneous

3. **SPECIAL REPORT:** A service, material or supply that is rarely provided, unusual, variable or new may require a special report in determining medical appropriateness for reimbursement purposes. Pertinent information should include an adequate definition or description of the nature, extent, and need for the service, material or supply.

4. **MODIFIERS:** Listed services may be modified under certain circumstances. When appropriate, the modifying circumstance is identified by adding a modifier to the basic procedure code. CPT and HCPCS National Level II modifiers may be used with CPT and HCPCS National Level II procedure codes. Modifiers commonly used with VISION SERVICES are as follows:

-AP   Determination of refractive state was not performed in the course of diagnostic ophthalmological examination

-CC   Procedure code change (use "CC" when the procedure code submitted was changed either for administrative reasons or because an incorrect code was filed)

-LS   FDA-monitored intraocular lens implant

-LT   Left side (used to identify procedures performed on the left side of the body)

-PL   Progressive addition lenses

-RT   Right side (used to identify procedures performed on the right side of the body)

-SF   Second opinion ordered by a professional review organization (PRO) per section 9401, P.L. 99-272. (100 percent reimbursement; no Medicare deductible or coinsurance)

-TC   Technical component. Under certain circumstances, a charge may be made for the technical component alone. Under those circumstances, the technical component charge is identified by adding modifier -TC to the usual procedure number. Technical component charges are institutional charges and are not billed separately by physicians. However, portable x-ray suppliers bill only for the technical component and should use modifier -TC. The charge data from portable x-ray suppliers will then be used to build customary and prevailing profiles.

-VP   Aphakic patient

5. **CPT CODE CROSS-REFERENCE:** See sections for equivalent CPT code(s) for all listings in this section.

Vision Services

FRAMES

V2020 Frames, purchases

V2025 Deluxe frame

SPECTACLE LENSES

NOTE: If CPT code 92390 or 92395 is reported, recode with the specific lens type listed below. For aphakic temporary spectacle correction, see CPT code 92358.

SINGLE VISION, GLASS OR PLASTIC

V2100 Sphere, single vision; plano to plus or minus 4.00, per lens

V2101 plus or minus 4.12 to plus or minus 7.00d, per lens

V2102 plus or minus 7.12 to plus or minus 20.00d, per lens

V2103 Spherocylinder, single vision, plano to plus or minus 4.00d sphere; .12 to 2.00d cylinder, per lens

V2104 2.12 to 4.00d cylinder, per lens

V2105 4.25 to 6.00d cylinder, per lens

V2106 over 6.00d cylinder, per lens

V2107 Spherocylinder, single vision, plus or minus 4.25d to plus or minus 7.00d sphere; .12 to 2.00d cylinder, per lens

V2108 2.12 To 4.00d cylinder, per lens

V2109 4.25 to 6.00d cylinder, per lens

V2110 over 6.00d cylinder, per lens

V2111 Spherocylinder, single vision, plus or minus 7.25 to plus or minus 12.00d sphere; .25 to 2.25d cylinder, per lens

V2112 2.25d to 4.00d cylinder, per lens

V2113   4.25 to 6.00d cylinder, per lens

V2114   Spherocylinder, single vision, sphere over plus or minus 12.00d per lens

V2115   Lenticular, (myodisc), per lens, single vision

V2116   Lenticular lens, nonaspheric, per lens, single vision

V2117   Lenticular, aspheric, per lings, single vision

V2118   Aniseikonic lens, single vision

V2199   Not otherwise classified, single vision lens

BIFOCAL, GLASS OR PLASTIC

(Up to and including 28mm seg width, add power up to and including 3.25d)

V2200   Sphere, bifocal, plano to plus or minus 4.00d, per lens

V2201   Sphere, bifocal, plus or minus 4.12 to plus or minus 7.00d, per lens

V2202   Sphere, bifocal, plus or minus 7.12 to plus or minus 20.00d, per lens

V2203   Spherocylinder, bifocal, plano to plus or minus 4.00d sphere; .12 to 2.00d cylinder, per lens

V2204   2.12 to 4.00d cylinder, per lens

V2205   4.25 to 6.00d cylinder, per lens

V2206   over 6.00d cylinder, per lens

V2207   Spherocylinder, bifocal, plus or minus 4.25 to plus or minus 7.00d sphere; .12 to 2.00d cylinder, per lens

V2208   2.12 to 4.00d cylinder, per lens

V2209   4.25 to 6.00d cylinder, per lens

V2210   over 6.00d cylinder, per lens

V2211 Spherocylinder, bifocal, plus or minus 7.25 to plus or minus 12.00d sphere; .25 to 2.25d cylinder, per lens

V2212 2.25 to 4.00d cylinder, per lens

V2213 4.25 to 6.00d cylinder, per lens

V2214 Spherocylinder, bifocal, sphere over plus or minus 12.00d, per lens

V2215 Lenticular (myodisc), per lens, bifocal

V2216 Lenticular, nonaspheric, per lens, bifocal

V2217 Lenticular, aspheric lens, bifocal

V2218 Aniseikonic, per lens, bifocal

V2219 Bifocal seg width over 28mm

V2220 Bifocal add over 3.25d

V2299 Specialty bifocal (by report)

TRIFOCAL, GLASS OR PLASTIC

(Up to and including 28mm seg width, add power up to and including 3.25d)

V2300 Sphere, trifocal, plano to plus or minus 4.00d, per lens

V2301 Sphere, trifocal, plus or minus 4.12 to plus or minus 7.00d, per lens

V2302 Sphere, trifocal, plus or minus 7.12 to plus or minus 20.00, per lens

V2303 Spherocylinder, trifocal, plano to plus or minus 4.00d sphere; .12 to 2.00d cylinder, per lens

V2304 2.25 to 4.00d cylinder, per lens

V2305 4.25 to 6.00d cylinder, per lens

V2306 over 6.00d cylinder, per lens

V2307	Spherocylinder, trifocal, plus or minus 4.25 to plus or minus 7.00d sphere; .12 to 2.00d cylinder, per lens
V2308	2.12 to 4.00d cylinder, per lens
V2309	4.25 to 6.00d cylinder, per lens
V2310	over 6.00d cylinder, per lens
V2311	Spherocylinder, trifocal, plus or minus 7.25 to plus or minus 12.00d sphere; .25 to 2.25d cylinder, per lens
V2312	2.25 to 4.00d cylinder, per lens
V2313	4.25 to 6.00d cylinder, per lens
V2314	Spherocylinder, trifocal, sphere over plus or minus 12.00d, per lens
V2315	Lenticular, (myodisc), per lens, trifocal
V2316	Lenticular, nonaspheric, per lens, trifocal
V2317	Lenticular, aspheric lens, trifocal
V2318	Aniseikonic lens, trifocal
V2319	Trifocal seg width over 28mm
V2320	Trifocal add over 3.25d
V2399	Specialty trifocal (by report)

VARIABLE ASPHERICITY

(Welsh 4-drop, hyperaspheric, double drop, etc.)

V2410	Variable asphericity lens; single vision, full field, glass or plastic, per lens
V2430	bifocal, full field, glass or plastic, per lens
V2499	other type

CONTACT LENSES (CPT 92391 OR 92396)

NOTE: If CPT code 92391 or 92396 is reported, recode with specific lens type listed below, per lens.

V2500 Contact lens, PMMA; spherical, per lens

V2501 toric or prism ballast, per lens

V2502 bifocal, per lens

V2503 color vision deficiency, per lens

V2510 Contact lens, gas permeable; spherical, per lens

V2511 toric, prism ballast, per lens

V2512 bifocal, per lens

V2513 extended wear, per lens

V2520 Contact lens hydrophilic; spherical, per lens

V2521 toric, or prism ballast, per lens

V2522 bifocal, per lens

V2523 extended wear, per lens

V2530 Contact lens, scleral, gas impermeable, per lens (for contact lens modification, see 92325)

V2531 Contact lens, scleral, gas permeable, per lens (for contact lens modification, see 92325)

V2599 Contact lens, other type

LOW VISION AIDS (CPT 92392)

NOTE: If CPT code 92392 is reported, record with specific systems listed below.

V2600 Hand held low vision aids and other nonspectacle mounted aids

V2610 Single lens spectacle mounted low vision aids

| | Not valid for Medicare | | Non-covered by Medicare | | Special coverage instructions | | Carrier discretion | **317** |

V2615   Telescopic and other compound lens system, including distance vision telescopic, near vision telescopes and compound microscopic lens system

EYE PROSTHESIS

PROSTHETIC EYE (CPT 92330 OR 92393)

V2623   Prosthetic, eye; plastic, custom

V2624   Polishing/resurfacing or ocular prosthesis

V2625   Enlargement of ocular prosthesis

V2626   Reduction of ocular prosthesis

V2627   Scleral cover shell

V2628   Fabrication and fitting of ocular conformer

V2629   Prosthetic eye, other type

INTRAOCULAR LENSES

V2630   Anterior chamber intraocular lens

V2631   Iris supported intraocular lens

V2632   Posterior chamber intraocular lens

MISCELLANEOUS

V2700   Balance lens, per lens

V2710   Slab off prism, glass or plastic, per lens

V2715   Prism, per lens

V2718   Press-on lens, fresnell prism, per lens

V2730   Special base curve, glass or plastic, per lens

V2740   Tint; plastic, rose 1 or 2, per lens

V2741   plastic, other than rose 1 or 2, per lens

V2742	glass rose 1 or 2, per lens
V2743	glass other than rose 1 or 2, per lens
V2744	photochromatic, per lens
V2750	Anti-reflective coating, per lens
V2755	U-V lens, per lens
V2760	Scratch resistant coating, per lens
V2770	Occluder lens, per lens
V2780	Oversize lens, per lens
V2781	Progressive lens, per lens
V2785	Processing, preserving and transporting corneal tissue
V2790	Amniotic membrane for surgical reconstruction, per procedure
V2799	Vision service, miscellaneous

● New code ▲ Revised code ( ) Deleted code

HEARING SERVICES

Guidelines

In addition to the information presented in the INTRODUCTION, several other items unique to this section are defined or identified here:

1. **PROSTHETIC DEVICES:** Prosthetic devices that replace all or part of an internal body organ or the function of a permanently inoperative or malfunctioning internal body organ are covered when furnished on a physician's order. If the medical record and attending physician indicate the condition will be indefinite, the test of permanence is met.

2. **SPEECH PATHOLOGY:** Services necessary for diagnosing and treating speech disorders that result in communication disabilities, and swallowing disorders, regardless of the presence of a disability, are covered Medicare services if reasonable and necessary. The services must be considered to be an effective treatment for the patient's condition, and the patient's condition must be at a level of severity that requires the service of a qualified speech pathologist.

3. **UNLISTED SERVICE OR PROCEDURE:** A service or procedure may be provided that is not listed in this edition of HCPCS. When reporting such a service, the appropriate "unlisted procedure" code may be used to indicate the service, identifying it by "special report" as defined below. HCPCS terminology is inconsistent in defining unlisted procedures. The procedure definition may include the term(s) "unlisted", "not otherwise classified", "unspecified", "unclassified", "other" and "miscellaneous". Prior to using these codes, try to determine if a Local Level III code or CPT code is available. The "unlisted procedures" and accompanying codes for HEARING SERVICES are as follows:

   V5299   Hearing service, miscellaneous

4. **SPECIAL REPORT:** A service, material or supply that is rarely provided, unusual, variable or new may require a special report in determining medical appropriateness for reimbursement purposes. Pertinent information should include an adequate definition or description of the nature, extent, and need for the service, material or supply.

5. **MODIFIERS:** Listed services may be modified under certain circumstances. When appropriate, the modifying circumstance is identified by adding a modifier to the basic procedure code. CPT

Not valid   Non-covered   Special   Carrier   **321**
for Medicare   by Medicare   coverage   discretion
                                 instructions

and HCPCS National Level II modifiers may be used with CPT and HCPCS National Level II procedure codes. Modifiers commonly used with HEARING SERVICES are as follows:

-CC   Procedure code change (use "CC" when the procedure code submitted was changed either for administrative reasons or because an incorrect code was filed)

-LT   Left side (used to identify procedures performed on the left side of the body)

-RT   Right side (used to identify procedures performed on the right side of the body)

-SF   Second opinion ordered by a professional review organization (PRO) per sectoin 9401, P.L. 99-272 (100 percent reimbursement; no Medicare deductible or coinsurance)

-TC   Technical component. Under certain circumstances, a charge may be made for the technical component alone. Under those circumstances, the technical component charge is identified by adding modifier -TC to the usual procedure number. Technical component charges are institutional charges and are not billed separately by physicians. However, portable x-ray suppliers bill only for the technical component and should use modifier -TC. The charge data from portable x-ray suppliers will then be used to build customary and prevailing profiles.

6. **CPT CODE CROSS-REFERENCE:** See sections for equivalent CPT code(s) for all listings in this section.

Hearing Services

V5008   Hearing screening

V5010   Assessment for hearing aid

V5011   Fitting/orientation/checking of hearing aid

V5014   Repair/modification of a hearing aid

V5020   Conformity evaluation

V5030   Hearing aid, monaural; body worn, air conduction

V5040   body worn, bone conduction

V5050	in the ear
V5060	behind the ear
V5070	Glasses; air conduction
V5080	bone conduction
V5090	Dispensing fee, unspecified hearing aid
V5100	Hearing aid, bilateral, body worn
V5110	Dispensing fee, bilateral
V5120	Binaural; body
V5130	in the ear
V5140	behind the ear
V5150	glasses
V5160	Dispensing fee, binaural
V5170	Hearing aid, CROS; in the ear
V5180	behind the ear
V5190	glasses
V5200	Dispensing fee, CROS
V5210	Hearing aid, bicros; in the ear
V5220	behind the ear
V5230	glasses
V5240	Dispensing fee, bicros
● **V5241**	Dispensing fee, monaural hearing aid, any type
● **V5242**	Hearing aid, analog, monaural, cic (completely in the ear canal)
● **V5243**	Hearing aid, analog, monaural, itc (in the canal)

● **V5244**   Hearing aid, digitally programmable analog, monaural, cic

● **V5245**   Hearing aid, digitally programmable, analog, monaural, itc

● **V5246**   Hearing aid, digitally programmable analog, monaural, ite (in the ear)

● **V5247**   Hearing aid, digitally programmable analog, monaural, bte (behind the ear)

● **V5248**   Hearing aid, analog, binaural, cic

● **V5249**   Hearing aid, analog, binaural, itc

● **V5250**   Hearing aid, digitally programmable analog, binaural, cic

● **V5251**   Hearing aid, digitally programmable analog, binaural, itc

● **V5252**   Hearing aid, digitally programmable, binaural, ite

● **V5253**   Hearing aid, digitally programmable, binaural, bte

● **V5254**   Hearing aid, digital, monaural, cic

● **V5255**   Hearing aid, digital, monaural, itc

● **V5256**   Hearing aid, digital, monaural, ite

● **V5257**   Hearing aid, digital, monaural, bte

● **V5258**   Hearing aid, digital, binaural, cic

● **V5259**   Hearing aid, digital, binaural, itc

● **V5260**   Hearing aid, digital, binaural, ite

● **V5261**   Hearing aid, digital, binaural, bte

● **V5262**   Hearing aid, disposable, any type, monaural

● **V5263**   Hearing aid, disposable, any type, binaural

● **V5264**   Ear mold/insert, not disposable, any type

● **V5265**   Ear mold/insert, disposable, any type

● **V5266**   Battery for use in hearing device

● **V5267**   Hearing aid supplies/accessories

● **V5268**   Assistive listening device, telephone amplifier, any type

● **V5269**   Assistive listening device, alerting, any type

● **V5270**   Assistive listening device, television amplifier, any type

● **V5271**   Assistive listening device, television caption decoder

● **V5272**   Assistive listening device, TDD

● **V5273**   Assistive listening device, for use with cochlear implant

● **V5274**   Assistive learning device, not otherwise specified

● **V5275**   Ear impression, each

V5299   Hearing service, miscellaneous

SPEECH-LANGUAGE PATHOLOGY SERVICES

V5336   Repair/modification of augmentative communicative system or device (excludes adaptive hearing aid)

V5362   Speech screening

V5363   Language screening

V5364   Dysphagia screening

● New code ▲ Revised code ( ) Deleted code

APPENDIX A

HCPCS National Level II Modifiers

The following list is the complete list of HCPCS National Level II modifiers and descriptions.

-AA   Anesthesia services performed personally by anesthesiologist

(-AB)   Modifier deleted 2000

(-AC)   Modifier deleted 2000

-AD   Medical supervision by a physician; more than four concurrent anesthesia procedures

(-AE)   Modifier deleted 2000

(-AF)   Modifier deleted 2000

(-AG)   Modifier deleted 2000

-AH   Clinical psychologist

-AJ   Clinical social worker

(-AK)   Modifier deleted 1999

(-AL)   Modifier deleted 1999

-AM   Physician, team member service

(-AN)   Modifier deleted 1999

-AP   Determination of refractive state was not performed in the course of diagnostic ophthalmological examination

-AS   Physician assistant, nurse practitioner or clinical nurse specialist services for assistant at surgery

---

-AT	Acute treatment (this modifier should be used when reporting service 98940, 98941, 98942)
(-AU)	Modifier deleted 1999
(-AV)	Modifier deleted 1999
(-AW)	Modifier deleted 1999
(-AY)	Modifier deleted 1999
-BP	The beneficiary has been informed of the purchase and rental options and has elected to purchase the item
-BR	The beneficiary has been informed of the purchase and rental options and has elected to rent the item
-BU	The beneficiary has been informed of the purchase and rental options and after 30 days has not informed the supplier of his/her decision
-CC	Procedure code change (use -CC when the procedure code submitted was changed either for administrative reasons or because an incorrect code was filed)
-E1	Upper left, eyelid
-E2	Lower left, eyelid
-E3	Upper right, eyelid
-E4	Lower right, eyelid
-EJ	Subsequent claims for a defined course of therapy, e.g., EPO, sodium hyaluronate, infliximab
-EM	Emergency reserve supply (for ESRD benefit only)
-EP	Service provided as part of Medicaid early periodic screening, diagnosis, and treatment (EPSDT) program
▲**-ET**	Emergency services

-F1   Left hand, second digit

-F2   Left hand, third digit

-F3   Left hand, fourth digit

-F4   Left hand, fifth digit

-F5   Right hand, thumb

-F6   Right hand, second digit

-F7   Right hand, third digit

-F8   Right hand, fourth digit

-F9   Right hand, fifth digit

-FA   Left hand, thumb

-FP   Service provided as part of Medicaid family planning program

-G1   Most recent URR reading of less than 60

-G2   Most recent URR reading of 60 to 64.9

-G3   Most recent URR reading of 65 to 69.9

-G4   Most recent URR reading of 70 to 74.9

-G5   Most recent URR reading of 75 or greater

-G6   ESRD patient for whom less than six dialysis sessions have been provided in a month

-G7   Pregnancy resulted from rape or incest or pregnancy certified by physician as life threatening

-G8   Monitored anesthesia care (MAC) for deep complex, complicated, or markedly invasive surgical procedure

-G9	Monitored anesthesia care for patient who has history of severe cardio-pulmonary condition
-GA	Wiaver of liability statement on file
●**-GB**	Claim being re-submitted for payment because it is no longer covered under a global payment demonstration
-GC	This service has been performed in part by a resident under the direction of a teaching physician
-GE	This service has been performed by a resident without the presence of a teaching physician under the primary care exception
●**-GG**	Performance and payment of a screening mammogram and diagnostic mammogram on the same patient, same day
-GH	Diagnostic mammogram converted from screening mammogram on same day
-GJ	"Opt Out" physician or practitioner emergency or urgent service
●**-GK**	Actual item/service ordered by physician, item associated with -GA or -GZ modifier
●**-GL**	Medically unnecessary upgrade provided instead of standard item, no charge, no advance beneficiary notice (ABN)
●**-GM**	Multiple patients on one ambulance trip
-GN	Service delivered personally by a speech-language pathologist or under an outpatient speech-language pathology plan of care
-GO	Service delivered personally by an occupational therapist or under an outpatient occupational therapy plan of care
-GP	Service delivered personally by a physical therapist or under an outpatient physical therapy plan of care
●**-GQ**	Via asynchronous telecommunications system

-GT   Via interactive audio and video telecommunication systems

(-GU)   Modifier deleted 2002

● -GV   Attending physician not employed or paid under arrangement by the patient's hospice provider

● -GW   Service not related to the hospice patient's terminal condition

(-GX)   Modifier deleted 2002

● -GY   Item or service statutorily excluded or does not meet the definition of any medicare benefit

● -GZ   Item or service expected to be denied as not reasonable and necessary

-K0   Lower extremity prosthesis functional level 0: Does not have the ability or potential to ambulate or transfer safely with or without assistance and a prosthesis does not enhance their quality of life or mobility

-K1   Lower extremity prosthesis functional level 1: Has the ability or potential to use a prosthesis for transfers or ambulation on level surfaces at fixed cadence. Typical of the limited and unlimited household ambulator.

-K2   Lower extremity prosthesis functional level 2: Has the ability or potential for ambulation with the ability to traverse low-level environmental barriers such as curbs, stairs or uneven surfaces. Typical of the limited community ambulator.

-K3   Lower extremity prosthesis functional level 3: Has the ability or potential for ambulation with variable cadence. Typical of the community ambulator who has the ability to traverse most environmental barriers and may have vocational, therapeutic or exercise activity that demands prosthetic utilization beyond simple locomotion.

-K4   Lower prosthesis functional level 4: Has the ability or potential for prosthetic ambulation that exceeds the basic ambulation skills, exhibiting high impact, stress or energy levels, typical of the prosthetic demands of the child, active adult, or athlete.

-KA   Add on option/accessory for wheelchair

-KH   DMEPOS item, initial claim, purchase or first month rental

-KI   DMEPOS item, second or third month rental

-KJ   DMEPOS item, parenteral enteral nutrition (PEN) pump or capped rental, months four to fifteen

(-KK)   Modifier deleted 2001

(-KL)   Modifier deleted 2001

-KM   Replacement of facial prosthesis including new impression/ moulage

-KN   Replacement of facial prosthesis using previous master model

-KO   Single drug unit dose formulation

-KP   First drug of a multiple drug unit dose formulation

-KQ   Second or subsequent drug of a multiple drug unit dose formulation

●**-KR**   Rental item, billing for partial month

-KS   Glucose monitor supply for diabetic beneficiary not treated with insulin

-LC   Left circumflex coronary artery

-LD   Left anterior descending coronary artery

-LL   Lease/rental (use the -LL modifier when DME equipment rental is to be applied against the purchase price)

-LR   Laboratory round trip

-LS   FDA-monitored intraocular lens implant

-LT   Left side (used to identify procedures performed on the left side of the body)

-MS   Six-month maintenance and servicing fee for reasonable and necessary parts and labor which are not covered under any manufacturer or supplier warranty

-NR   New when rented (use the -NR modifier when DME which was new at the time of rental is subsequently purchased)

-NU   New equipment

-PL   Progressive addition lenses

-Q2   HCFA/ORD demonstration project procedure/service

-Q3   Live kidney donor: services associated with postoperative medical complications directly related to the donation

-Q4   Service for ordering/referring physician qualifies as a service exemption

-Q5   Service furnished by a substitute physician under a reciprocal billing arrangement

-Q6   Service furnished by a locum tenens physician

-Q7   One class A finding

-Q8   Two class B findings

-Q9   One class B and two class C findings

-QA   FDA investigational device exemption

-QB   Physician providing service in a rural HPSA

-QC   Single channel monitoring

-QD   Recording and storage in solid state memory by a digital recorder

-QE   Prescribed amount of oxygen is less than one liter per minute (LPM)

-QF   Prescribed amount of oxygen exceeds 4 liters per minute (LPM) and portable oxygen is prescribed

-QG   Prescribed amount of oxygen is greater than four liters per minute (LPM)

-QH   Oxygen conserving device is being used with an oxygen delivery system

-QK   Medical direction of two, three or four concurrent anesthesia procedures involving qualified individuals

-QL   Patient pronounced dead after ambulance called

-QM   Ambulance service provided under arrangement by a provider of services

-QN   Ambulance service furnished directly by a provider of service

-QP   Documentation is on file showing that the laboratory test(s) was ordered individually or ordered as a CPT-recognized panel other than automated profile codes 80002-80019, G0058, G0059, and G0060.

-QQ   Claim submitted with a written statement of intent

(-QR) Modifier deleted 2000; use CPT Level I HCPCS modifier -91

-QS   Monitored anesthesia care service

-QT   Recording and storage on tape by an analog tape recorder

-QU   Physician providing services in an urban HPSA

-QV   Item or service provided as routine care in a medical qualifying clinical trial

-QW   CLIA waived test

-QX CRNA service: with medical direction by a physician

-QY Medical direction of one Certified Registered Nurse Anesthetist by an anesthesiologist

-QZ CRNA service: without medical direction by a physician

-RC Right coronary artery

-RP Replacement and repair (may be used to indicate replacement of DME, orthotic, and prosthetic devices which have been in use for some time. The claim shows the code for the part, followed by the -RP modifier and the charge for the part)

-RR Rental (use the -RR modifier when DME is to be rented)

-RT Right side (used to identify procedures performed on the right side of the body)

● **-SA** Nurse practitioner rendering service in collaboration with a physician

● **-SB** Nurse midwife

● **-SC** Medically necessary service or supply

● **-SD** Services provided by registered nurse with specialized, highly technical home infusion training

● **-SE** State and/or federally funded programs/services

-SF Second opinion ordered by a professional review organization (PRO) per section 9401, P.L. 99-272 (100% reimbursement — no Medicare deductible or coinsurance)

-SG Ambulatory surgical center (ASC) facility service

● **-SH** Second concurrently administered infusion therapy

● **-SJ** Third or more concurrently administered infusion therapy

-T1 Left foot, second digit

-T2 Left foot, third digit

-T3 Left foot, fourth digit

-T4 Left foot, fifth digit

-T5 Right foot, great toe

-T6 Right foot, second digit

-T7 Right foot, third digit

-T8 Right foot, fourth digit

-T9 Right foot, fifth digit

-TA Left foot, great toe

-TC Technical component. Under certain circumstances, a charge may be made for the technical component alone. Under those circumstances the technical component charge is identified by adding modifier -TC to the usual procedure number. Technical component charges are institutional charges and not billed separately by physicians. However, portable x-ray suppliers only bill for technical component and should utilize modifier -TC. The charge data from portable x-ray suppliers will then be used to build customary and prevailing profiles.

● **-TD** RN

● **-TE** LPN/LVN

● **-TF** Intermediate level of care

● **-TG** Complex/high tech level of care

● **-TH** Obstetrical treatment/services, prenatal or postpartum

● **-TJ** Program group, child and/or adolescent

-UE Used durable medical equipment

-VP   Aphakic patient

AMBULANCE SERVICE MODIFIERS

For ambulance service, one-digit modifiers are combined to form a two-digit modifier that identifies the ambulance's place of origin with the first digit, and ambulance's destination with the second digit. They are used in items 12 and 13 on the HCFA Form 1491.

One digit modifiers:

-D   Diagnostic or therapeutic site other than -P or -H when these are used as origin codes

-E   Residential, domiciliary, custodial facility (other than an 1819 facility)

-H   Hospital

-N   Skilled nursing facility (SNF) (1819 facility)

-P   Physician's office

-R   Residence

-S   Scene of accident or acute event

-X   (Destination code only) Intermediate stop at physician's office on the way to the hospital

● New modifier ▲ Revised modifier ( ) Deleted modifier

APPENDIX B

Summary of HCPCS Additions, Changes and Deletions 2002

-ET   Emergency services
Description Changed

-GB   Claim being re-submitted for payment because it is no longer covered under a global payment demonstration
Code Added

-GG   Performance and payment of a screening mammogram and diagnostic mammogram on the same patient, same day
Code Added

-GK   Actual item/service ordered by physician, item associated with -GA or -GZ modifier
Code Added

-GL   Medically unnecessary upgrade provided instead of standard item, no charge, no advance beneficiary notice (ABN)
Code Added

-GM   Multiple patients on one ambulance trip
Code Added

-GQ   Via asynchronous telecommunications system
Code Added

-GU   Procedure performed in non fee schedule place of service
Code Deleted

-GV   Attending physician not employed or paid under arrangement by the patient's hospice provider
Code Added

-GW   Service not related to the hospice patient's terminal condition
Code Added

-GX   Service not covered by Medicare
Code Deleted

-GY Item or service statutorily excluded or does not meet the definition of any medicare benefit
Code Added

-GZ Item or service expected to be denied as not reasonable and necessary
Code Added

-KR Rental item, billing for partial month
Code Added

-SA Nurse practitioner rendering service in collaboration with a physician
Code Added

-SB Nurse midwife
Code Added

-SC Medically necessary service or supply
Code Added

-SD Services provided by registered nurse with specialized, highly technical home infusion training
Code Added

-SE State and/or federally funded programs/services
Code Added

-SH Second concurrently administered infusion therapy
Code Added

-SJ Third or more concurrently administered infusion therapy
Code Added

-TD RN
Code Added

-TE LPN/LVN
Code Added

-TF Intermediate level of care
Code Added

-TG Complex/high tech level of care
Code Added

-TH Obstetrical treatment/services, prenatal or postpartum
Code Added

-TJ Program group, child and/or adolescent
Code Added

A4257   Replacement lens shield cartridge for use with laser skin piercing device, each
Code Added

A4300   Implantable access catheter, (e.g., venous, arterial, epidural subarachnoid, or peritoneal, etc) external access
Description Changed

A4301   Implantable access total system; catheter, port/reservoir (e.g., venous, arterial, epidural, or subarachnoid, etc) percutaneous access
Description Changed

A4329   External catheter starter set, male/female, includes catheters/urinary collection device, bag/pouch and accessories (tubing, clamps, etc.), 7 day supply
Code Deleted

A4351   Intermittent urinary catheter; straight tip, with or without coating (teflon, silicone, silicone elastomer, or hydrophilic, etc), each
Description Changed

A4352   Intermittent urinary catheter; coude (curved) tip, with or without coating (teflon, silicone, silicone elastomeric, or hydrophilic, etc), each
Description Changed

A4358   Urinary drainage bag, leg or abdomen, vinyl, with or without tube, with straps, each
Description Changed

A4360   Adult incontinence garment (e.g., brief, diaper), each
Code Added

A4650   Centrifuge (includes calibrated microcapillary tubes and sealease)
Code Deleted

A4651   Calibrated microcapillary tube, each
Code Added

A4652   Microcapillary tube sealant
Code Added

A4655   Needles and syringes for dialysis
Code Deleted

A4656   Needle, any size, for dialysis, each
Code Added

A4657 Syringe, with or without needle, for dialysis, each
Code Added

A4660 Sphygmomanometer/blood pressure apparatus with cuff and stethoscope, for dialysis
Description Changed

A4663 Blood pressure cuff only, for dialysis
Description Changed

A4670 Automatic blood pressure monitor, for dialysis
Description Changed

A4680 Activated carbon filter for hemodialysis, each
Description Changed

A4690 Dialyzer (artificial kidneys), all types, all sizes, for hemodialysis, each
Description Changed

A4700 Standard dialysate solution, each
Code Deleted

A4705 Bicarbonate dialysate solution, each
Code Deleted

A4706 Bicarbonate concentrate, solution, for hemodialysis, per gallon
Code Added

A4707 Bicarbonate concentrate, powder, for hemodialysis, per packet
Code Added

A4708 Acetate concentrate solution, for hemodialysis, per gallon
Code Added

A4709 Acid concentrate, solution, for hemodialysis, per gallon
Code Added

A4712 Water, sterile, for injection for dialysis, per 10 ml
Description Changed

A4714 Treated water (deionized, distilled, or reverse osmosis) for peritoneal dialysis, per gallon
Description Changed

A4719 Y set tubing for peritoneal dialysis
Code Added

A4720 Dialysate solution, any concentration of dextrose, fluid volume greater than 249cc, but less than or equal to 999cc, for peritoneal dialysis
Code Added

A4721 Dialysate solution, any concentration of dextrose, fluid volume greater than 999cc, but less than or equal to 1999cc, for peritoneal dialysis
Code Added

A4722 Dialysate solution, any concentration of dextrose, fluid volume greater than 1999cc, but less than or equal to 2999cc, for peritoneal dialysis
Code Added

A4723 Dialysate solution, any concentration of dextrose, fluid volume greater than 2999cc, but less than or equal to 3999cc, for peritoneal dialysis
Code Added

A4724 Dialysate solution, any concentration of dextrose, fluid volume greater than 3999cc, but less than or equal to 4999cc, for peritoneal dialysis
Code Added

A4725 Dialysate solution, any concentration of dextrose, fluid volume greater than 4999cc, but less than or equal to 5999cc, for peritoneal dialysis
Code Added

A4726 Dialysate solution, any concentration of dextrose, fluid volume greater than 5999cc, for peritoneal dialysis
Code Added

A4730 Fistula cannulation set for hemodialysis, each
Description Changed

A4735 Local/topical anesthetics for dialysis only
Code Deleted

A4736 Topical anesthetic, for dialysis, per gram
Code Added

A4737 Injectable anesthetic, for dialysis, per 10 ml
Code Added

A4740 Shunt accessory, for hemodialysis, any type, each
Description Changed

A4750 Blood tubing, arterial or venous, for hemodialysis, each
Description Changed

A4755 Blood tubing, arterial and venous combined, for hemodialysis, each
Description Changed

A4760 Dialysate solution test kit, for peritoneal dialysis, any type, each
Description Changed

A4765 Dialysate concentrate, powder, additive for peritoneal dialysis, per packet
Description Changed

A4766 Dialysate concentrate, solution, additive for peritoneal dialysis, per 10 ml
Code Added

A4770 Blood collection tube, vacuum, for dialysis, per 50
Description Changed

A4771 Serum clotting time tube, for dialysis, per 50
Description Changed

A4772 Blood glucose test strips, for dialysis, per 50
Description Changed

A4773 Occult blood test strips, for dialysis, per 50
Description Changed

A4774 Ammonia test strips, for dialysis, per 50
Description Changed

A4780 Sterilizing agent for dialysis equipment, per gallon
Code Deleted

A4790 Cleansing agents for equipment for dialysis only
Code Deleted

A4800 Heparin for dialysis and antidote, any strength, porcine or beef, up to 1000
Code Deleted

A4801 Heparin, any type, for hemodialysis, per 1000 units
Code Added

A4802 Protamine sulfate, for hemodialysis, per 50 mg
Code Added

A4820 Hemodialysis kit supplies
Code Deleted

A4850 Hemostats with rubber tips for dialysis
Code Deleted

A4860 Disposable catheter tips for peritoneal dialysis, per 10
Description Changed

A4870 Plumbing and/or electrical work for home hemodialysis equipment
Description Changed

A4880 Storage tanks utilized in connection with water purification system,
Code Deleted

A4890 Contracts, repair and maintenance, for hemodialysis equipment
Description Changed

A4900 Continuous ambulatory peritoneal dialysis (capd) supply kit
Code Deleted

A4901 Continuous cycling peritoneal dialysis (ccpd) supply kit
Code Deleted

A4905 Intermittent peritoneal dialysis (ipd) supply kit
Code Deleted

A4910 Non-medical supplies for dialysis, (i.e., Scale, scissors, stopwatch, etc.)
Code Deleted

A4911 Drain bag/bottle, for dialysis, each
Code Added

A4912 Gomco drain bottle
Code Deleted

A4913 Miscellaneous dialysis supplies, not otherwise specified
Description Changed

A4914 Preparation kits
Code Deleted

A4918 Venous pressure clamp, for hemodialysis, each
Description Changed

A4919   Dialyzer holder, each
Code Deleted

A4920   Harvard pressure clamp, each
Code Deleted

A4921   Measuring cylinder, any size, each
Code Deleted

A4927   Gloves, non-sterile, for dialysis, per 100
Description Changed

A4928   Surgical mask, for dialysis, per 20
Code Added

A4929   Tourniquet for dialysis, each
Code Added

A5064   Pouch, drainable, with faceplate attached; plastic or rubber
Code Deleted

A5074   Pouch, urinary, with faceplate attached; plastic or rubber
Code Deleted

A5075   Pouch, urinary, for use on faceplate; plastic or rubber
Code Deleted

A5502   For diabetics only, multiple density insert(s), per shoe
Code Deleted

A5509   For diabetics only, direct formed, molded to foot with external heat source (ie heat gun) multiple density insert(s), prefabricated, per shoe
Code Added

A5510   For diabetics only, direct formed, compression molded to patient's foot without external heat source, multiple-density insert(s) prefabricated, per shoe
Code Added

A5511   For diabetics only, custom-molded from model of patient's foot, multiple density insert(s), custom-fabricated, per shoe
Code Added

A6000   Non-contact wound warming wound cover for use with the non-contact wound warming device and warming card
Code Added

A6010 Collagen based wound filler, dry form, per gram of collagen
Code Added

A6196 Alginate or other fiber gelling dressing, wound cover, pad size 16 sq in Or less, each dressing
Description Changed

A6197 Alginate or other fiber gelling dressing, wound cover, pad size more than 16 sq in But less than or equal to 48 sq in, each dressing
Description Changed

A6198 Alginate or other fiber gelling dressing, wound cover, pad size more than 48 sq in, each dressing
Description Changed

A6199 Alginate or other fiber gelling dressing, wound filler, per 6 inches
Description Changed

A9160 Non-covered svc. By podiatrist
Code Deleted

A9170 Non-covered svc. By chiropractor
Code Deleted

A9190 Personal comfort item
Code Deleted

A9511 Supply of radiopharmaceutical diagnostic imaging agent, technetium tc 99m, depreotide, per mci
Code Added

B4084 Gastrostomy/jejunostomy tubing
Code Deleted

B4085 Gastrostomy tube, silicone with sliding ring, each
Code Deleted

B4086 Gastrostomy/jejunostomy tube, any material, any type, (standard or low profile), each
Code Added

C1000 Closure, arterial vascular device, perclose closer arterial vascular closure device, prostar arterial vascular closure device, closer s arterial vascular device
Code Deleted

C1001   Catheter, diagnostic ultrasound, acunav diagnostic
          ultrasound catheter
          Code Deleted

C1003   Catheter, livewire tc ablation catheter 402132, 402133,
          402134, 402135, 402136, 402137, 402145, 402146,
          402147, 402148, 402149, 402150, 402151, 402152,
          402153, 402154, 402155, 402156, 7 fr csm livewire ep
          catheter (model 401935), 5fr decapolar (models 401938,
          401939, 401940, 401941), livewire tc compass ablation
          catheter (models 402205, 402006, 402207, 402208)
          Code Deleted

C1004   Fast-cath, swartz, safl, csta, sept, ramp guiding introducer
          Code Deleted

C1005   Intraocular lens, sensar soft acrylic ultraviolet light
          absorbing posterior chamber intraocular lens
          Code Added

C1006   Intraocular lens, array multifocal silicone posterior
          chamber intraocular lens
          Code Deleted

C1007   Prosthesis, penile, ams 700 penile prosthesis, ams
          ambicor penile prosthesis, dura ii penile prosthesis, ams
          malleable 650 penile prosthesis. Note: only the ams
          ambicor penile prosthesis is effective October 1, 2000
          Code Deleted

C1008   Stent, urolume, cook harrison fetal bladder stent
          Code Deleted

C1009   Plasma, cryoprecipitate reduced, each unit
          Code Deleted

C1019   Platelet, leukoreduced, irradiated, apheresis/pheresis, each
          unit
          Code Deleted

C1024   Quinopristin/dalfopristin, 10ml, synercid iv
          Code Deleted

C1025   Catheter, marinr cs catheter
          Code Deleted

C1026   Catheter ablation, rf performr, 5f rf marinr
          Code Deleted

C1027   Stent, coronary, magic wallstent extra short or short coronary self-expanding stent with delivery system, radius 14mm self expanding stent with over the wire delivery system
Code Deleted

C1028   Sling fixation system for treatment of stress urinary incontinence, precision twist transvaginal anchor system, precision tack transvaginal anchor system, vesica press-in anchor system, capio cl (tvb/s) transvaginal suturing device
Code Deleted

C1029   Catheter, balloon dilatation, controlled radial expansion (cre) balloon dilatation catheter wire guided and fixed wire, quantum dilation balloon, ms classique balloon dilation catheter
Code Deleted

C1030   Catheter, balloon dilatation, marshal, blue max 20, ultra-thin diamond, ultra-thin balloon dilatation catheter, ultra-thin st balloon dilatation catheter, ultra-thin balloon dilatation catheter with glidex hydrophilic coated balloon, ultra-thin st balloon dilatation catheter with glidex hydrophilic coated balloon
Code Deleted

C1033   Catheter, imaging, sonicath ultra model 37-410 ultrasound imaging catheter, sonicath ultra 9 mhz ultrasound imaging catheter
Code Deleted

C1034   Catheter, coronary angioplasty, surpass superfusion catheter, long 30 surpass superfusion catheter
Code Deleted

C1035   Catheter, intracardiac echocardiography, ultra ice 6f, 12.5 Mhz catheter (with disposable sheath), ultra ice 9f, 9 mhz catheter (with disposable sheath)
Code Deleted

C1036   Port/reservoir, venous access device, vaxcel implantable vascular access system, r port premier vascular access system (model 45-100), bard port implanted port, bard rosenblatt lumen port, bard ultra low profile port, bardport titanium implanted port, bardport x-port implanted port, bardport m.R.I. Dual implanted port, bardport m.R.I. Hard-base implanted port
Code Deleted

C1037   Catheter, vaxcel chronic dialysis catheter, medcomp bio flex tesio catheter, medcomp silicone tesio catheter, medcomp hemo-cath long term silicone catheter, bard niagara dual lumen catheter, bard opti-flow dual lumen catheter, medcomp ash split catheter
Code Deleted

C1038   Catheter, imaging, ultracross 2.9F 30mhz coronary imaging catheter, ultracross 3.2F mhz coronary imaging catheter
Code Deleted

C1039   Stent, tracheobronchial, wallstent tracheobronchial endoprosthesis (covered), wallstent tracheobronchial endoprosthesis with permalume covering and unistep plus delivery system, wallstent rp tracheobronchial endoprosthesis with unistep plus delivery system note: only the wallstent rp tracheobronchial endoprosthesis with unistep plus delivery system is effective October 1, 2000. The wallstent tracheobronchial was effective August 1, 2000
Code Deleted

C1040   Stent, self-expandable for creation of intrahepatic shunts, wallstent transjugular intrahepatic portosystemic shunt (tips) with unistep plus delivery system (40/42/60/68mm in length), wallstent rp endoprosthesis with unistep plus delivery system (42/68mm in length) note: only the wallstent rp tips endoprosthesis with unistep plus delivery system is effective October 1, 2000. The wallstent tips endoprosthesis with unistep plus delivery system was effective August 1, 2000
Code Deleted

C1042   Stent, biliary, wallstent biliary endoprosthesis with unistep plus delivery system, wallstent biliary endoprosthesis with unistep delivery system (biliary stent and catheter), wallstent rp biliary endoprosthesis with unistep plus delivery system, ultraflex diamond biliary stent system, new microvasive biliary stent and delivery system note: only the wallstent rp biliary endoprosthesis with unistep plus delivery system is effective October 1, 2000. The wallstent, ultraflex diamond, new microvasive biliary stent systems were effective August 1, 2000
Code Deleted

C1043   Atherectomy system, coronary, rotablator rotalink atherectomy catheter and burr, rotablator rotalink rotational atherectomy system advancer and guide wire, atherocath-gto atherectomy catheter, interventional technologies transluminal extraction coronary (tec) atherectomy system
Code Deleted

C1045   Supply of radiopharmaceutical diagnostic imaging agent, I-131 mibg [iobenguane sulfate I-131], per 0.5 Mci
Code Deleted

C1047   Catheter, diagnostic, navi-star diagnostic deflectable tip catheter, noga-star diagnostic deflectable tip catheter
Code Deleted

C1048   Generator, bipolar pulse, cyberonics neurocybernetic prosthesis generator
Code Deleted

C1050   Protein a immunoadsorption, prosorba column
Code Deleted

C1051   Catheter, thrombectomy, oasis thrombectomy catheter, fogarty adherent clot catheter (4 fr, 5 fr, 6 fr), 6 fr thrombex pmt catheter (60cm, 120cm)
Code Deleted

C1053   Catheter, diagnostic, ensite 3000 catheter
Code Deleted

C1054   Catheter, thrombectomy, hydrolyser 6f mechanical thrombectomy catheter, hydrolyser 7f mechanical thrombectomy catheter
Code Deleted

C1055   Catheter, transesophageal 210 atrial pacing catheter, transesophageal 210-s atrial pacing catheter, flex-ez balloon dilator, ez resolution balloon dilator (models 3802, 3804, 3806)
Code Deleted

C1056   Catheter, gynecare thermachoice ii catheter, cook intrauterine insemination catheter, cook jansen-anderson insemination set, cook ob/gyn suprapubic balloons, cook urological o'brien suprapubic access set, cook urological suprapubic balloons, product health induct breast microcatheter, cook chorionic villus sampling set
Code Deleted

C1057   Tissue marker, 11-gauge micromark ii tissue marker
Code Deleted

C1058   Supply of radiopharmaceutical diagnostic imaging agent,
technetium tc 99m oxidronate, per vial
Code Added

C1059   Autologous cultured chondrocytes, implantation, carticel
Code Deleted

C1060   Stent, coronary, acs multi-link tristar coronary stent
system and delivery system, acs multi-link ultra coronary
stent system note: acs multi-link ultra is effective
01/01/01. Acs multi-link tristar was effective 08/01/00
Code Deleted

C1061   Catheter, coronary guide, acs viking guiding catheter,
cardima vueport balloon occlusion guiding catheter, merit
medical systems performa vessel sizing catheter, merit
medical systems pediatric/adult pigtail catheter
Code Deleted

C1063   Lead, defibrillator, endotak endurance ez, endotak
endurance rx, endotak endurance 0134, 0135, 0136 note:
endotak endurance is effective 01/01/01. Endotak
endurance ez and rx were effective 08/01/00
Code Deleted

C1064   Supply of radiopharmaceutical therapeutic imaging agent,
sodium iodide i-131, capsule, each additional mci
Code Added

C1065   Supply of radiopharmaceutical therapeutic imaging agent,
sodium iodide i-131, solution, each additional mci
Code Added

C1066   Supply of radiopharmaceutical diagnostic imaging agent,
indium 111 satumomab pendetide, per vial
Code Added

C1067   Stent, biliary, megalink biliary stent, palmaz balloon
expandable stent and delivery system, spiral z biliary
metal expandable stent, za biliary metal expandable stent,
wallstent transhepatic biliary endoprosthesis
Code Deleted

C1068   Pacemaker, dual chamber, pulsar ddd, unity vddr (model
292-07)
Code Deleted

C1069   Pacemaker, dual chamber, discovery dr
Code Deleted

C1071   Pacemaker, single chamber, pulsar max sr, pulsar sr, vigor ssi
Code Deleted

C1072   Catheter, balloon dilatation, coronary, rx esprit, rx gemini, rx solaris, otw photon, otw solaris
Code Deleted

C1073   Morcellator, laparoscopic, gynecare x-tract laparascopic morcellator
Code Deleted

C1074   Catheter, peripheral dilatation, rx viatrac 14 peripheral dilatation catheter, otw viatrac 18 peripheral dilatation catheter
Code Deleted

C1075   Lead, pacemaker, selute picotip, selute, sweet picotip rx, sweet tip rx, fineline, fineline ez, thinline, thinline ez
Code Deleted

C1076   Defibrillator, single chamber, automatic, implantable, ventak mini iv, ventak mini iv+ (models 1793, 1796), ventak mini iii he, ventak mini iii he+ (models 1788, 1789), ventak mini iii, ventak mini iii + (models 1783, 1786) note: only the ventak mini iv+, ventak mini iii he+ and ventak mini iii+ are effective 01/01/01. Ventak mini iv, ventak mini iii he, and ventak mini iii were effective 08/01/00
Code Deleted

C1077   Defibrillator, single chamber, automatic, implantable, ventak prizm vr, ventak vr
Code Deleted

C1078   Defibrillator, dual chamber, automatic, implantable, ventak prizm, ventak av iii dr
Code Deleted

C1079   Supply of radiopharmaceutical diagnostic imaging agent, cyanocobalamin co 57/58, per 0.5 microcurie
Description Changed

C1084   Denileukin diftitox, 300 mcg, ontak iv
Code Deleted

C1086 Temozolomide, 5 mg, temodar
Code Deleted

C1087 Supply of radiopharmaceutical diagnostic imaging agent, sodium iodide 1-123 per 100 microcuries
Description Changed

C1089 Supply of radiopharmaceutical diagnostic imaging agent, cyanocobalamin co 57, 0.5 mci, capsule
Code Deleted

C1090 Supply of radiopharmaceutical diagnostic imaging agent, indium in 111 chloride, per mci
Code Deleted

C1091 Supply of radiopharmaceutical diagnostic imaging agent, indium 111 oxyquinoline, per 0.5 millicurie
Description Changed

C1092 Supply of radiopharmaceutical diagnostic imaging agent, indium 111 pentetate, per 0.5 millicurie
Description Changed

C1094 Supply of radiopharmaceutical diagnostic imaging agent, technetium tc 99m albumin aggregated, per 10 millicurie
Description Changed

C1095 Supply of radiopharmaceutical diagnostic imaging agent, technetium tc 99m depreotide, per vial
Code Deleted

C1100 Guide wire, percutaneous transluminal coronary angioplasty, medtronic ave gt1 guide wire, medtronic ave gt2 fusion guide wire, interventional technologies trackwire, interventional technologies trackwire support, interventional technologies trackwire extra support
Code Deleted

C1101 Catheter, percutaneous transluminal coronary angioplasty guide, medtronic ave 5f, 6f, 7f, 8f, 9f zuma guide catheter, medtronic ave z2 5f, 6f, 7f, 8f, 9f zuma guide catheter, medtronic ave vector guide catheter, medtronic ave vector x guide catheter. Note: only the medtronic ave z2 zuma guide catheters are effective October 1, 2000. The medtronic ave zuma guide catheters were effective August 1, 2000
Code Deleted

C1102   Generator, pulse, neurostimulator, medtronic synergy
neurostimulator generator and extension
Code Deleted

C1103   Defibrillator, implantable, micro jewel, micro jewel ii
Code Deleted

C1104   Catheter, ablation, rf conductr mc 4mm, rf conductr mc
5mm (models 6042, 7544) note: rf conductr mc 5mm is
effective 01/01/01. Rf conductr mc 4mm was effective
08/01/00. Catheter, ablation, rf conductr mc--ext (with
stiffer tip) 07864447, 078754447
Code Deleted

C1105   Pacemaker, dual chamber, sigma 300 vdd
Code Deleted

C1106   Neurostimulator, patient programmer, synergy ez patient
programmer
Code Deleted

C1107   Catheter, diagnostic, electrophysiology, torqr, soloist,
dynamic xt decapolar catheter
Code Deleted

C1109   Anchor, implantable, mitek gii anchor, mitek knotless,
mitek tacit, mitek rotator cuff, mitek gls, mitek mini,
mitek fastin, mitek super, mitek panalok, mitek micro,
mitek panalok rc, mitek fastin rc, innovasive roc ez,
innovasive miniroc, innovasive bioroc, innovasive roc xs,
innovasive contack, biomet 3.5Mm cortical screw, biomet
4.5Mm cortical screw (fully threaded), biomet 6.5Mm
cancellous lag screw (32mm thread length), biomet
6.5Mm cannulated cancellous screw (20mm thread length)
Code Deleted

C1110   Catheter, diagnostic, electrophysiology, stable mapper
Code Deleted

C1111   Stent graft system, aneurx aorto-uniiliac-stent graft system
Code Deleted

C1112   Stent graft system, aneurx stent graft system
Code Deleted

C1113   Stent graft system, talent endoluminal spring stent graft
system
Code Deleted

C1114 Stent graft system, talent spring stent graft system
Code Deleted

C1115 Lead, pacemaker, 5038s, 5038, 5038l, 2188 coronary
sinus lead, 4057m, 4058m, 4557m, 4558m, 5058, 6416
pacemaker lead, innomedica sutureless myocardial
(models 4045, 4046, 4047, 4058), unipass (models
425-02, 425-04, 425-06)
Code Deleted

C1116 Lead, pacemaker, capsure sp novus, capsure sp, capsure,
excellence +, s+, ps+, capsure z novus, capsure z, impulse
Code Deleted

C1117 Endograft system, ancure endograft delivery system
Code Deleted

C1118 Pacemaker, dual chamber, sigma 300 dr, legacy ii dr,
legacy ii s
Code Deleted

C1119 Lead, defibrillator, sprint 6932, sprint 6943
Code Deleted

C1120 Lead, defibrillator, sprint 6942, sprint 6945
Code Deleted

C1121 Defibrillator, implantable, gem
Code Deleted

C1123 Defibrillator, implantable, gem ii vr, gem iii vr (model
7231)
Code Deleted

C1124 Lead, neurostimulator, kit, interstim test stimulation lead
kit
Code Deleted

C1125 Pacemaker, single chamber, kappa 400 sr, topaz ii sr,
topaz3/topaz sr (model 540)
Code Deleted

C1126 Pacemaker, dual chamber, kappa 700 dr (all models),
clarity dr (models 860, 862, 865), diamond 3/diamond dr
(model 840)
Code Deleted

C1127 Pacemaker, single chamber, kappa 700 sr, clarity sr
(models 560, 562, 565)
Code Deleted

C1128 Pacemaker, dual chamber, kappa 700 d, ruby ii d, ruby 3/ruby 3 d (model 740), vita 2 dr (model 830)
Code Deleted

C1129 Pacemaker, kappa 700 vdd
Code Deleted

C1130 Pacemaker, dual chamber, sigma 200 d, legacy ii d
Code Deleted

C1131 Pacemaker, dual chamber, sigma 200 dr
Code Deleted

C1132 Pacemaker, single chamber, sigma 200 sr, legacy ii sr
Code Deleted

C1133 Pacemaker, single chamber, sigma 300 sr, vita sr, vita 2 sr (model 530)
Code Deleted

C1134 Pacemaker, dual chamber, sigma 300 d
Code Deleted

C1135 Pacemaker, dual chamber, rate-responsive, entity dr 5326l, entity dr 5326r, entity dr 5326 note: only the entity dr 5326 is effective 01/01/01. Entity dr 5326l and 5326r were effective 08/01/00
Code Deleted

C1136 Pacemaker, dual chamber, rate-responsive, affinity dr 5330l, affinity dr 5330r, affinity dr 5330 note: only the affinity dr 5330 is effective 01/01/01. Affinity dr 5330l and 5330r were effective 08/01/00
Code Deleted

C1137 Septal defect implant system, cardioseal septal occlusion system, cardioseal occluder delivery catheter, aga medical amplatzer pfo occluder
Code Deleted

C1143 Pacemaker, dual chamber, addvent 2060bl, paragon iii (models 2314l, 2315 m/s)
Code Deleted

C1144 Pacemaker, single chamber, rate-responsive, affinity sr 5130, affinity sr 5130l, affinity sr 5130r, integrity sr 5142, integrity u sr 5136. Note: only the affinity sr 5130 is effective 01/01/01. Affinity sr 5130l, affinity sr 5130r, and integrity sr 5142 were effective 08/01/00
Code Deleted

C1145   Vascular closure device, angio-seal 6 french vascular closure device (model 610091), angio-seal 8 french vascular closure device (610089, 610097), angio-seal 6 fr ev vascular closure device, angio-seal 8 fr ev vascular closure device (models 610099, 610101). Note: model 610097 is effective 01/01/01. Models 610091 and 610089 were effective 08/01/00
Code Deleted

C1147   Lead, pacemaker, av plus dx 1368/52, av plus dx 1368/58, av plus dx 1368/65 note: the av plus dx 1368/65 is effective 01/01/01. Models 1368/52 and 1368/58 were effective 08/01/00
Code Deleted

C1148   Defibrillator, single chamber, implantable, contour md v-175, contour md v-175a, contour md v-175ac, contour md v-175b, contour md v-175c, contour md v-175d, contour ii (models v-185ac, v-185b, v-185c)
Code Deleted

C1149   Pacemaker, dual chamber, non-rate responsive, entity dc 5226r, entity dc 5226 note: model 5226 is effective 01/01/01. Model 5226r was effective 08/01/00
Code Deleted

C1151   Lead, pacemaker, passive plus dx 1343k/46, passive plus dx 1343k/52, passive plus dx 1345k/52, passive plus dx 1345k/58, passive plus dx 1336t/52, passive plus dx 1336t/58, passive plus dx 1342t/46, passive plus dx 1342t/52, passive plus dx 1346t/52, passive plus dx 1346t/58, passive plus tin (model 1242t)
Code Deleted

C1152   Access system, dialysis, lifesite access system
Code Deleted

C1153   Pacemaker, single chamber, regency sc+ 2402l
Code Deleted

C1154   Lead, defibrillator, spl sp01, sp02, spl sp04, 6721l, 6721m, 6721s, 6939 oval patch lead, capsure 4965, dp-3238, endotak dsp, transvene 6933, transvene 6937
Code Deleted

C1155   Repliform tissue regeneration matrix, per 8 square centimeters
Code Deleted

C1156 Pacemaker, single chamber, affinity sr 5131m/s, tempo vr 1102, trilogy sr+ 2260l, trilogy sr+ 2264l, solus ii (models 2006l, 2007 m/s)
Code Deleted

C1157 Pacemaker, dual chamber, trilogy dc+2318l, synchrony iii (models 2028l, 2029 m/s)
Code Deleted

C1158 Lead, defibrillator, tvl sv01, tvl sv02, tvl sv04
Code Deleted

C1159 Lead, defibrillator, tvl rv02, tvl rv06, tvl rv07
Code Deleted

C1160 Lead, defibrillator, tvl-adx 1559/65
Code Deleted

C1161 Lead, pacemaker, tendril dx 1388k/46, tendril dx 1388k/52, tendril dx 1388k/58, tendril dx 1388t/46, tendril dx 1388t/52, tendril dx 1388t/58, tendril dx 1388t/85, tendril dx 1388t/100, tendril dx 1388tc/46, tendril dx 1388tc/52, tendril dx 1388t/58
Code Deleted

C1162 Pacemaker, dual-chamber, affinity dr 5331 m/s, tempo dr 2102, trilogy dr+ 2360l, trilogy dr+ 2364l
Code Deleted

C1163 Lead, pacemaker, tendril sdx 1488t/46, tendril sdx 1488t/52, tendril sdx 1488t/58, tendril sdx 1488tc/46, tendril sdx 1488tc/52, tendril sdx 1488tc/58
Code Deleted

C1164 Brachytherapy seed, i-125 seed
Code Deleted

C1171 Site marker device, disposable, auto suture site marker device
Code Deleted

C1172 Balloon, tissue dissector, spacemaker tissue dissection balloon, spacemaker 1000cc hernia balloon dissector note: the hernia balloon dissector is effective 01/01/01. The spacemaker tissue dissection balloon is effective 08/01/00
Code Deleted

C1173   Stent, coronary, s540 over-the-wire coronary stent system, s670 with discrete technology over-the-wire coronary stent system, s670 with discrete technology rapid exchange coronary stent system
Code Deleted

C1174   Needle, brachytherapy, bard brachystar brachytherapy needle
Code Deleted

C1180   Pacemaker, single chamber, vigor sr
Code Deleted

C1181   Pacemaker, single chamber, meridian ssi
Code Deleted

C1182   Pacemaker, single chamber, pulsar ssi
Code Deleted

C1183   Pacemaker, single chamber, jade ii s, sigma 300 s, jade 3/jade 3s (model 340)
Code Deleted

C1184   Pacemaker, single chamber, sigma 200 s, sigma 100 s
Code Deleted

C1188   Supply of radiopharmaceutical therapeutic imaging agent, sodium iodide i-131, capsule, per initial 1-5 mci
Description Changed

C1203   Injection, visudyne (verteporfin)
Code Deleted

C1205   Supply of radiopharmaceutical diagnostic imaging agent, technetium tc 99m disofenin, per vial
Code Deleted

C1302   Lead, defibrillator, tvl sq01
Code Deleted

C1303   Lead, defibrillator, capsure fix 6940, capsure fix 4068-110
Code Deleted

C1304   Catheter, imaging, sonicath ultra model 37-416 ultrasound imaging catheter, sonicath ultra model 37-418 ultrasound imaging catheter
Code Deleted

C1306   Lead, neurostimulator, cyberonics neurocybernetic
        prosthesis lead, octad lead 3898-33/389861, on-point
        model 3987, pisces-quad plus model 3888, resume tl
        model 3986, pisces-quad model 3487a, resume ii model
        3587a, symmix lead 3982
        Code Deleted

C1311   Pacemaker, dual chamber, trilogy dr+/dao
        Code Deleted

C1312   Stent, coronary, magic wallstent mini coronary self
        expanding stent with delivery system
        Code Deleted

C1313   Stent, coronary, magic wallstent medium coronary self
        expanding stent with delivery system, radius 31mm self
        expanding stnet with over the wire delivery system
        Code Deleted

C1314   Stent, coronary, magic wallstent long coronary self
        expanding stent with delivery system
        Code Deleted

C1315   Pacemaker, dual chamber, vigor dr, meridian dr, vigor
        ddd, vista ddd
        Code Deleted

C1316   Pacemaker, dual chamber, meridian ddd
        Code Deleted

C1317   Pacemaker, single chamber, discovery sr
        Code Deleted

C1318   Pacemaker, single chamber, meridian sr
        Code Deleted

C1319   Stent, enteral, wallstent enteral endoprosthesis and
        unistep delivery system (60mm in length), enteral
        wallstent endoprosthesis and unistep plus delivery
        system/single-use colonic and duodenal endoprosthesis
        with unistep plus delivery system (60mm in length),
        esophageal z metal expandable stent with dua anti-reflux
        valve, esophageal z metal expandable stent with uncoated
        flanges, ultraflex esophageal stent system, wallstent
        esophageal prosthesis (double), wallstent esophageal
        prosthesis with delivery system, wilson-cook esophageal z
        metal expandable stent, bard memotherm esophageal
        stent. Note: only the enteral walsltent endoprosthesis and
        unistep plus delivery system is effective October 1, 2000.

The wallstent enteral endoprosthesis and unistep delivery system was effective August 1, 2000
Code Deleted

C1320   Stent, iliac, wallstent iliac endoprosthesis with unistep plus delivery system, wallstent rp iliac endoprosthesis with unistep plus delivery system note: only the wallstent rp iliac endoprosthesis with unistep plus delivery system is effective October 1, 2000. The wallstent iliac endoprosthesis with unistep plus delivery system was effective August 1, 2000
Code Deleted

C1325   Brachytherapy seed, palladium-103 seed
Code Deleted

C1326   Catheter, thrombectomy, angiojet rheolytic thrombectomy catheter
Code Deleted

C1328   External transmitter, neurostimulation system, ans renew spinal cord stimulator system
Code Deleted

C1333   Stent, biliary, palmaz corinthian transhepatic biliary stent and delivery system, cook oasis one action stent introductory system, cook z stent gianturco-rosch biliary design, cordis palmaz xl transhepatic biliary stent, large palmaz balloon expandable stent with delivery system
Code Deleted

C1334   Stent, coronary, palmaz-schatz crown stent, mini-crown stent, crossflex lc stent, cook gianturco-roubin flex-stent coronary stent
Code Deleted

C1335   Mesh, hernia, prolene polypropylene hernia system, prolene soft mesh (polypropylene), trelex natural mesh
Code Deleted

C1336   Infusion pump, implantable, non-programmable, constant flow implantable pump with bolus safety valve model 3000, model 3000-16 (16ml), model 3000-50 (50ml) note: constant flow implantable pump model 3000 was effective August 1, 2000. Models 3000-16 and 3000-50 are effective October 1, 2000
Code Deleted

C1337   Infusion pump, implantable, non-programmable, isomed infusion pump model 8472-20, 8472-35, 8472-60
Code Deleted

C1348   Supply of radiopharmaceutical therapeutic imaging agent, sodium iodide i-131, solution, per initial 1-6 mci
Description Changed

C1350   Brachytherapy, per source, prostaseed i-125
Code Deleted

C1351   Lead, pacemaker, capsurefix, surefix, pirouet +, s+
Code Deleted

C1352   Defibrillator, dual chamber, implantable, gem ii dr
Code Deleted

C1353   Neurostimulator, implantable, itrel ii/soletra implantable neurostimulator and extension, itrel iii implantable neurostimulator and extension, interstim neurostimulator (implantable) and extension, neurocontrol stim system
Code Deleted

C1354   Pacemaker, dual chamber, kappa 400 dr, diamond ii 820 dr
Code Deleted

C1355   Pacemaker, dual chamber, kappa 600 dr, vita dr
Code Deleted

C1356   Defibrillator, single chamber, implantable, profile md v-186hv3
Code Deleted

C1357   Defibrillator, single chamber, implantable, angstrom md v-190hv3
Code Deleted

C1358   Pacemaker, dual chamber, non-rate responsive, affinity dc 5230r, affinity dc 5230 note: model 5230 is effective 01/01/01. Model 5230r was effective 08/01/00
Code Deleted

C1359   Pacemaker, dual chamber, pulsar dr, pulsar max dr
Code Deleted

C1360   Ocular photodynamic therapy
Code Deleted

C1361   Recorder, cardiac event, implantable, reveal, reveal plus
Code Deleted

C1362   Stent, biliary, rx herculink 14 biliary stent, otw megalink
sds biliary stent
Code Deleted

C1363   Defibrillator, implantable, dual chamber, gem dr, gem iii
dr (model 7275)
Code Deleted

C1364   Defibrillator, dual chamber, photon dr v-230hv3
Code Deleted

C1365   Guide wire, peripheral, hi-torque spartacore 14 guide
wire, hi-torque memcore firm 14 guide wire, hi-torque
steelcore 18 guide wire, hi-torque steelcore 18 lt guide
wire, hi-torque supra core 35 guide wire, doc wire,
hi-torque extra balance, hi-torque extra s|port, hi-torque
extra support, hi-torque floppy ii, hi-torque intermediate,
hi-torque standard, hi-torque traverse, tad ii guide wire
system (145cm, 200cm, 260cm, 300cm), tad guide wire
system (145cm), wholey hi-torque modified j guide wire
system (145cm, 175cm, 260cm, 300cm), wholey
hi-torque floppy guide wire system (145cm, 175cm,
260cm), wholey hi-torque standard guide wire system
(145cm, 300cm), loc guide wire extension (115cm),
hobbs medical flex-ex guide wire (models 3406, 3408,
3410, 3412, 3413). Note: only the hi-torque steelcore 18
lt guide wire is effective October 1, 2000. The other
guide wires were effective August 1, 2000
Code Deleted

C1366   Guide wire, percutaneous transluminal coronary
angioplasty, hi-torque iron man, hi-torque balance
middleweight, hi-torque all star, hi-torque balance
heavyweight, hi-torque balance trek
Code Deleted

C1367   Guide wire, percutaneous transluminal coronary
angioplasty, hi-torque cross it, hi-torque cross-it 100xt,
hi-torque cross-it 200xt, hi-torque cross-it 300xt,
hi-torque wiggle
Code Deleted

C1369   Internal receiver, neurostimulation system, ans renew
spinal cord stimulator system, medtronic mattrix
receiver/transmitter
Code Deleted

C1370   Single use device for treatment of female stress urinary incontinence, tension-gree vaginal tape single use device
Code Deleted

C1371   Stent, biliary, symphony nitinol stent transhepatic biliary system, nir biliary stent system
Code Deleted

C1372   Stent, biliary, smart cordis nitinol stent and delivery system, cordis smart .018 Nitinol transhepatic biliary stent
Code Deleted

C1375   Stent, coronary, nir on ranger stent delivery system, nir w/sox stent system, nir primo premounted stent system
Code Deleted

C1376   Lead, neurostimulator, ans renew spinal cord stimulation system lead (with or without extension)
Code Deleted

C1377   Lead, neurostimulator, specify 3988 lead
Code Deleted

C1378   Lead, neurostimulator, inerstim therapy 3080 lead, interstim therapy 3886 lead
Code Deleted

C1379   Lead, neurostimulator, pisces-quad compact 3887 lead
Code Deleted

C1420   Anchor system, stapletac2 bone anchor system with dermis, stapletac2 bone anchor system with dermis, biosorb fx system
Code Deleted

C1421   Anchor system, stapletac2 bone anchor system without dermis
Code Deleted

C1450   Orthosphere spherical interpositional arthroplasty
Code Deleted

C1451   Orthosphere spherical interpositional arthroplasty kit
Code Deleted

C1500   Atherectomy system, peripheral, rotablator rotational angioplasty system with rotalink exchangeable catheter, advancer, and guide wire
Code Deleted

C1531   Stent, colorectal, Bard Memotherm colorectal stent model
S30R060
Code Added

C1700   Needle, brachytherapy, authentic mick tp brachytherapy
needle, cook urological brachytherapy needle
Code Deleted

C1701   Needle, brachytherapy, medtec mt-bt-5201-25
brachytherapy needle, avid medical metal hub pre-load
style brachytherapy seeding insertion needle, mick style
brachytherapy seeding insertion needle
Code Deleted

C1702   Needle, brachytherapy, wwmt brachytherapy needle,
nucletron pancreas flexible brachytherapy needle
Code Deleted

C1703   Needle, brachytherapy, mentor prostate brachytherapy
needle
Code Deleted

C1704   Needle, brachytherapy, medtec mt-bt-5001-25,
mt-bt-5051-25
Code Deleted

C1705   Needle, brachytherapy, best flexi needle brachytherapy
seed implantation (13g, 14g, 15g, 16g, 17g, 18g), best
industries prostate brachytherapy needle, nycomed
amersham mick applicator style brachytherapy needle,
nycomed amersham brachytherapy needle
Code Deleted

C1706   Needle, brachytherapy, indigo prostate seeding needle
Code Deleted

C1707   Needle, brachytherapy, varisource interstitial implant
needle
Code Deleted

C1708   Needle, brachytherapy, uromed prostate seeding needle
Code Deleted

C1709   Needle, brachytherapy, remington medical brachytherapy
needle
Code Deleted

C1710   Needle, brachytherapy, us biopsy prostate seeding needle
Code Deleted

C1711   Needle, brachytherapy, md tech p.S.S. Prostate seeding
set (needle)
Code Deleted

C1712   Needle, brachytherapy, imagyn medical technologies
isostar prostate brachytherapy needle
Code Deleted

C1713   Anchor/screw for opposing bone-to-bone or soft
tissue-to-bone (implantable)
Code Added

C1714   Catheter, transluminal atherectomy, directional
Code Added

C1715   Brachytherapy needle
Code Added

C1716   Brachytherapy seed, gold 198
Code Added

C1717   Brachytherapy seed, high dose rate iridium 192
Code Added

C1718   Brachytherapy seed, iodine 125
Code Added

C1719   Brachytherapy seed, non-high dose rate iridium 192
Code Added

C1720   Brachytherapy seed, palladium 103
Code Added

C1721   Cardioverter-defibrillator, dual chamber (implantable)
Code Added

C1722   Cardioverter-defibrillator, single chamber (implantable)
Code Added

C1723   Catheter, ablation, non-cardiac
Code Deleted

C1724   Catheter, transluminal atherectomy, rotational
Code Added

C1725   Catheter, transluminal angioplasty, non-laser (may include
guidance, infusion/perfusion capability)
Code Added

C1726   Catheter, balloon dilatation, non-vascular
Code Added

C1727   Catheter, balloon tissue dissector, non-vascular (insertable)
Code Added

C1728   Catheter, brachytherapy seed administration
Code Added

C1729   Catheter, drainage
Code Added

C1730   Catheter, electrophysiology, diagnostic, other than 3D mapping (19 or fewer electrodes)
Code Added

C1731   Catheter, electrophysiology, diagnostic, other than 3D mapping (20 or more electrodes)
Code Added

C1732   Catheter, electrophysiology, diagnostic/ablation, 3D or vector mapping
Code Added

C1733   Catheter, electrophysiology, diagnostic/ablation, other than 3D or vector mapping, other than cool-tip
Code Added

C1750   Catheter, hemodialysis, long-term
Code Added

C1751   Catheter, infusion, inserted peripherally, centrally or midline (other than hemodialysis)
Code Added

C1752   Catheter, hemodialysis, short-term
Code Added

C1753   Catheter, intravascular ultrasound
Code Added

C1754   Catheter, intradiscal
Code Added

C1755   Catheter, intraspinal
Code Added

C1756   Catheter, pacing, transesophageal
Code Added

C1757   Catheter, thrombectomy/embolectomy
Code Added

C1758   Catheter, ureteral
Code Added

C1759   Catheter, intracardiac echocardiography
Code Added

C1760   Closure device, vascular (implantable/insertable)
Code Added

C1762   Connective tissue, human (includes fascia lata)
Code Added

C1763   Connective tissue, non-human (includes synthetic)
Code Added

C1764   Event recorder, cardiac (implantable)
Code Added

C1765   Adhesion barrier
Code Added

C1766   Introducer/sheath, guiding, intracardiac
electrophysiological, steerable, other than peel-away
Code Added

C1767   Generator, neurostimulator (implantable)
Code Added

C1768   Graft, vascular
Code Added

C1769   Guide wire
Code Added

C1770   Imaging coil, magnetic resonance (insertable)
Code Added

C1771   Repair device, urinary, incontinence, with sling graft
Code Added

C1772   Infusion pump, programmable (implantable)
Code Added

C1773   Retrieval device, insertable (used to retrieve fractured
medical devices)
Code Added

C1776   Joint device (implantable)
Code Added

C1777   Lead, cardioverter-defibrillator, endocardial single coil (implantable)
Code Added

C1778   Lead, neurostimulator (implantable)
Code Added

C1779   Lead, pacemaker, transvenous vdd single pass
Code Added

C1780   Lens, intraocular (new technology)
Code Added

C1781   Mesh (implantable)
Code Added

C1782   Morcellator
Code Added

C1784   Ocular device, intraoperative, detached retina
Code Added

C1785   Pacemaker, dual chamber, rate-responsive (implantable)
Code Added

C1786   Pacemaker, single chamber, rate-responsive (implantable)
Code Added

C1787   Patient programmer, neurostimulator
Code Added

C1788   Port, indwelling (implantable)
Code Added

C1789   Prosthesis, breast (implantable)
Code Added

C1790   Brachytherapy seed, nucletron iridium 192 hdr, mds nordion therasphere (yttrium-90) brachytherapy seed, mds nordion gamma med iridium-192 hdr brachytherapy seed
Code Deleted

C1791   Brachytherapy seed, nycomed amersham i-125 (oncoseed, rapid strand)
Code Deleted

C1792   Brachytherapy seed, uromed symmetra i-125
Code Deleted

C1793   Brachytherapy seed, bard intersource-103 palladium seed 1031l, 1031c, international brachytherapy intersource-103 (palladium 103)
Code Deleted

C1794   Brachytherapy seed, bard isoseed 103 palladium seed pd3s111l, pd3s111p
Code Deleted

C1795   Brachytherapy seed, bard brachysource-125 iodine seed 1251l, 1251c, international brachytherapy intersource-125
Code Deleted

C1796   Brachytherapy seed, source tech medical i-125 seed model stm 1251
Code Deleted

C1797   Brachytherapy seed, draximage i-125 seed model ls-1
Code Deleted

C1798   Brachytherapy seed, syncor i-125 pharmaseed model bt-125-1
Code Deleted

C1799   Brachytherapy seed, i-plant iodine 125 model 3500
Code Deleted

C1800   Brachytherapy seed, mentor pdgold pd-103
Code Deleted

C1801   Brachytherapy seed, mentor iogold i-125
Code Deleted

C1802   Brachytherapy seed, best iridium 192, best dummy ribbon brachytherapy seed (model 3 dr, 4 dr series)
Code Deleted

C1803   Brachytherapy seed, best industries iodine 125
Code Deleted

C1804   Brachytherapy seed, best industries palladium 103
Code Deleted

C1805   Brachytherapy seed, imagyn isostar iodine-125 interstitial brachytherapy seed
Code Deleted

C1806   Brachytherapy seed, best industries gold 198
Code Deleted

C1810   Catheter, balloon dilatation, d114s over-the-wire balloon
        dilatation catheter
        Code Deleted

C1811   Anchor, surgical dynamics anchorsew, surgical dynamics
        s.D. Sorb ez tac, surgical dynamics s.D. Sorb suture
        anchor 2.0Mm, surgical dynamics s.D. Sorb suture
        anchor 3.0Mm, biomet bone mulch screw, biomet
        washerloc screw and washerloc washer, wright medical
        technology hammertoe implant (swanson type) weil
        design, wright medical technology swanson titanium great
        toe implant, wright medical technology sta - peg (subtalar
        arthrosis implant - smith design), wright medical
        technology spin snap-off screw, wright medical
        technology bold cannulated titanium compression screw,
        wright medical technology i.C.O.S. Ideal compression
        screw, wright medical technology swanson finger joint
        implant with grommets, wright medical technology
        swanson basal thumb implant, wright medical technology
        swanson titanium carpal scaphoid implant, wright medical
        technology swanson trapezium implant, biomet becton
        colles| fracture plate, biomet repicci ii unicondylar knee
        sytem, wright medical technology osteoset bone graft
        substitute (5cc, 10cc, 20cc, 50cc), wright medical
        technology uni-clip compression staple
        Code Deleted

C1812   Anchor, obl 2.0Mm mini tac achor, obl 2.8Mm hs
        anchor, obl 2.8Mm s anchor, obl 3.5Mm ti anchor, obl
        rc5 anchor, obl prc5 anchor, arthrex anterior cruciate
        ligament (acl) avulsion lag screw with sheath, arthrex
        chrondral dart, arthrex bio-absorbable corkscrew, arthrex
        bio-fastak suture anchor, arthrex headed bio-absorbable
        corkscrew, arthrex bio-interference screw, arthrex
        cannulated interference screw, arthrex suture anchor
        screw, arthrex fastak suture anchor, arthrex parachute
        corkscrew anchor, arthrex tissuetak, bionx bankart tack
        plla implant, bionx cannulated smartscrew plla implant,
        bionx contour labral nail plla implant, bionx smartnail
        plla implant, bionx smartscrew plla implant, bionx
        smartpin plla and pga implant, bionx wedge pla implant,
        bionx biocuff pla implant, bionx meniscus arrow pla
        implant, bionx smartscrew acl interference screw pla
        implant, depuy neuflex pip finger, medtronic xomed
        epidisc otologic lamina (model 14-17000)
        Code Deleted

C1813   Prosthesis, penile, inflatable
        Code Added

C1815   Prosthesis, urinary sphincter (implantable)
Code Added

C1816   Receiver and/or transmitter, neurostimulator (implantable)
Code Added

C1817   Septal defect implant system, intracardiac
Code Added

C1850   Repliform tissue regeneration matrix, per 14 or 21 square
centimeters
Code Deleted

C1851   Repliform tissue regeneration matrix, per 24 or 28 square
centimeters
Code Deleted

C1852   Transcyte, per 247 square centimeters
Code Deleted

C1853   Suspend tutoplast processed fascia lata, per 8 or 14
square centimeters
Code Deleted

C1854   Suspend tutoplast processed fascia lata, per 24 or 28
square centimeters
Code Deleted

C1855   Suspend tutoplast processed fascia lata, per 36 square
centimeters
Code Deleted

C1856   Suspend tutoplast processed fascia lata, per 48 square
centimeters
Code Deleted

C1857   Suspend tutoplast processed fascia lata, per 84 square
centimeters
Code Deleted

C1858   Duraderm acellular allograft, per 8 or 14 square
centimeters
Code Deleted

C1859   Duraderm acellular allograft, per 21, 24, or 28 square
centimeters
Code Deleted

C1860   Duraderm acellular allograft, per 48 square centimeters
Code Deleted

C1861 Duraderm acellular allograft, per 36 square centimeters
Code Deleted

C1862 Duraderm acellular allograft, per 72 square centimeters
Code Deleted

C1863 Duraderm acellular allograft, per 84 square centimeters
Code Deleted

C1864 Bard sperma tex mesh, per 13.44 Square centimeters
Code Deleted

C1865 Bard faslata allograft tissue, per 8 or 14 square centimeters
Code Deleted

C1866 Bard faslata allograft tissue, per 24 or 28 square centimeters
Code Deleted

C1867 Bard faslata allograft tissue, per 36 or 48 square centimeters
Code Deleted

C1868 Bard faslata allograft tissue, per 96 square centimeters
Code Deleted

C1869 Gore thyroplasty device, per 8, 12, 30, or 37.5 Square centimeters (0.6Mm)
Code Deleted

C1870 Dermmatrix surgical mesh, per 16 square centimeters
Code Deleted

C1871 Dermmatrix surgical mesh, per 32 or 64 square centimeters
Code Deleted

C1872 Dermagraft, per 37.5 Square centimeters
Code Deleted

C1873 Bard 3dmax mesh, medium or large size
Code Deleted

C1874 Stent, coated/covered, with delivery system
Code Added

C1875 Stent, coated/covered, without delivery system
Code Added

C1876 Stent, non-coated/non-covered, with delivery system
Code Added

C1877 Stent, non-coated/non-covered, without delivery system
Code Added

C1878 Material for vocal cord medialization, synthetic
(implantable)
Code Added

C1879 Tissue marker (implantable)
Code Added

C1880 Vena cava filter
Code Added

C1881 Dialysis access system (implantable)
Code Added

C1882 Cardioverter-defibrillator, other than single or dual
chamber (implantable)
Code Added

C1883 Adaptor/extension, pacing lead or neurostimulator lead
(implantable)
Code Added

C1885 Catheter, transluminal angioplasty, laser
Code Added

C1887 Catheter, guiding (may include infusion/perfusion
capability)
Code Added

C1891 Infusion pump, non-programmable, permanent
(implantable)
Code Added

C1892 Introducer/sheath, guiding, intracardiac
electrophysiological, fixed-curve, peel-away
Code Added

C1893 Introducer/sheath, guiding, intracardiac
electrophysiological, fixed-curve, other than peel-away
Code Added

C1894 Introducer/sheath, other than guiding, intracardiac
electrophysiological, non-laser
Code Added

C1895 Lead, cardioverter-defibrillator, endocardial dual coil (implantable)
Code Added

C1896 Lead, cardioverter-defibrillator, other than endocardial single or dual coil (implantable)
Code Added

C1897 Lead, neurostimulator test kit (implantable)
Code Added

C1898 Lead, pacemaker, other than transvenous vdd single pass
Code Added

C1899 Lead, pacemaker/cardioverter-defibrillator combination (implantable)
Code Added

C1929 Catheter, maverick monorail ptca catheter, maverick over-the-wire ptca catheter
Code Deleted

C1930 Catheter, percutaneous transluminal coronary angioplasty, coyote dilatation catheter 20mm/30mm/40mm
Code Deleted

C1931 Catheter, talon balloon dilatation catheter
Code Deleted

C1932 Catheter, scimed remedy coronary balloon dilatation infusion catheter (20mm), dispatch coronary infusion catheter, ultra fuse 4mm, ultra fuse 8mm, ultra fuse-x, angiodynamics pulse spray infusion catheter, angiodynamics unifuse infusion catheter, cordis commodore temporary occlusion balloon catheter, cordis rapidtransit infusion catheter, cordis regatta flow guided infusion catheter, cordis prowler plus microcatheter, cordis prowler small profile infusion microcatheter, cordis plus microcatheter, cordis masstransit max id microcatheter, cordis transit microcatheter, merit medical systems mistique infusion catheter
Code Deleted

C1933 Catheter, opti-plast centurion 5.5F pta catheter (shaft length 50 cm to 120 cm), opti-plast xl 5.5F pta catheter (shaft length 75 cm to 120 cm), opti-plast pta catheter (5.5 Fr), tru trac 5fr percutaneous transluminal angioplasty balloon dilatation catheter, optiplast xt 5 fr

percutaneous transluminal angioplasty catheter (various sizes)
Code Deleted

C1934   Catheter, ultraverse 3.5F balloon dilatation catheter, interventional technologies cutting balloon
Code Deleted

C1935   Catheter, workhorse pta balloon catheter
Code Deleted

C1936   Catheter, uromax ultra high pressure balloon dilatation catheter with hydroplus coating, urethramax high pressure urethral balloon dilatation catheter, carson zero tip balloon dilatation catheters with hydroplus coating, passport balloon on a wire dilatation catheters with hydroplus coating, tandem thin-shaft transureteroscopic balloon dilatation catheter with hydroplus coating, trilogy low profile balloon dilatation catheters with hydroplus coating, ureteral dilators with hydroplus coating and procedural sheath, amplatz renal dilator set
Code Deleted

C1937   Catheter, synergy balloon dilatation catheter, explorer st (6 fr), explorer 360 jr., Explorer 360, explorer st, symmetry small vessel balloon dilatation catheter with glidex hydrophilic coating, symmetry stiff shaft small vessel balloon dilatation catheter with glidex hydrophilic coating, xxl large balloon dilatation catheter
Code Deleted

C1938   Catheter, bard uroforce balloon dilatation catheter, cook urological urodynamic catheter
Code Deleted

C1939   Catheter, ninja ptca dilatation catheter, raptor ptca dilatation catheter, nc raptor ptca dilatation catheter, charger ptca dilatation catheter, titan ptca dilatation catheter, titan mega ptca dilatation catheter note: only the nc raptor, charger, titan, and titan mega ptca dilatation catheters are effective 01/01/01. The ninja and raptor ptca dilatation catheters were effective 10/01/00
Code Deleted

C1940   Catheter, cordis powerflex extreme pta balloon catheter, cordis powerflex plus pta balloon catheter, cordis opta lp pta balloon catheter, cordis opta 5 pta balloon catheter, cordis powerflex p3 pta balloon catheter
Code Deleted

C1941   Catheter, jupiter pta balloon dilatation catheter, cordis
          opta propta dilatation catheter, cordis slalom pta
          dilatation catheter
          Code Deleted

C1942   Catheter, cordis maxi ld pta balloon catheter
          Code Deleted

C1943   Catheter, rx crosssail coronary dilatation catheter, otw
          opensail coronary dilatation catheter
          Code Deleted

C1944   Catheter, rapid exchange single-use biliary balloon
          dilatation catheter, maxforce single-use biliary balloon
          dilatation catheter
          Code Deleted

C1945   Catheter, cordis savvy pta dilatation catheter
          Code Deleted

C1946   Catheter, r1s rapid exchange pre-dilatation balloon catheter
          Code Deleted

C1947   Catheter, gazelle balloon dilatation catheter
          Code Deleted

C1948   Catheter, pursuit balloon angioplasty catheter, cook accent
          balloon angioplasty catheter
          Code Deleted

C1949   Catheter, endosonics oracle megasonics five-64 f/x ptca
          catheter
          Code Deleted

C1979   Catheter, endosonics visions pv 8.2F intravascular
          ultrasound imaging catheter, endosonics avanar f/x
          intravascular ultrasound imaging catheter
          Code Deleted

C1980   Catheter, atlantis sr coronary imaging catheter
          Code Deleted

C1981   Catheter ,coronary angioplasty balloon, adante, bonnie,
          bonnie 15mm, bonnie monorail 30mm or 40mm, bonnie
          sliding rail, bypass speedy, chubby, chubby sliding rail,
          coyote 20mm, coyote 9/15/25mm, maxxum, nc ranger, nc
          ranger 9mm, ranger 20mm, long ranger 30mm or 40mm,
          nc ranger 16/18mm, nc ranger 22/25/30mm, nc big
          ranger, quantum ranger, quantum ranger 1/4 sizes,
          quantum ranger 9/16/18mm, quantum ranger 22/30mm,

quantum ranger 25mm, ranger lp 20/30/40, viva/long viva, ace - 1cm, ace - 2cm, ace graft, long ace, pivot cobra (10, 14, 18, 30, 40mm in lengths) note: only the bonnie monorail 30mm or 40mm, long ranger 30mm or 40mm, and ranger 20mm are effective 01/01/01. The other catheters were effective 08/01/00
Code Deleted

C2000 Catheter, orbiter st steerable electrode catheter
Code Deleted

C2001 Catheter, constellation diagnostic catheter
Code Deleted

C2002 Catheter, irvine inquiry steerable electrophysiology 5f catheter, livewire steerable electrophysiology catheter, livewire ep catheter, 7 fr duo-decapolar (model 401932), marinr rf marinr mc
Code Deleted

C2003 Catheter, irvine inquiry steerable electrophysiology 6f catheter
Code Deleted

C2004 Catheter, electrophysiology, biosense webster deflectable tip electrophysiology catheter
Code Deleted

C2005 Catheter, electrophysiology, ep deflectable tip catheter (hexapolar small anatomy models only)
Code Deleted

C2006 Catheter, electrophysiology, ep deflectable tip catheter (decapolar small anatomy models only)
Code Deleted

C2007 Catheter, electrophysiology, irvine luma-cath 6f fixed curve electrophysiology catheter, ibi-1000 inquiry fixed curve ep catheter (5 fr), ibi-1000 inquiry fixed curve ep catheter (6 fr, bipolar), ibi-1000 inquiry fixed curve ep catheter (6 fr, decapolar), ibi-1000 inquiry fixed curve ep catheter (6 fr, octapolar), ibi-1000 inquiry fixed curve ep catheter (6 fr, quadrapolar), santoro fixed curve catheter, ismus cath deflectable 20-pole catheter/crista cath ii deflectable 20-pole catheter
Code Deleted

C2008   Catheter, electrophysiology, irvine luma-cath 7f steerable electrophysiology catheter model 81910, model 81912, model 81915
Code Deleted

C2009   Catheter, electrophysiology, irvine luma-cath 7f steerable electrophysiology catheter model 81920
Code Deleted

C2010   Catheter, diagnostic, electrophysiology, response fixed curve catheter, supreme fixed curve catheter, torqr cs, biosense webster fixed curve diagnostic electrophysiology catheter
Code Deleted

C2011   Catheter, electrophysiology, deflectable tip catheter (quadrapolar small anatomy models only)
Code Deleted

C2012   Catheter, ablation, biosense webster celsius braided tip ablation catheter, biosense webster celsius 5mm temperature ablation catheter, biosense webster celsius temperature sensing diagnostic/ablation tip catheter, biosense webster celsius long reach ablation catheter note: only the celsius long reach ablaiton catheter is effective 01/01/01. The other ablation catheters were effective 10/01/00
Code Deleted

C2013   Catheter, ablation, biosense webster celsius large dome ablation catheter
Code Deleted

C2014   Catheter, ablation, biosense webster celsius ii asymmetrical ablation catheter
Code Deleted

C2015   Catheter, ablation, biosense webster celsius ii symmetrical ablation catheter
Code Deleted

C2016   Catheter, ablation, navi-star ds diagnostic/ablation catheter, navi-star thermo-cool temperature diagnostic/ablation catheter
Code Deleted

C2017   Catheter, ablation, navi-star diagnostic/ablation deflectable tip catheter
Code Deleted

C2018   Catheter, ablation, polaris t ablation catheter, meca ablation catheter, steerocath-a, steerocath-t, polaris le (7 fr), polaris dx
Code Deleted

C2019   Catheter, ep medsystems deflectable electrophysiology catheter, ep medsystems non-deflectable platinum electrophysiology catheter, cardima naviport deflectable tip guiding catheter, cardima venaport guiding catheter
Code Deleted

C2020   Catheter, ablation, blazer ii xp, blazer ii 6f, blazer ii high torque distal (htd), blazer ii (7 fr)
Code Deleted

C2021   Catheter, ep medsystems silverflex electrophysiology catheter, non-deflectable
Code Deleted

C2022   Catheter, ablation, cardiac pathways chilli cooled ablation catheter models 41422, 41442, 45422, 45442, 43422, 43442
Code Deleted

C2023   Catheter, ablation, cardiac pathways chilli cooled ablation catheter, standard curve 3005 or large curve 3006
Code Deleted

C2100   Catheter, electrophysiology, cardiac pathways cs reference catheter, boston scientific special procedure steero dx octa, boston scientific map pacing catheter
Code Deleted

C2101   Catheter, electrophysiology, cardiac pathways rv reference catheter, boston scientific ept-dx steerable
Code Deleted

C2102   Catheter, electrophysiology, cardiac pathways 7f radii catheter
Code Deleted

C2103   Catheter, electrophysiology, cardiac pathways 7f radii catheter with tracking, boston scientific valve mapper steerodx
Code Deleted

C2104   Catheter, electrophysiology, lasso deflectable circular tip mapping catheter, cardima tracer over-the-wire mapping microcatheter, cardima pathfinder microcatheter, cardima revelation microcatheter
Code Deleted

C2151   Catheter, veripath peripheral guiding catheter
Code Deleted

C2152   Catheter, cordis 5f, 6f, 7f, 8f, 9f, 10f vista brite tip guiding catheter, cordis 0.056 Vista brite tip guiding catheter (5 fr), cordis vista brite tip ig introducer guiding catheter (7 fr), cordis vista brite tip ig introducer guiding catheter (8 fr), cordis vista brite tip supra-aortic guiding catheter (8 fr), cordis vista brite tip supra-aortic guiding catheter (9 fr), cordis envoy large lumen guiding catheter (5 fr), cordis envoy large lumen guiding catheter (6 fr)
Code Deleted

C2153   Catheter, electrophysiology, bard viking fixed curve catheter (bipolar, quadrapolar, and asp models only)
Code Deleted

C2200   Catheter, arrow-trerotola percutaneous thrombolytic device catheter
Code Deleted

C2300   Catheter, varisource standard catheter, nucletron nasopharyngeal brachytherapy catheter
Code Deleted

C2597   Clinicath peripherally inserted midline catheter (picc) dual-lumen polyflow polyurethane catheter 18g (includes catheter and introducer), clinicath peripherally inserted central catheter (picc) dual-lumen polyflow polyurethane 16g/18g (includes catheter and introducer), clinicath peripherally inserted central catheter (picc) single-lumen polyflow polyurethane 16g (includes catheter and introducer), bd first midcath catheter (3 fr, 4 fr, 5 fr, 20cm/4 fr, 20cm/5 fr), dual lumen silicone midline catheter, dual lumen silicone midline catheter (5 fr/5fr, 20 cm), bdl single-lumen polyurethane picc, bdl single-lumen polyurethane midline catheter (catheter and introducer only), bard per-q-cath, bard per-q-cath plus, bard radpicc, bard groshong peripherally inserted central catheter (picc), ethicon endo-surgery 18g/20g single lumen biovue midline catheter starter set (catheter and introducer only), ethicon endo-surgery 18g dual lumen

biovue midline catheter starter set (catheter and introducer only)
Code Deleted

C2598   Catheter, clinicath peripherally inserted central catheter (picc) single-lumen polyflow polyurethane catheter 18g/20g/24g (catheter and introducer), clinicath peripherally inserted midline catheter (picc) single-lumen polyflow polyurethane catheter 20g/24g (catheter and introducer), bd first picc catheter, 5fr dual lumen silicone picc (catheter and introducer only), bdl 16g/18g/20g dual lumen cath catheter (catheter and introducer only)
Code Deleted

C2599   Clinicath peripherally inserted central catheter (picc) single-lumen polyflow polyurethane catheter 16g/18g/19g (includes catheter and introducer), bd first picc catheter, 1.9 Fr, 2.8 Fr, 3 fr, 4 fr, 5 fr single-lumen silicone picc (catheter and introducer only), boston scientific vaxcel peripherally inserted central catheter (picc), cook peripherally inserted central venous catheter, ethicon endo-surgery 18g/20g/24g single lumen biovue peripherally inserted central catheter starter set (catheter and introducer only), ethicon endo-surgery 16g/18g dual lumen biovue peripherally inserted central catheter starter set (catheter and introducer only)
Code Deleted

C2601   Catheter, bard dual lumen ureteral catheter, cook urological ureteral dilatation balloon, flexima ureteral catheter, axxcess ureteral catheter (6 fr), c-flex ureteral catheter, boston scientific dual lumen ureteral catheter
Code Deleted

C2602   Catheter, spectranetics 1.4/1.7Mm vitesse concentric laser catheter, spectranetics 0.9 Mm vitesse c concentric laser catheter (model 110-003)
Code Deleted

C2603   Catheter, spectranetics 2.0Mm vitesse cos concentric laser catheter
Code Deleted

C2604   Catheter, spectranetics 2.0Mm vitesse e eccentric laser catheter
Code Deleted

C2605   Catheter, spectranetics extreme laser catheter, spectranetics extreme 0.9Mm coronary angioplasty catheter (model 110-001)
Code Deleted

C2606   Catheter, oratec spinecath xl intradiscal catheter
Code Deleted

C2607   Catheter, oratec spinecath intradiscal catheter
Code Deleted

C2608   Catheter, scimed 6f wiseguide guide catheter, cyber guide catheter, merit medical systems trax interventional guide catheter (7 fr), merit medical systems trax cavern interventional guide catheter (8 fr), mighty max guide catheter (7 fr), triguide-flex guide catheter (10 fr)
Code Deleted

C2609   Catheter, flexima biliary drainage catheter with locking pigtail, flexima biliary drainage catheter with twist loc hub, flexima bilary drainage catheters with temp tip
Code Deleted

C2610   Catheter, arrow flex tip plus intraspinal catheter kit
Code Deleted

C2611   Catheter, medtronic ps medical algoline intraspinal catheter system/kit 81102, 81192
Code Deleted

C2612   Catheter, medtronic indura intraspinal catheter, myelotec video guided catheter, ebi vuecath steerable spinal catheter, synchromed vascular catheter (models 8702, 8700a, 8700v)
Code Deleted

C2615   Sealant, pulmonary, liquid
Code Added

C2616   Brachytherapy seed, yttrium-90
Code Added

C2617   Stent, non-coronary, temporary, without delivery system
Code Added

C2618   Probe, cryoablation
Code Added

C2619   Pacemaker, dual chamber, non rate-responsive
(implantable)
Code Added

C2620   Pacemaker, single chamber, non rate-responsive
(implantable)
Code Added

C2621   Pacemaker, other than single or dual chamber
(implantable)
Code Added

C2622   Prosthesis, penile, non-inflatable
Code Added

C2625   Stent, non-coronary, temporary, with delivery system
Code Added

C2626   Infusion pump, non-programmable, temporary
(implantable)
Code Added

C2627   Catheter, suprapubic/cystoscopic
Code Added

C2628   Catheter, occlusion
Code Added

C2629   Introducer/sheath, other than guiding, intracardiac
electrophysiological, laser
Code Added

C2630   Catheter, electrophysiology, diagnostic/ablation, other than
3D or vector mapping, cool-tip
Code Added

C2631   Repair device, urinary, incontinence, without sling graft
Code Added

C2676   Catheter, response cv catheter
Code Deleted

C2700   Defibrillator, single chamber, implantable, mycrophylax
plus
Code Deleted

C2701   Defibrillator, single chamber, implantable, phylax xm
Code Deleted

C2702 Defibrillator, single chamber, implantable, ventak prizm 2 vr 1860
Code Deleted

C2703 Defibrillator, single chamber, implantable, ventak prizm vr he 1857, 1858
Code Deleted

C2704 Defibrillator, single chamber, implantable, ventak mini iv+ 1793, 1796
Code Deleted

C2801 Defibrillator, dual chamber, implantable, ela medical defender iv dr model 612
Code Deleted

C2802 Defibrillator, dual chamber, implantable, phylax av
Code Deleted

C2803 Defibrillator, dual chamber, implantable, ventak prizm dr he models 1853, 1858, biotronik tachos dr
Code Deleted

C2804 Defibrillator, dual chamber, implantable, ventak prizm 2 dr 1861
Code Deleted

C2805 Defibrillator, dual chamber, implantable, jewel af 7250
Code Deleted

C2806 Defibrillator, implantable, gem vr 7227
Code Deleted

C2807 Defibrillator, implantable, contak cd 1823
Code Deleted

C2808 Defibrillator, implantable, contak tr 1241
Code Deleted

C3001 Lead, defibrillator, implantable, kainox sl, kainox rv
Code Deleted

C3002 Lead, defibrillator, implantable, easytrak 4510, 4511, 4512, 4513
Code Deleted

C3003   Lead, defibrillator, implantable, endotak sq array xp (model 0085), endotak sq array (models 0048, 0049), endotak sq patch (models 0047, 0063) endotak reliance (models 0147, 0148, 0149, s-0127, s-0128, s-0129)
Code Deleted

C3004   Lead, defibrillator, implantable, intervene 497-23, 497-24
Code Deleted

C3400   Prosthesis, breast, mentor saline-filled contour profile, mentor siltex spectrum mammary prosthesis, mentor siltex gel-filled mammary prosthesis, smooth-surface gel-filled mammary prosthesis, mcghan biodimensional anatomical tissue expander saline-filled (biospan textured, style 133, 133fv, 133mv, 133lv), mentor tissue expander, mentor contour profile tissue expander, mentor siltex becker expander/mammary prosthesis
Code Deleted

C3401   Prosthesis, breast, mentor saline-filled spectrum, mcghan biocurve round, biocell textured, saline-filled moderate profile (style 168), mcghan biocurve round, smooth saline-filled moderate profile (style 68), mcghan biodimensional biocurve shaped (biocell textured full height, saline filled, style 163), mcghan breast implant smooth silicone-filled intrashiel barrier (moderate profile, round, style 110), mcghan biocell textured silicone-filled intrashiel barrier (standard profile, round, style 40)
Code Deleted

C3500   Prosthesis, penile, mentor alpha I inflatable penile prosthesis, mentor alpha I narrow-base inflatable penile prosthesis, mentor acu-form malleable penile prosthesis, mentor malleable penile prosthesis note: the mentor alpha I narrow-base inflatable penile prosthesis is effective oct 1, 2000. The mentor alpha I inflatable penile prosthesis was effective aug 1, 2000
Code Deleted

C3510   Prosthesis, ams sphincter 800 urinary prosthesis
Code Deleted

C3551   Guide wire, percutaneous transluminal coronary angioplasty, choice, luge, patriot, pt graphix intermediate, trooper, mailman 182/300 cm, glidewire gold guidewire, platinum plus guidewire, platinum plus guidewire with glidex hydrophilic coating, jagwire single-use high performance guide wire, merit medical systems extender

guidewire, merit medical systems tomcat ptca guidewire, platinum plus guidewire (0.014 And 0.018 In diameters)
Code Deleted

C3552   Guide wire, hi-torque whisper, zebra single-use exchange guidewire
Code Deleted

C3553   Guide wire, cordis stabilizer marker wire steerable guidewire, cordis wizdom marker wire steerable guidewire, cordis atw marker wire steerable guidewire, cordis shinobi steerable guidewire, cordis atw steerable guidewire, cordis cinch qr steerable guidewire extension, cordis stor q guidewire, cordis essence steerable guidewire, cordis instinct steerable guidewire, cordis agility 10 hydrophilic steerable guidewire, cordis agility 14 hydrophilic steerable guidewire, cordis stabilizer balanced performance guidewire, cordis stabilizer plus steerable guidewire, cordis shinobi plus steerable guidewire (models 547-214, 547-214x), cordis stabilizer xs steerable guidewire (models 527-914, 527-914j, 527-914x, 527-914y), cordis sv guidewire--5cm distal taper configuration (models 503-558, 503-558x), 8cm distal taper configuration (models 503-658, 503-658x), 14cm distal taper configuration (models 503-758, 503-758x), cordis wisdom st steerable guidewire (models 537-114, 537-114j, 537-114x, 537-114y)
Code Deleted

C3554   Guide wire, jindo tapered peripheral guidewire
Code Deleted

C3555   Guide wire, wholey hi-torque plus guide wire system, 145cm, 190cm, 300cm
Code Deleted

C3556   Guide wire, endosonics cardiometrics wavewire pressure guide wire, cardiometrics flowire doppler guide wire
Code Deleted

C3557   Guidewire, hytek guidewire, biotronik galeo hydro guide wire, microvena ultra select nitinol guidewire, wilson-cook axcess 21 wire guide, wilson-cook roadrunner extra support wire guide, wilson-cook tracer wire guide, wilson-cook tracer hybrid wire guide, wilson-cook tracer metro wire guide, wilson-cook protector wire guides
Code Deleted

C3800   Infusion pump, implantable, programmable, synchromed
el infusion pump, synchromed infusion pump
Code Deleted

C3801   Infusion pump, arrow/microject pca system
Code Deleted

C3851   Intraocular lens, staar elastic ultraviolet-absorbing silicone
posterior chamber intraocular lens with toric optic model
aa-4203t, model aa-4203tf, model aa-4203tl
Code Deleted

C4000   Pacemaker, single chamber, ela medical opus g model
4621, 4624
Code Deleted

C4001   Pacemaker, single chamber, ela medical opus s model
4121, 4124
Code Deleted

C4002   Pacemaker, single chamber, ela medical talent model 113
Code Deleted

C4003   Pacemaker, single chamber, kairos sr
Code Deleted

C4004   Pacemaker, single chamber, actros sr+, actros sr-b+
Code Deleted

C4005   Pacemaker, single chamber, philos sr, philos sr-b
Code Deleted

C4006   Pacemaker, single chamber, pulsar max ii sr 1180, 1181
Code Deleted

C4007   Pacemaker, single chamber, marathon sr 291-09, 292-09r,
292-09x
Code Deleted

C4008   Pacemaker, single chamber, discovery ii ssi 481
Code Deleted

C4009   Pacemaker, single chamber, discovery ii sr 1184, 1185,
1186, 1187
Code Deleted

C4300   Pacemaker, dual chamber, integrity afx dr model 5342,
integrity u dr 5336
Code Deleted

C4301   Pacemaker, dual chamber, integrity afx dr model 5346
Code Deleted

C4302   Pacemaker, dual chamber, affinity vdr 5430
Code Deleted

C4303   Pacemaker, dual chamber, ela brio model 112 pacemaker
system
Code Deleted

C4304   Pacemaker, dual chamber, ela medical brio model 212,
talent model 213, talent model 223
Code Deleted

C4305   Pacemaker, dual chamber, ela medical brio model 222
Code Deleted

C4306   Pacemaker, dual chamber, ela medical brio model 220
Code Deleted

C4307   Pacemaker, dual chamber, kairos dr
Code Deleted

C4308   Pacemaker, dual chamber, inos 2, inos 2+
Code Deleted

C4309   Pacemaker, dual chamber, actros dr+, actros d+, actros
dr-a+, actros slr+
Code Deleted

C4310   Pacemaker, dual chamber, actros dr-b+
Code Deleted

C4311   Pacemaker, dual chamber, philos dr, philos dr-b, philos slr
Code Deleted

C4312   Pacemaker, dual chamber, pulsar max ii dr 1280
Code Deleted

C4313   Pacemaker, dual chamber, marathon dr 293-09, 294-09,
294-09r, 294-10
Code Deleted

C4314   Pacemaker, dual chamber, momentum dr 294-23
Code Deleted

C4315   Pacemaker, dual chamber, selection afm 902 slc 902c
Code Deleted

C4316 Pacemaker, dual chamber, discovery ii dr 1283, 1284, 1285, 1286
Code Deleted

C4317 Pacemaker, dual chamber, discovery ii ddd 981
Code Deleted

C4600 Lead, pacemaker, synox, polyrox, elox, retrox, sl-bp, elc, pr-b permanent implantable pacing lead (models pr 44 b, pr 48 b, pr 52 b, pr 58 b), pr-s permanent implantable pacing lead (models pr 44 s, pr 48 s, pr 52 s, pr 58 s), py-psbv permanent implantable pacing lead (models py 44 psbv, py 48 psbv, py 52 psbv, py 58 psbv), py-pv permanent implantable pacing lead (models py 48 pv, py 52 pv, py 58 pv), zy-pbv permanent implantable pacing lead (models zy 52 pbv, zy 58 pbv), zy-pjbv permanent implantable pacing lead (models zy 48 pjbv, zy 52 pjbv, zy-pjusbv permanent implantable pacing lead (models zy 44 pjusbv, zy 48 pjusbv, zy 52 pjusbv) zy-pjuv permanent implantable pacing lead (models zy 48 pjuv, zy 52 pjuv), zy-pjv permanent implantable pacing lead (models zy 48 pjv, zy 52 pjv), zy pusbv permanent implantable pacing lead (models zy 52 pusbv, zy 58 pusbv), zy-puv permanent implantable pacing lead (models zy 52 puv, zy 58 puv), zy-pv permanent implantable pacing lead (models zy 52 pv, zy 58 pv)
Code Deleted

C4601 Lead, pacemaker, aescula lv 1055k
Code Deleted

C4602 Lead, pacemaker, tendril sdx 1488k/46, tendril sdx 1488k/52, tendril sdx 1488k/58
Code Deleted

C4603 Lead, pacemaker, oscor pr 4015, 4016, 4017, 4018, flexion 4015, 4016, 4017, 4018, ela medical stela pacing lead (models bj44, bj45), ela medical stelid ii pacing lead (model btfr26d), ela medical stelix pacing lead (model br45d), ht-pb permanent implantable pacing lead (models ht 48 pb, ht 52 pb, ht 58 pb), oscor py (models 4439, 4440, 4441), oscor zy (models 4036, 4037, 4038, 4039, 4042, 4056, 4057), rt-tjv permanent implantable pacing lead (models rt 48 tjv, rt 52 tjv), rt-tv permanent implantable pacing lead (models rt 52 tv, rt 58 tv), ru-tbv permanent implantable pacing lead (models ru 52 tbv, ru 58 tbv, ru 70 tbv), ru-tjsbv permanent implantable pacing lead (models ru 44 tjsbv, ru 48 tjsbv, ru 52 tjsbv), ru-tjv permanent implantable pacing lead (models ru 48 tjv, ru 52 tjv), ru-tsbv permanent implantable pacing lead

(models ru 52 tsbv, ru 58 tsbv, ru 70 tsbv), ru-tv permanent implantable pacing lead (models ru 52 tv, ru 58 tv)
Code Deleted

C4604   Lead, pacemaker, crystalline actfix icf09, capsurefix novus 5076
Code Deleted

C4605   Lead, pacemaker, capsure epi 4968
Code Deleted

C4606   Lead, pacemaker, flextend 4080, 4081, 4082
Code Deleted

C4607   Lead, pacemaker, fineline ii 4452, 4453, 4454, 4455, 4477, 4478, fineline ii ez 4463, 4464, 4465, 4466, 4467, 4468, thinline ii 430-25, 430-35, 432-35, thinline ii ez 438-25, 438-35, fineline ii ez sterol (models 4469, 4470, 4471, 4472, 4473, 4474), fineline ii sterox (models 4456, 4457, 4459, 4479, 4480) thinline ii ez sterox (models 438-25s, 438-35s), thinline ii sterox (models 430-25s, 430-35s, 432-35s)
Code Deleted

C5000   Stent, biliary, bx velocity with hepacoat on raptor stent system (28 or 33mm in length)
Code Deleted

C5001   Stent, biliary, bard memotherm-flex biliary stent (small/medium diameter)
Code Deleted

C5002   Stent, biliary, bard memotherm-flex biliary stent, large diameter
Code Deleted

C5003   Stent, biliary, bard memotherm-flex biliary stent, x-large diameter
Code Deleted

C5004   Stent, biliary, cordis palmaz corinthian iq transhepatic biliary stent
Code Deleted

C5005   Stent, biliary, cordis palmaz corinthian iq transhepatic biliary stent and delivery system
Code Deleted

C5006 Stent, biliary, cordis medium palmaz transhepatic biliary stent and delivery system
Code Deleted

C5007 Stent, biliary, cordis palmaz xl transhepatic biliary stent (40mm length)
Code Deleted

C5008 Stent, biliary, cordis palmaz xl transhepatic biliary stent (50mm length)
Code Deleted

C5009 Stent, biliary, biliary vistaflex stent
Code Deleted

C5010 Stent, biliary, rapid exchange single-use biliary stent system
Code Deleted

C5011 Stent, biliary, intrastent, intrastent lp,, wilson-cook st2 soehendra tannenbaum
Code Deleted

C5012 Stent, biliary, intrastent doublestrut ld, intrastent double strut para mount biliary stent, olympus double layer biliary stent
Code Deleted

C5013 Stent, biliary, intrastent doublestrut, intrastent doublestrut xs
Code Deleted

C5014 Stent, biliary, medtronic ave bridge stent system--biliary indication (10mm, 17mm, 28mm)
Code Deleted

C5015 Stent, biliary, medtronic ave bridge stent system--biliary indication (40-60mm, 80-100mm), medtronic ave bridge x3 biliary stent system (17mm)
Code Deleted

C5016 Stent, biliary, wallstent single-use covered biliary endoprosthesis with unistep plus delivery system, gore biliary endoprosthesis
Code Deleted

C5017 Stent, biliary, wallstent rp biliary endoprosthesis with unistep plus delivery system (20/40/42/60/68 mm in length)
Code Deleted

C5018   Stent, biliary, wallstent rp biliary endoprosthesis with unistep plus delivery system (80/94 mm in length)
Code Deleted

C5019   Stent, biliary, flexima single-use biliary stent system
Code Deleted

C5020   Stent, biliary, cordis smart nitinol stent transhepatic biliary system (20mm in length)
Code Deleted

C5021   Stent, biliary, cordis smart nitinol stent transhepatic biliary system (40 or 60mm in length)
Code Deleted

C5022   Stent, biliary, cordis smart nitinol stent transhepatic biliary system (80mm in length)
Code Deleted

C5023   Stent, biliary, bx velocity transhepatic biliary stent and delivery system (8 or 13mm in length)
Code Deleted

C5024   Stent, biliary, bx velocity transhepatic biliary stent and delivery system (18mm in length)
Code Deleted

C5025   Stent, biliary, bx velocity transhepatic biliary stent and delivery system (23mm in length)
Code Deleted

C5026   Stent, biliary, bx velocity transhepatic biliary stent and delivery system (28 0r 33mm in length)
Code Deleted

C5027   Stent, biliary, bx velocity with hepacoat on raptor stent system (8 or 13mm in length), bx velocity e.5/5.0 Balloon expandable stent with raptor over-the-wire delivery system
Code Deleted

C5028   Stent, biliary, bx velocity with hepacoat on raptor stent system (18mm in length)
Code Deleted

C5029   Stent, biliary, bx velocity with hepacoat on raptor stent system (23mm in length)
Code Deleted

C5030   Stent, coronary, s660 discrete technology over-the-wire coronary stent system (9mm, 12mm), s660 with discrete technology rapid exchange coronary stent system (9mm, 12mm), biodivysio as pc coated coronary stent delivery system (11 mm)
Code Deleted

C5031   Stent, coronary, s660 discrete technology over-the-wire coronary stent system (15mm, 18mm), s660 with discrete technology rapid exchange coronary stent system (15mm, 18mm), biodivysio as pc coated coronary stent delivery system (15 mm)
Code Deleted

C5032   Stent, coronary, s660 discrete technology over-the-wire coronary stent system 24mm, 30mm s660 with discrete technology rapid exchange coronary stent system 24mm, 30mm
Code Deleted

C5033   Stent, coronary, niroyal advance premounted stent system (9mm), tenax-xr stent and delivery system
Code Deleted

C5034   Stent, coronary, niroyal advance premounted stent system (12mm/15mm)
Code Deleted

C5035   Stent, coronary, niroyal advance premounted stent system (18mm)
Code Deleted

C5036   Stent, coronary, niroyal advance premounted stent system (25mm)
Code Deleted

C5037   Stent, coronary, niroyal advance premounted stent system (31mm)
Code Deleted

C5038   Stent, coronary, bx velocity balloon-expandable stent with raptor over-the-wire delivery system
Code Deleted

C5039   Stent, peripheral, intracoil peripheral stent (40mm stent length), dynalink peripheral self-expanding stent system
Code Deleted

C5040 Stent, peripheral, intracoil peripheral stent (60mm stent length)
Code Deleted

C5041 Stent, coronary, medtronic bestent 2 over-the-wire coronary stent system (24mm, 30mm), medtronic bestent 2 rapid exchange coronary stent system (24mm, 30mm)
Code Deleted

C5042 Stent, coronary, medtronic bestent 2 over-the-wire coronary stent system (18mm), medtronic bestent 2 rapid exchange (18mm)
Code Deleted

C5043 Stent, coronary, medtronic bestent 2 over-the-wire coronary stent system (15mm), medtronic bestent 2 rapid exchange (15mm)
Code Deleted

C5044 Stent, coronary, medtronic bestent 2 over-the-wire coronary stent system (9mm, 12mm), medtronic bestent 2 rapid exchange coronary stent system (9mm, 12mm)
Code Deleted

C5045 Stent, coronary, multilink tetra coronary stent system
Code Deleted

C5046 Stent, coronary, radius 20mm self expanding stent with over the wire delivery system
Code Deleted

C5047 Stent, coronary, niroyal elite premounted stent system 15mm, 25mm, or 31mm
Code Deleted

C5048 Stent, coronary, gr ii coronary stent
Code Deleted

C5130 Stent, colon, wilson-cook colonic z-stent
Code Deleted

C5131 Stent, colorectal, bard memotherm colorectal stent model s30r060
Code Deleted

C5132 Stent, colorectal, bard memotherm colorectal stent model s30r080
Code Deleted

C5133 Stent, colorectal, bard memotherm colorectal stent model s30r100
Code Deleted

C5134 Stent, enteral, wallstent enteral endoprosthesis and unistep delivery system (90mm in length), enteral wallstent endoprosthesis with unistep plus delivery system (90mm in length) note: only the enteral wallstent endoprosthesis with unistep plus delivery system is effective October 1, 2000. The wallstent enteral and unistep delivery system was effective August 1, 2000
Code Deleted

C5279 Stent, ureteral, boston scientific contour soft percuflex stent with hydroplus coating (braided), contour soft percuflex stent with hydroplus coating, contour vl variable length percuflex stent with hydroplus coating, percuflex plus stent with hydroplus coating, percuflex stent (braided), contour closed soft percuflex stent with hydroplus coating, contour injection soft percuflex stent with hydroplus coating, soft percuflex stent, percuflex tail plus tapered ureteral stent, contour polaris ureteral stent with hydroplus coating, mardis firm stent with hydroplus coating, mardis soft stent with hydroplus coating, mardis soft variable length stent with hydroplus coating, nottingham one-step tapered dilators with hydroplus coating, stretch vl variable length flexima stent with hydroplus coating, percuflex urinary diversion stent note: the contour closed soft percuflex stent, conour injection soft percuflex stent, soft percuflex, and percuflex tail plus tapered ureteral stent are effective 01/01/01. The other ureteral stents were effective 10/01/00
Code Deleted

C5280 Stent, ureteral, bard inlay double pigtail ureteral stent, cook klein rectal tamponade balloon, cook urological cystostomy catheter, cook urological ureteral dilator set, cook urological fascial dilator set, circon surgitek classic double pigtail ureteral stent, circon surgitek classic double pigtail hydrophilic coated ureteral stent, circon surgitek quadracoil ureteral stent, circon surgitek double j ii ureteral stent, circon surgitek lithostent ureteral stent, circon surgitek soft-curl ureteral stent, cook urological lse double pigtail ureteral stent, cook urological lse multi length ureteral stent, cook urological multi length ureteral stent, cook urological double pigtail ureteral stent, cook urological double pigtail ureteral stent with aq (hydrophilic) coating, cook urological mazer antegrade double pigtail ureteral stent set
Code Deleted

C5281   Stent, tracheobronchial, wallgraft tracheobronchial
         endoprosthesis with unistep delivery system (70mm in
         length)
         Code Deleted

C5282   Stent, tracheobronchial, wallgraft tracheobronchial
         endoprosthesis with unistep delivery system (20mm,
         30mm, 50mm in length)
         Code Deleted

C5283   Stent, self-expandable for creation of intrahepatic shunts,
         wallstent transjugular intrahepatic protosystemic shunt
         (tips) with unistep plus delivery system (90/94mm in
         length), wallstent rp tips endoprosthesis with unistep plus
         delivery system (94mm in length) note: only the wallstent
         rp tips endoprosthesis with unistep plus delivery system
         is effective October 1, 2000. The wallstent tips with
         unistep plust delivery system was effective August 1, 2000
         Code Deleted

C5284   Stent, tracheobronchial, ultraflex tracheobronchial
         endoprosthesis (covered and non-covered)
         Code Deleted

C5600   Vascular closure device, vasoseal es (extravascular
         security) device
         Code Deleted

C5601   Vascular closure device, vascular solutions duett sealing
         device 1000
         Code Deleted

C6001   Mesh, hernia, bard composix mesh, per 8 or 21 inches,
         atrium hernia/surgical mesh, bard composix e/x mesh,
         bard kugel hernia patch (large circle, 12 cm x 12 cm),
         bard kugel hernia patch (small circle, 8 cm x 8 cm), bard
         kugel hernia patch (large oval, 14 cm x 18 cm), bard
         kugel hernia patch (medium oval, 11 cm x 14 cm), bard
         kugel hernia patch (small oval, 8 cm x 12 cm), bard
         mesh perfix plug, bard visilex mesh (3 in x 6 in), bard
         visilex mesh (4.5 In x 6 in)
         Code Deleted

C6002   Mesh, hernia, bard composix mesh, per 32 inches
         Code Deleted

C6003   Mesh, hernia, bard composix mesh, per 48 inches
         Code Deleted

C6004   Mesh, hernia, bard composix mesh, per 80 inches
Code Deleted

C6005   Mesh, hernia, bard composix mesh, per 140 inches
Code Deleted

C6006   Mesh, hernia, bard composix mesh, per 144 inches
Code Deleted

C6012   Pelvicol acellular collagen matrix, per 8 or 14 quare
centimeters, contigen bard collagen implant (contigen
implant)
Code Deleted

C6013   Pelvicol acellular collagen matrix, per 21, 24, or 28
square centimeters
Code Deleted

C6014   Pelvicol acellular collagen matrix, per 40 square
centimeters
Code Deleted

C6015   Pelvicol acellular collagen matrix, per 48 square
centimeters
Code Deleted

C6016   Pelvicol acellular collagen matrix, per 96 square
centimeters
Code Deleted

C6017   Gore-tex dualmesh biomaterial, per 75 or 96 square
centimeters (1mm thick)
Code Deleted

C6018   Gore-tex dualmesh biomaterial, per 150 square
centimeters oval shaped (1mm thick)
Code Deleted

C6019   Gore-tex dualmesh biomaterial, per 285 square
centimeters oval shaped (1mm thick)
Code Deleted

C6020   Gore-tex dualmesh biomaterial, per 432 square
centimeters (1mm thick)
Code Deleted

C6021   Gore-tex dualmesh biomaterial, per 600 square
centimeters (1mm thick)
Code Deleted

C6022   Gore-tex dualmesh biomaterial, per 884 square centimeters (1mm thick)
Code Deleted

C6023   Gore-tex dualmesh plus biomaterial, per 75 or 96 square centimeters (1mm thick)
Code Deleted

C6024   Gore-tex dualmesh plus biomaterial, per 150 square centimeters oval shaped (1mm thick)
Code Deleted

C6025   Gore-tex dualmesh plus biomaterial, per 285 square centimeters oval shaped (1mm thick)
Code Deleted

C6026   Gore-tex dualmesh plus biomaterial, per 432 square centimeters (1mm thick)
Code Deleted

C6027   Gore-tex dualmeshplus biomaterial, per 600 square centimeters (1mm thick)
Code Deleted

C6028   Gore-tex dualmesh plus biomaterial, per 884 square centimeters oval shaped (1mm thick)
Code Deleted

C6029   Gore-tex dualmesh plus biomaterial, per 150 square centimeters oval shaped (2mm thick)
Code Deleted

C6030   Gore-tex dualmesh plus biomaterial, per 285 square centimeters oval shaped (2mm thick)
Code Deleted

C6031   Gore-tex dualmesh plus biomaterial, per 432 square centimeters (2mm thick)
Code Deleted

C6032   Gore-tex dualmesh plus biomaterial, per 600 square centimeters (2mm thick)
Code Deleted

C6033   Gore-tex dualmesh plus biomaterial, per 884 square centimeters (2mm thick)
Code Deleted

C6034 Bard reconix eptfe reconstruction patch 150 square
centimeters (2mm thick)
Code Deleted

C6035 Bard reconix eptfe reconstruction patch 150 square
centimeters (1mm thick), 75 square centimeters (2mm
thick)
Code Deleted

C6036 Bard reconix eptfe reconstruction patch 50/75 square
centimeters (1mm thick), 50 square centimeters (2mm
thick)
Code Deleted

C6037 Bard reconix eptfe reconstruction patch 300 square
centimeters (1 mm thick)
Code Deleted

C6038 Bard reconix eptfe reconstruction patch 600 square
centimeters (1mm thick), 300 square centimeters (2mm
thick)
Code Deleted

C6039 Bard reconix eptfe reconstruction patch 884 square
centimeters oval shaped (1mm thick)
Code Deleted

C6040 Bard reconix eptfe reconstruction patch 600 square
centimeters (2mm thick)
Code Deleted

C6041 Bard reconix eptfe reconstruction patch 884 square
centimeters oval shaped (2mm thick)
Code Deleted

C6050 Sling fixation system for treatment of stress urinary
incontinence, female in-fast sling fixation system with
electric inserter with sling material, female in-fast sling
fixation system with electric inserter without sling
material, advanced uroscience acyst
Code Deleted

C6051 Depuy orthotech restore, stratasis urethral sling, 20/40 cm
Code Deleted

C6052 Stratasis urethral sling, 60 cm
Code Deleted

C6053 Surgisis soft tissue graft, per 70cm, 105cm, or 140cm
Code Deleted

C6054 Surgisis enhanced strength soft tissue graft, per 4.2Cm, 20cm, 28cm or 40cm
Code Deleted

C6055 Surgisis enhanced strength soft tissue graft, per 52.5Cm, 60cm, or 70cm
Code Deleted

C6056 Surgisis enhanced strength soft tissue graft, per 105cm, 140cm
Code Deleted

C6057 Surgisis hernia graft, per 195cm
Code Deleted

C6058 Sugipro hernia mate plug, medium or large
Code Deleted

C6080 Sling fixation system for treatment of stress urinary incontinence, male straight-in fixation system with electric inserter with sling material and disposable pressure sensor, male straight-in fixation system with electric inserter without sling material and disposable pressure sensor
Code Deleted

C6200 Vascular graft, exxcel soft eptfe vascular graft, exxcel eptfe vascular graft (6mm or greater in diameter), b. Braun vena tech lgm vena cava filter (dual approach--model #31328, jugular approach--model #31326, femoral approach--model #31327), cordis trapease permanent vena cava filter, stainless steel green field vena cava filter with 12 fr introducer system
Code Deleted

C6201 Vascular graft, impra venaflo vascular graft with carbon (straight graft, 10cm or 20cm in length), atrium hybrid ptfe vascular graft
Code Deleted

C6202 Vascular graft, impra venaflo vascular graft with carbon, straight graft 30cm or 40cm in length
Code Deleted

C6203 Vascular graft, impra venaflo vascular graft with carbon, straight graft (50cm in length) or centerflex venaflo stepped graft (45cm in length)
Code Deleted

C6204 Vascular graft, impra venaflo vascular graft with carbon, stepped graft 20cm, 25cm, 30cm, 35cm, 40cm, or 45cm in length
Code Deleted

C6205 Vascular graft, impra carboflo vascular graft (straight graft, 10cm in length), atrium advanta ptfe vascular graft
Code Deleted

C6206 Vascular graft, impra carboflo vascular graft, straight graft 20cm in length
Code Deleted

C6207 Vascular graft, impra carboflo vascular graft, straight graft 30cm, 35cm or 40cm in length
Code Deleted

C6208 Vascular graft, impra carboflo vascular graft, straight graft (50cm in length), access tapered graft (40cm in length), or stepped graft (45 or 50cm in length)
Code Deleted

C6209 Vascular graft, impra carboflo vascular graft, centerflex straight graft (40cm or 50cm in length) or centerflex stepped graft (40cm, 45cm, or 50cm in length)
Code Deleted

C6210 Exxcel eptfe vascular graft (less than 6mm in diameter), hemashield woven double velour fabric, hemashield finesse ultra-thin, knitted cardiovascular patch
Code Deleted

C6300 Stent graft system, vanguard iii bifurcated endovascular aortic graft
Code Deleted

C6500 Sheath, guiding, preface braided guiding sheat (anterior curve, multipurpose curve, posterior curve)
Code Deleted

C6501 Sheath, soft-tip sheaths
Code Deleted

C6502 Sheath, electrophysiology, perry exchange dilator
Code Deleted

C6525 Spectranetics laser sheath 12f 500-001, 14f 500-012, 16f 500-013
Code Deleted

C6600   Probe, microvasive swiss f/g lithoclast flexible probe
         .89Mm, microvasive swiss f/g lithoclast flexible probe ii
         .89Mm
         Code Deleted

C6650   Introducer, guiding, fast-cath two-piece guiding introducer
         (models 406869, 406892, 406893, 406904), accustick ii
         with ro marker introducer system, cook extra large
         check-flo introducer, cook keller-timmermans introducer,
         fast-cath hemostasis introducer, maximum hemostasis
         introducer, fast-cath duo sl1 guiding introducer fast-cath
         duo sl2 guiding introducer
         Code Deleted

C6651   Introducer, guiding, seal-away cs guiding introducer
         407508, 407510
         Code Deleted

C6652   Introducer, bard safety excalibur introducer, bard radstic
         microintroducer, bard universal microintroducer
         Code Deleted

C6700   Synthetic absorbable sealant, focal seal-l, perfluoron (per
         2ml vial, 5ml vial or 7ml vial)
         Code Deleted

C8099   Spectranetics lead locking device (models 518-018,
         518-019, 518-020), oscor c/vs permanent implantable
         pacing lead adaptor (models c/vs-10, c/vs-40), oscor m/vs
         permanent implantable pacing lead adaptor (models
         m/vs-10, m/vs-40), oscor vs/m permanent implantable
         pacing lead adaptor (model vs/m-10), oscor vv permanent
         implantable pacing lead extension (models vv-10, vv-40)
         Code Deleted

C8100   Adhesion barrier, adcon-l
         Code Deleted

C8102   Surgi-vision esophageal stylet internal coil
         Code Deleted

C8103   Capio suture capturing device, standard or open access
         Code Deleted

C8500   Catheter, atherectomy, atherocath-gto atherectomy catheter
         Code Deleted

C8501   Pacemaker, single chamber, vigor ssi
         Code Deleted

C8502 Catheter, diagnostic, electrophysiology, livewire steerable electrophysiology catheter
Code Deleted

C8503 Catheter, synchromed vascular catheter model 8702
Code Deleted

C8504 Closure device, vasoseal vascular hemostasis device
Code Deleted

C8505 Infusion pump, implantable, programmable, synchromed infusion pump
Code Deleted

C8506 Lead, pacemaker, 4057m, 4058m, 4557m, 4558m,5058
Code Deleted

C8507 Lead, pacemaker,6721l, 6721m, 6721s, 6939 oval patch lead
Code Deleted

C8508 Lead, defibrillator, capsure 4965
Code Deleted

C8509 Lead, defibrillator, transvene 6933, transvene 6937
Code Deleted

C8510 Lead, defibrillator, dp-3238
Code Deleted

C8511 Lead, defibrillator, endotak dsp
Code Deleted

C8512 Lead, neurostimulation, on-point model 3987, pisces-quad plus model 3888, resume tl model 3986
Code Deleted

C8513 Lead, neurostimulation, pisces-quad model 3487a, resume ii model 3587a
Code Deleted

C8514 Prosthesis, penile, dura ii penile prosthesis
Code Deleted

C8515 Prosthesis, penile, Mentor Alpha I narrow-base inflatable penile prosthesis
Code Added

C8516 Prosthesis, penile, mentor acu-form malleable penile prosthesis, mentor malleable penile prosthesis
Code Deleted

C8517   Prosthesis, penile, Ambicor penile prosthesis
Code Added

C8518   Pacemaker, dual chamber, vigor ddd
Code Deleted

C8519   Pacemaker, dual chamber, vista ddd
Code Deleted

C8520   Pacemaker, single chamber, legacy ii s
Code Deleted

C8521   Receiver/transmitter, neurostimulator, medtronic mattrix
Code Deleted

C8522   Stent, biliary, palmaz balloon expandable stent
Code Deleted

C8523   Stent, biliary, wallstent transhepatic biliary endoprosthesis
Code Deleted

C8524   Stent, esophageal, wallstent esophageal prosthesis
Code Deleted

C8525   Stent, esophageal, wallstent esophageal prosthesis (double)
Code Deleted

C8526   Optiplast xt 5f percutaneous transluminal angioplasty
catheter (various sizes)
Code Deleted

C8528   Ms classique balloon dilatation catheter
Code Deleted

C8529   Ismus cath deflectable 20-pole catheter/crista cath ii
deflectable 20-pole catheter
Code Deleted

C8530   Mentor siltex gel-filled mammary prosthesis,
smooth-surface gel-filled mammary prosthesis
Code Deleted

C8531   Wilson-cook esophageal z metal expandable stent
Code Deleted

C8532   Stent, esophageal, ultraflex esophageal stent system
Code Deleted

C8533   Catheter, synchromed vascular catheter model 8700a,
model 8700v
Code Deleted

C8534   Prosthesis, penile, ams malleable 650 penile prosthesis
Code Deleted

C8535   Stent, biliary, spiral z biliary metal expandable stent, za
biliary metal expandable stent
Code Deleted

C8536   Stent, esophageal, esophageal z metal expandable stent
with dua anti-reflux valve, esophageal z metal expandable
stent with uncoated flanges
Code Deleted

C8539   Wilson-cook quantum dilatation balloon
Code Deleted

C8540   Flex-ez (esophageal) balloon dilator 3302, 3304, 3306
Code Deleted

C8541   Carson zero tip balloon dilatation catheters with
hydroplus coating kit, passport balloon on a wire
dilatation catheters with hydroplus coating kit
Code Deleted

C8542   Urethramax high pressure urethral balloon dilatation
catheter/kit
Code Deleted

C8543   Amplatz renal dilator set
Code Deleted

C8550   Catheter, livewire ep catheter, 7f csm 401935, 5f
decapolar 401938, 401939, 401940, 401941
Code Deleted

C8551   Catheter, livewire ep catheter, 7f duo-decapolar 401932
Code Deleted

C8552   Catheter, santuro fixed curve catheter
Code Deleted

C8597   Guide wire, cordis wisdom st steerable guidewire
537-114, 537-114j, 537-114x, 537-114y
Code Deleted

C8598   Guide wire, cordis sv guidewire 5cm distal taper
configuration (models 503-558, 503-558x), 8cm distal
taper configuration (models 503-658, 503-658x), 14cm
distal taper configuration (models 503-758, 503-758x)
Code Deleted

C8599   Guide wire, cordis stabilizer xs steerable guidewire 527-914, 527-914j, 527-914x, 527-914y
Code Deleted

C8600   Guide wire, cordis shinobi plus steerable guidewire 547-214, 547-214x
Code Deleted

C8650   Introducer, cook extra large check-flo introducer
Code Deleted

C8724   Lead, neurostimulation, octad lead 3898-33/389861
Code Deleted

C8725   Lead, neurostimulation, symmix lead 3982
Code Deleted

C8748   Lead, defibrillator, endotak sq patch 0047, 0063
Code Deleted

C8749   Lead, defibrillator, endotak sq array 0048, 0049
Code Deleted

C8750   Pacemaker, dual chamber, unity vddr 292-07
Code Deleted

C8775   Lead, pacemaker, 2188 coronary sinus lead
Code Deleted

C8776   Lead, pacemaker, innomedica sutureless myocardial 4045, 4058, 4046, 4047
Code Deleted

C8777   Lead, pacemaker, unipass 425-02, 425-04, 425-06
Code Deleted

C8800   Stent, biliary, large palmaz balloon expandable stent with delivery system
Code Deleted

C8801   Stent, biliary, cook z stent gianturco-rosch biliary design
Code Deleted

C8802   Stent, biliary, cook oasis one action stent introductory system
Code Deleted

C8830   Stent, coronary, cook gianturco-roubin flex-stent coronary stent
Code Deleted

C8890   Perfluoron, per 2ml
Code Deleted

C8891   Perfluoron, per 5ml vial or 7ml vial
Code Deleted

C8900   Magnetic resonance angiography with contrast, abdomen
Code Added

C8901   Magnetic resonance angiography without contrast, abdomen
Code Added

C8902   Magnetic resonance angiography without contrast followed by with contrast, abdomen
Code Added

C8903   Magnetic resonance imaging with contrast, breast; unilateral
Code Added

C8904   Magnetic resonance imaging without contrast, breast; unilateral
Code Added

C8905   Magnetic resonance imaging without contrast followed by with contrast, breast; unilateral
Code Added

C8906   Magnetic resonance imaging with contrast, breast; bilateral
Code Added

C8907   Magnetic resonance imaging without contrast, breast; bilateral
Code Added

C8908   Magnetic resonance imaging without contrast followed by with contrast, breast; bilateral
Code Added

C8909   Magnetic resonance angiography with contrast, chest (excluding myocardium)
Code Added

C8910   Magnetic resonance angiography without contrast, chest (excluding myocardium)
Code Added

C8911   Magnetic resonance angiography without contrast followed by with contrast, chest (excluding myocardium)
Code Added

C8912   Magnetic resonance angiography with contrast, lower extremity
Code Added

C8913   Magnetic resonance angiography without contrast, lower extremity
Code Added

C8914   Magnetic resonance angiography without contrast followed by with contrast, lower extremity
Code Added

C9001   Linezolid injection, per 200mg
Code Deleted

C9002   Tenecteplase, per 50mg/vial
Code Deleted

C9004   Injection, gemtuzumab ozogamicin, per 5 mg
Code Deleted

C9005   Injection, reteplase, 18.8 Mg (one single-use vial)
Code Deleted

C9006   Injection, tacrolimus, per 5 mg (1 amp)
Code Deleted

C9011   Injection, caffeine citrate, per 1ml
Code Deleted

C9012   Injection, arsenic trioxide, per 1 mg/kg
Code Deleted

C9013   Supply of co 57 cobaltous chloride, radiopharmaceutical diagnostic imaging agent
Code Added

C9017   Lomustine, 10 mg
Code Deleted

C9018   Botulinum toxin type b, per 100 units
Code Deleted

C9019   Injection, caspofungin acetate, 5 mg
Code Added

C9020   Sirolimus tablet, 1 mg
Code Added

C9104   Anti-thymocyte globulin, per 25 mg
Code Deleted

C9106   Sirolimus, per 1 mg/ml
Code Deleted

C9107   Injection, tinzaparin sodium, per 2ml vial
Code Deleted

C9108   Injection, thyrotropin alpha, 11 mg
Code Added

C9109   Injection, tirofiban hydrochloride, 625 mg
Code Added

C9110   Alemtuzumab, per 10 mg/ml
Code Added

C9111   Injection, bivalirudin, 250 mg per vial
Code Added

C9112   Injection, perflutren lipid microsphere, per 2 ml vial
Code Added

C9113   Injection, pantoprazole sodium, per vial
Code Added

C9114   Injection, nesiritide, per 15 mg vial
Code Added

C9115   Injection, zoledronic acid, per 2 mg
Code Added

C9200   Orcel, per 36 square centimeters
Code Added

C9201   Dermagraft, per 375 square centimeters
Code Added

C9500   Platelets, irradiated, each unit
Code Deleted

C9501   Platelets, pheresis, each unit
Code Deleted

C9502   Platelets, pheresis, irradiated, each unit
Code Deleted

C9504   Red blood cells, deglycerolized, ea unit
Code Deleted

C9505   Red blood cells, irradiated, each unit
Code Deleted

C9506   Granulocytes, pheresis, each unit
Code Deleted

C9700   Water induced thermotherapy
Code Deleted

C9702   Checkmate intravascular brachytherapy system, novoste beta-cath intravascular brachytherapy system, galileo intravascular radiotherapy system
Code Deleted

C9703   Bard endoscopic suturing system
Code Added

C9708   Preview treatment planning software
Code Added

C9711   HELP Apheresis system
Code Added

E0169   Commode chair with seat lift mechanism
Code Added

E0221   Infrared heating pad system
Code Added

E0231   Non-contact wound warming device (temperature control unit, ac adapter and power cord) for use with warming card and wound cover
Code Added

E0232   Warming card for use with the non-contact wound warming device and non contact wound warming wound cover
Code Added

E0298   Hospital bed, heavy duty, extra wide, with any type side rails, with mattress
Code Deleted

E0316   Safety enclosure frame/canopy for use with hospital bed, any type
Code Added

E0481   Intrapulmonary percussive ventilation system and related accessories
Code Added

E0482   Cough stimulating device, alternating positive and negative airway pressure
Code Added

E0600   Respiratory suction pump, home model, portable or stationary, electric
Description Changed

E0602   Breast pump, manual, any type
Description Changed

E0603   Breast pump, electric (AC and/or DC), any type
Code Added

E0604   Breast pump, heavy duty, hospital grade, piston operated, pulsatile vacuum suction/release cycles, vacuum regulator, supplies, transformer, electric (AC and/or DC)
Code Added

E0609   Blood glucose monitor with special features (eg., Voice synthesizers automatic timers, etc.)
Code Deleted

E0620   Skin piercing device for collection of capillary blood, laser, each
Code Added

E0752   Implantable neurostimulator electrode, each
Code Added

E0753   Implantable neurostimulator electrodes, per group of four
Code Deleted

E0754   Patient programmer (external) for use with implantable programmable neurostimulator pulse generator
Code Added

E0759   Radiofrequency transmitter (external) for use with implantable sacral root neurostimulator receiver for bowel and bladder management, replacement
Code Added

E1500   Centrifuge, for dialysis
Code Added

E1520 Heparin infusion pump for hemodialysis
Description Changed

E1530 Air bubble detector for hemodialysis, each, replacement
Description Changed

E1540 Pressure alarm for hemodialysis, each, replacement
Description Changed

E1550 Bath conductivity meter for hemodialysis, each
Description Changed

E1560 Blood leak detector for hemodialysis, each, replacement
Description Changed

E1575 Transducer protectors/fluid barriers, for hemodialysis, any size, per 10
Description Changed

E1580 Unipuncture control system for hemodialysis
Description Changed

E1600 Delivery and/or installation charges for hemodialysis equipment
Description Changed

E1610 Reverse osmosis water purification system, for hemodialysis
Description Changed

E1615 Deionizer water purification system, for hemodialysis
Description Changed

E1620 Blood pump for hemodialysis, replacement
Description Changed

E1625 Water softening system, for hemodialysis
Description Changed

E1632 Wearable artificial kidney, each
Description Changed

E1636 Sorbent cartridges, for hemodialysis, per 10
Description Changed

E1637 Hemostats, for dialysis, each
Code Added

E1638 Heating pad, for peritoneal dialysis, any size, each
Code Added

E1639   Scale, for dialysis, each
Code Added

E1640   Replacement components for hemodialysis and/or peritoneal dialysis machines that are owned or being purchased by the patient
Code Deleted

E1699   Dialysis equipment, not otherwise specified
Description Changed

E1800   Dynamic adjustable elbow extension/flexion device, includes soft interface material
Description Changed

E1801   Bi-directional static progressive stretch elbow device with range of motion adjustment, includes cuffs
Code Added

E1805   Dynamic adjustable wrist extension/flexion device, includes soft interface material
Description Changed

E1806   Bi-directional static progressive stretch wrist device with range of motion adjustment, includes cuffs
Code Added

E1810   Dynamic adjustable knee extension/flexion device, includes soft interface material
Description Changed

E1811   Bi-directional static progressive stretch knee device with range of motion adjustment, includes cuffs
Code Added

E1815   Dynamic adjustable ankle extension/flexion device, includes soft interface material
Description Changed

E1816   Bi-directional static progressive stretch ankle device with range of motion adjustment, includes cuffs
Code Added

E1818   Bi-directional static progressive stretch forearm pronation/supination device with range of motion adjustment, includes cuffs
Code Added

E1820   Replacement soft interface material, dynamic adjustable extension/flexion device
Description Changed

E1821   Replacement soft interface material/cuffs for bi-directional static progressive stretch device
Code Added

E1825   Dynamic adjustable finger extension/flexion device, includes soft interface material
Description Changed

E1830   Dynamic adjustable toe extension/flexion device, includes soft interface material
Description Changed

E1840   Dynamic adjustable shoulder flexion/abduction/rotation device, includes soft interface material
Code Added

E1900   Synthesized speech augmentative communication device with dynamic display
Code Deleted

E1902   Communication board, non-electronic augmentative or alternative communication device
Code Added

E2000   Gastric suction pump, home model, portable or stationary, electric
Code Added

E2100   Blood glucose monitor with integrated voice synthesizer
Code Added

E2101   Blood glucose monitor with integrated lancing/blood sample
Code Added

G0016   Post-symptom telephonic transmission of electrocardiogram rhythm strips(s) and 24 hour attended monitoring, per 30 day period; physician review and interpretation only
Code Deleted

G0117   Glaucoma screening for high risk patients furnished by an optometrist or ophthalmologist
Code Added

G0118 Glaucoma screening for high risk patient furnished under the direct supervision of an optometrist or ophthalmologist
Code Added

G0126 Pet lung imaging of solitary pulmonary nodules, using 2-(fluorine-18)-fluoro-2-deoxy-d-glucose (fdg), following ct (71250/71260 or 71270); initial staging of pathologically diagnosed non-small cell lung cancer
Code Deleted

G0163 Positron emission tomography (pet), whole body, for recurrence of colorectal metastatic cancer
Code Deleted

G0164 Positron emission tomography (pet), whole body, for staging and characterization of lymphoma
Code Deleted

G0165 Positron emission tomography (pet), whole body, for recurrence of melanoma or melanoma metastatic cancer
Code Deleted

G0174 Intensity modulated radiation therapy (imrt) delivery to one or more treatment areas, multiple couch angles/fields/arc, custom collimated pencil-beams with treatment setup and verification images, complete course of therapy requiring more than one session, per session
Code Deleted

G0178 Intensity modulated radiation therapy (imrt) plan, including dose volume histograms for target and critical structure partial tolerances, inverse plan optimization performed for highly conformal distributions, plan positional accuracy and dose verification, per course of treatment
Code Deleted

G0184 Ocular photodynamic therapy treatment, second eye; destruction of localized lesion of choroid (includes intravenous infusion)
Code Deleted

G0188 Full length radiography of lower extremity, which includes hip, knee and ankle
Code Deleted

G0190   Immunization administration (includes percutaneous, intradermal, subcutaneous, intramuscular and jet injections; each additional vaccine (single or combination vaccine/toxoid)
Code Deleted

G0191   Immunization administration (includes percutaneous, intradermal, subcutaneous, intramuscular and jet injections); each additional vaccine (single or combination vaccine/toxoid) list separately in addition to code for primary procedure
Code Deleted

G0202   Screening mammography, producing direct digital image, bilateral, all views
Code Added

G0203   Screening mammography, film processed to produce digital images analyzed for
Code Deleted

G0204   Diagnostic mammography, producing direct digital image, bilateral, all views
Code Added

G0205   Diagnostic mammography, film processed to produce digital images analyzed for
Code deleted

G0206   Diagnostic mammography, producing direct digital image, unilateral, all views
Code Added

G0207   Diagnostic mammography, film processed to produce digital image analyzed for
Code Deleted

G0210   PET imaging whole body; full- and partial-ring PET scanners only, diagnosis, lung cancer, non-small cell
Code Added

G0211   PET imaging whole body; full- and partial-ring PET scanners only, initial staging, lung cancer, non-small cell
Code Added

G0212   PET imaging whole body, full- and partial-ring PET scanners only, restaging, lung cancer, non-small cell
Code Added

G0213 PET imaging whole body; full- and partial-ring PET scanners only, diagnosis, colorectal cancer
Code Added

G0214 PET imaging whole body; full- and partial-ring PET scanners only, initial staging, colorectal cancer
Code Added

G0215 PET imaging whole body; full- and partial-ring PET scanners only, restaging, colorectal cancer (replaces G0163)
Code Added

G0216 PET imaging whole body; full- and partial-ring PET scanners only, diagnosis, melanoma
Code Added

G0217 PET imaging whole body; full- and partial-ring PET scanners only, initial staging, melanoma
Code Added

G0218 PET imaging whole body; full- and partial-ring PET scanners only, restaging, melanoma (replaces G0165)
Code Added

G0219 PET imaging whole body; full and partial ring PET scanners only, for non-covered indications
Code Added

G0220 PET imaging whole body; full- and partial-ring PET scanners only, diagnosis, lymphoma
Code Added

G0221 PET imaging whole body; full- and partial-ring PET scanners only, initial staging, lymphoma (replaces G0164)
Code Added

G0222 PET imaging whole body; full- and partial-ring PET scanners only, restaging, lymphoma (replaces G0164)
Code Added

G0223 PET imaging whole body or regional; full- and partial-ring PET scanners only, diagnosis, head and neck cancer, excluding thyroid and CNS cancers
Code Added

G0224 PET imaging whole body or regional; full- and partial-ring PET scanners only, initial staging, head and neck cancer, excluding thyroid and CNS cancers
Code Added

G0225   PET imaging whole body or regional; full- and
partial-ring PET scanners only, restaging, head and neck
cancer, excluding thyroid and CNS cancers
Code Added

G0226   PET imaging whole body; full and partial ring PET
scanners only, diagnosis, esophageal cancer
Code Added

G0227   PET imaging whole body, full- and partial-ring PET
scanners only, initial staging, esophageal cancer
Code Added

G0228   PET imaging whole body, full- and partial-ring PET
scanners only, restaging, esophageal cancer
Code Added

G0229   PET imaging; metabolic brain imaging for pre-surgical
evaluation of refractory seizures, full- and partial-ring
PET scanners only
Code Added

G0230   PET imaging; metabolic assessment for myocardial
viability following inconclusive spect study, full- and
partial-ring PET scanners only
Code Added

G0231   PET, whole body, for recurrence of colorectal or
colorectal metastatic cancer; gamma cameras only
Code Added

G0232   PET, whole body, for staging and characterization of
lymphoma; gamma cameras only
Code Added

G0233   PET, whole body, for recurrence of melanoma or
melanoma metastatic cancer; gamma cameras only
Code Added

G0234   PET, regional or whole body, for solitary pulmonary
nodule following ct or for initial staging of pathologically
diagnosed nonsmall cell lung cancer; gamma cameras only
Code Added

G0236   Digitization of film radiographic images with computer
analysis for lesion detection and further physician review
for interpretation, diagnostic mammography (list
separately in addition to code for primary procedure)
Code Added

G0237 Therapeutic procedures to increase strength or endurance of respiratory muscles, face to face, one on one, each 15 minutes (includes monitoring)
Code Added

G0238 Therapeutic procedures to improve respiratory function, other than described by G0237, one on one, face to face, per 15 minutes (includes monitoring)
Code Added

G0239 Therapeutic procedures to improve respiratory function, other than services described by G0237, two or more (includes monitoring)
Code Added

G0240 Critical care service delivered by a physician, face to face; during interfacility transport of a critically ill or critically injured patient; first 30-74 minutes of active transport
Code Added

G0241 Each additional 30 minutes (list separately in addition to G0240)
Code Added

G0242 Multi-source photon stereotactic radiosurgery (cobalt 60 multi-source converging beams) plan, including dose volume histograms for target and critical structure tolerances, plan optimization performed for highly conformal distributions, plan positional accuracy and dose verification, all lesions treated, per course of treatment
Code Added

G0243 Multi-source photon stereotactic radiosurgery, delivery including collimator changes and custom plugging, complete course of treatment, all lesions
Code Added

G0244 Observation care provided by a facility to a patient with chf, chest pain, or asthma, minimum eight hours, maximum forty eight hours
Code Added

G9009 Coordinated care fee, risk adjusted maintenance, level 3
Code Added

G9010 Coordinated care fee, risk adjusted maintenance, level 4
Code Added

G9011 Coordinated care fee, risk adjusted maintenance, level 5
Code Added

G9012 Other specified case management service, not elsewhere classified
Code Added

H1000 Prenatal care, at-risk assessment
Code Added

H1001 Prenatal care, at-risk enhanced service; antepartum management
Code Added

H1002 Prenatal care, at risk enhanced service; care coordination
Code Added

H1003 Prenatal care, at-risk enhanced service; education
Code Added

H1004 Prenatal care, at-risk enhanced service; follow-up home visit
Code Added

H1005 Prenatal care, at-risk enhanced service package (includes H1001-H1004)
Code Added

J0340 Injection, nandrolone phenpropionate, up to 50 mg
Code Deleted

J0400 Injection, trimethaphan camsylate, up to 500 mg
Code Deleted

J0510 Injection, benzquinamide hcl, up to 50 mg
Code Deleted

J0587 Botulinum toxin type B, per 100 units
Code Added

J0590 Injection, ethylnorepinephrine hcl, 1 ml
Code Deleted

J0692 Injection, cefepime hydrochloride, 500 mg
Code Added

J0695 Injection, cefonicid sodium, 1 gram
Code Deleted

J0706 Injection, caffeine citrate, 5mg
Code Added

J0730   Injection, chlorpheniramine maleate, per 10 mg
Code Deleted

J0744   Injection, ciprofloxacin for intravenous infusion, 200 mg
Code Added

J0810   Injection, cortisone, up to 50 mg
Code Deleted

J1056   Injection, medroxyprogesterone acetate/estradiol
cypionate, 5mg/25mg
Code Added

J1090   Injection, testosterone cypionate, 1 cc, 50 mg
Code Deleted

J1270   Injection, doxercalciferol, 1 mcg
Code Added

J1362   Injection, erythromycin gluceptate, per 250 mg
Code Deleted

J1590   Injection, gatifloxacin, 10 mg
Code Added

J1655   Injection, tinzaparin sodium, 1000 IU
Code Added

J1690   Injection, prednisolone tebutate, up to 20 mg
Code Deleted

J1739   Injection, hydroxyprogesterone caproate 125 mg/ml
Code Deleted

J1741   Injection, hydroxyprogesterone caproate, 250 mg/ml
Code Deleted

J1755   Injection, iron sucrose, 20mg
Code Added

J1835   Injection, itraconazole, 50 mg
Code Added

J1930   Injection, propiomazine hcl, up to 20 mg
Code Deleted

J1970   Injection, methotrimeprazine, up to 20 mg
Code Deleted

J2020   Injection, linezolid, 200mg
Code Added

J2240 Injection, metocurine iodide, up to 2 mg
Code Deleted

J2330 Injection, thiothixene, up to 4 mg
Code Deleted

J2350 Injection, niacinamide, niacin, up to 100 mg
Code Deleted

J2480 Injection, hydrochlorides of opium alkaloids, up to 20 mg
Code Deleted

J2512 Injection, pentagastrin, per 2 ml
Code Deleted

J2640 Injection, prednisolone sodium phosphate, to 20 mg
Code Deleted

J2675 Injection, progesterone, per 50 mg
Code Deleted

J2860 Injection, secobarbital sodium, up to 250 mg
Code Deleted

J2940 Injection, somatrem, 1 mg
Code Added

J2941 Injection, somatropin, 1 mg
Code Added

J2970 Injection, methicillin sodium, up to 1 gm
Code Deleted

J3080 Injection, chlorprothixene, up to 50 mg
Code Deleted

J3100 Injection, tenecteplase, 50mg
Code Added

J3270 Injection, imipramine hcl, up to 25 mg
Code Deleted

J3390 Injection, methoxamine hcl, up to 20 mg
Code Deleted

J3395 Injection, verteporfin, 15mg
Code Added

J3450 Injection, mephentermine sulfate, up to 30 mg
Code Deleted

J7193   Factor IX (antihemophilic factor, purified, non-recombinant) per IU
Code Added

J7195   Factor IX (antihemophilic factor, recombinant) per IU
Code Added

J7302   Levonorgestrel-releasing intrauterine contraceptive system, 52 mg
Code Added

J7308   Aminolevulinic acid HCL for topical administration, 20%, single unit dosage form (354 mg)
Code Added

J7315   Sodium hyaluronate, 20 mg, for intra articular injection
Code Deleted

J7316   Sodium hyaluronate, 5 mg for intra-articular injection
Code Added

J7340   Dermal and epidermal, tissue of human origin, with or without bioengineered or processed elements, with metabolically active elements, per square centimeter
Code Added

J7504   Lymphocyte immune globulin, antithymocyte globulin, equine, parenteral, 250 mg
Description Changed

J7511   Lymphocyte immune globulin, antithymocyte globulin, rabbit, parenteral, 25 mg
Code Added

J7618   Albuterol, all formulations including separated isomers, inhalation solution administered through DME, concentrated form, per 1 mg (albuterol) or per 0.5 mg (levalbuterol)
Description Changed

J7619   Albuterol, all formulations including separated isomers, inhalation solution administered through DME, unit dose, per 1 mg (albuterol) or per 0.5 mg (levalbuterol)
Description Changed

J7622   Beclomethasone, inhalation solution administered through DME, unit dose form, per milligram
Code Added

J7624 Betamethasone, inhalation solution administered through DME, unit dose form, per milligram
Code Added

J7626 Budesonide inhalation solution, administered through DME, unit dose form, 0.25 mg
Code Added

J7641 Flunisolide, inhalation solution administered through DME, unit dose, per milligram
Code Added

J9017 Arsenic trioxide, 1 mg
Code Added

J9300 Gemtuzumab ozogamicin, 5 mg
Code Added

K0008 Custom manual wheelchair/base
Code Deleted

K0013 Custom motorized/power wheelchair base
Code Deleted

K0184 Nasal single piece interface, replacement for nasal application device, pair or single piece interface
Description Changed

K0541 Speech generating device, digitized speech, using pre-recorded messages, less than or equal to 8 minutes recording time
Description Changed

K0548 Injection, insulinn lispro, up to 50 units
Code Added

K0549 Hospital bed, heavy duty, extra wide, with weight capacity greater than 350 pounds but less than or equal to 600 pounds, with any type side rails, with mattress
Code Added

K0550 Hospital bed, extra heavy duty, extra wide, with weight capacity greater than 600 pounds, with any type side rails, with mattress
Code Added

K0551 Residual limb support system, solid base with adjustable drop hooks, mounts to wheelchair frame, each
Code Added

L0100   Cranial orthosis (helmet), with or without soft interface, molded to patient model
Description Changed

L0110   Cranial orthosis (helmet), with or without soft-interface, non-molded
Description Changed

L0321   TLSO, anterior-posterior control, with rigid or semi-rigid posterior panel, prefabricated (includes fitting and adjustment)
Code Added

L0331   TLSO, anterior-posterior-lateral control, with rigid or semi-rigid posterior panel, prefabricated (includes fitting and adjustment)
Code Added

L0391   TLSO, anterior-posterior-lateral-rotary control, with rigid or semi-rigid posterior panel, prefabricated (includes fitting and adjustment)
Code Added

L0515   LSO, anterior-posterior control, with rigid or semi-rigid posterior panel, prefabricated
Description Changed

L0561   LSO, anterior-posterior-lateral control, with rigid or semi-rigid posterior panel, prefabricated
Code Added

L0986   Addition to spinal orthosis, rigid or semi-rigid abdominal panel, prefabricated
Code Added

L1005   Tension based scoliosis orthosis and accessory pads, includes fitting and adjustment
Code Added

L1510   THKAO, standing frame, with or without tray and accessories
Description Changed

L1930   Ankle foot orthosis, plastic or other material, prefabricated, includes fitting and adjustment
Description Changed

L1940   Ankle foot orthosis, plastic or other material, custom-fabricated
Description Changed

L2415 Addition to knee lock with integrated release mechanism (bail, cable, or equal), any material, each joint
Description Changed

L2755 Addition to lower extremity orthosis, high strength, lightweight material, all hybrid lamination/prepreg composite, per segment
Description Changed

L2768 Orthotic side bar disconnect device, per bar
Code Added

L3677 Shoulder orthosis, hard plastic, shoulder stabilizer, pre-fabricated, includes fitting and adjustment
Code Added

L4000 Replace girdle for spinal orthosis (CTLSO or SO)
Description Changed

L4396 Static ankle foot orthosis, including soft interface material, adjustable for fit, for positioning, pressure reduction, may be used for minimal ambulation, prefabricated, includes fitting and adjustment
Description Changed

L5300 Below knee, molded socket, sach foot, endoskeletal system, including soft cover
Code Deleted

L5301 Below knee, molded socket, shin, each foot, endoskeletal system
Code Added

L5310 Knee disarticulation (or through knee), molded socket, sach foot endoskeletal
Code Deleted

L5311 Knee disarticulation (or through knee), molded socket, external knee joints, shin, sach foot, endoskeletal system
Code Added

L5320 Above knee, molded socket, open end, sach foot, endoskeletal system, single
Code Deleted

L5321 Above knee, molded socket, open end, sach foot, endoskeletal system, single axis knee
Code Added

L5330 Hip disarticulation, Canadian type; molded socket, endoskeletal system, hip
Code Deleted

L5331 Hip disarticulation, Canadian type, molded socket, endoskeletal system, hip joint, single axis knee, sach foot
Code Added

L5340 Hemipelvectomy, Canadian type; molded socket, endoskeletal system, hip joint
Code Deleted

L5341 Hemipelvectomy, Canadian type, molded socket, endoskeletal system, hip joint, single axis knee, sach foot
Code Added

L5667 Addition to lower extremity, below knee/above knee, socket insert, suction suspension with locking mechanism
Code Deleted

L5669 Addition to lower extremity, below knee/above knee, socket insert, suction
Code Deleted

L5671 Addition to lower extremity, below knee/above knee suspension locking mechanism (shuttle, lanyard or equal), excludes socket insert
Code Added

L5704 Custom shaped protective cover, below knee
Description Changed

L5705 Custom shaped protective cover, above knee
Description Changed

L5706 Custom shaped protective cover, knee disarticulation
Description Changed

L5707 Custom shaped protective cover, hip disarticulation
Description Changed

L5847 Addition, endoskeletal knee-shin system, microprocessor control feature, stance phase
Code Added

L5989 Addition to lower extremity prosthesis, endoskeletal system, pylon with integrated electronic force sensors
Code Added

L5990 Addition to lower extremity prosthesis, user adjustable heel height
Code Added

L6881 Automatic grasp feature, addition to upper limb prosthetic terminal device
Code Added

L6882 Microprocessor control feature, addition to upper limb prosthetic terminal device
Code Added

L8001 Breast prosthesis, mastectomy bra, with integrated breast prosthesis form, unilateral
Code Added

L8002 Breast prosthesis, mastectomy bra, with integrated breast prosthesis form, bilateral
Code Added

L8505 Artificial larynx replacement battery/accessory, any type
Code Added

L8507 Tracheo-esophageal voice prosthesis, patient inserted, any type, each
Code Added

L8509 Tracheo-esophageal voice prosthesis, inserted by a licensed health care provider, any type
Code Added

L8510 Voice amplifier
Code Added

M0302 Assessment of cardiac output by electrical bioimpedance
Code Deleted

P9042 Infusion, albumin (human), 25%, 10 ml
Code Deleted

P9045 Infusion, albumin (human), 5%, 250 ml
Code Added

P9046 Infusion, albumin (human), 25%, 20 ml
Code Added

P9047 Infusion, albumin (human), 25%, 50 ml
Code Added

P9048 Infusion, plasma protein fraction (human), 5%, 250 ml
Code Added

P9050 Granulocytes, pheresis, each unit
Code Added

Q0144 Azithromycin dihydrate, oral, capsules/powder, 1 gram
Code Deleted

Q0160 Factor ix (antihemophilic factor, purified, non-recombinant) per IU
Code Deleted

Q0161 Factor ix (antihemophilic factor, recombinant) per IU
Code Deleted

Q0185 Dermal and epidermal, tissue of human origin, with or without bioengineered or
Code Deleted

Q2015 Injection, somatrem, 5 mg
Code Deleted

Q2016 Injection, somatropin, 1 mg
Code Deleted

Q3013 Injection, verteporfin, 15 mg
Code Deleted

Q3014 Telehealth originating site facility fee
Code Added

Q3017 Ambulance service, advanced life support (ALS) assessment, no other ALS services provided
Code Added

Q4001 Cast supplies, body cast adult, with or without head, plaster
Code Added

Q4002 Cast supplies, body cast adult, with or without head, fiberglass
Code Added

Q4003 Cast supplies, shoulder cast, adult (11 years +), plaster
Code Added

Q4004 Cast supplies, shoulder cast, adult (11 years +), fiberglass
Code Added

Q4005 Cast supplies, long arm cast, adult (11 years +), plaster
Code Added

Q4006 Cast supplies, long arm cast, adult (11 years +), fiberglass
Code Added

Q4007 Cast supplies, long arm cast, pediatric (0-10 years), plaster
Code Added

Q4008 Cast supplies, long arm cast, pediatric (0-10 years), fiberglass
Code Added

Q4009 Cast supplies, short arm cast, adult (11 years +), plaster
Code Added

Q4010 Cast supplies, short arm cast, adult (11 years +), fiberglass
Code Added

Q4011 Cast supplies, short arm cast, pediatric (0-10 years), plaster
Code Added

Q4012 Cast supplies, short arm cast, pediatric (0-10 years), fiberglass
Code Added

Q4013 Cast supplies, gauntlet cast (includes lower forearm and hand), adult (11 years +), plaster
Code Added

Q4014 Cast supplies, gauntlet cast (includes lower forearm and hand), adult (11 years +), fiberglass
Code Added

Q4015 Cast supplies, gauntlet cast (includes lower forearm and hand), pediatric (0-10 years), plaster
Code Added

Q4016 Cast supplies, gauntlet cast (includes lower forearm and hand), pediatric (0-10 years), fiberglass
Code Added

Q4017 Cast supplies, long arm splint, adult (11 years +), plaster
Code Added

Q4018 Cast supplies, long arm splint, adult (11 years +), fiberglass
Code Added

Q4019 Cast supplies, long arm splint, pediatric (0-10 years), plaster
Code Added

Q4020   Cast supplies, long arm splint, pediatric (0-10 years), fiberglass
Code Added

Q4021   Cast supplies, short arm splint, adult (11 years +), plaster
Code Added

Q4022   Cast supplies, short arm splint, adult (11 years +), fiberglass
Code Added

Q4023   Cast supplies, short arm splint, pediatric (0-10 years), plaster
Code Added

Q4024   Cast supplies, short arm splint, pediatric (0-10 years), fiberglass
Code Added

Q4025   Cast supplies, hip spica (one or both legs), adult (11 years +), plaster
Code Added

Q4026   Cast supplies, hip spica (one or both legs), adult (11 years +), fiberglass
Code Added

Q4027   Cast supplies, hip spica (one or both legs), pediatric (0-10 years), plaster
Code Added

Q4028   Cast supplies, hip spica (one or both legs), pediatric (0-10 years), fiberglass
Code Added

Q4029   Cast supplies, long leg cast, adult (11 years +), plaster
Code Added

Q4030   Cast supplies, long leg cast, adult (11 years +), fiberglass
Code Added

Q4031   Cast supplies, long leg cast, pediatric (0-10 years), plaster
Code Added

Q4032   Cast supplies, long leg cast, pediatric (0-10 years), fiberglass
Code Added

Q4033   Cast supplies, long leg cylinder cast, adult (11 years +), plaster
Code Added

Q4034   Cast supplies, long leg cylinder cast, adult (11 years +), fiberglass
Code Added

Q4035   Cast supplies, long leg cylinder cast, pediatric (0-10 years), plaster
Code Added

Q4036   Cast supplies, long leg cylinder cast, pediatric (0-10 years), fiberglass
Code Added

Q4037   Cast supplies, short leg cast, adult (11 years +), plaster
Code Added

Q4038   Cast supplies, short leg cast, adult (11 years +), fiberglass
Code Added

Q4039   Cast supplies, short leg cast, pediatric (0-10 years), plaster
Code Added

Q4040   Cast supplies, short leg cast, pediatric (0-10 years), fiberglass
Code Added

Q4041   Cast supplies, long leg splint, adult (11 years +), plaster
Code Added

Q4042   Cast supplies, long leg splint, adult (11 years +), fiberglass
Code Added

Q4043   Cast supplies, long leg splint, pediatric (0-10 years), plaster
Code Added

Q4044   Cast supplies, long leg splint, pediatric (0-10 years), fiberglass
Code Added

Q4045   Cast supplies, short leg splint, adult (11 years +), plaster
Code Added

Q4046   Cast supplies, short leg splint, adult (11 years +), fiberglass
Code Added

Q4047 Cast supplies, short leg splint, pediatric (0-10 years), plaster
Code Added

Q4048 Cast supplies, short leg splint, pediatric (0-10 years), fiberglass
Code Added

Q4049 Finger splint, static
Code Added

Q4050 Cast supplies, for unlisted types and materials of casts
Code Added

Q4051 Splint supplies, miscellaneous (includes thermoplastics, strapping, fasteners, padding and other supplies)
Code Added

S0024 Injection, ciprofloxacin, 200 mg
Code Deleted

S0029 Injection, fluconazole, 400 mg
Code Deleted

S0079 Injection, octreotide acetate, 100 mcg (for doses over 1 mg use J2352 or C1207)
Code Added

S0086 Injection, verteporfin, 15 mg
Code Deleted

S0087 Injection, alemtuzumab, 30 mg
Code Added

S0088 Imatinib, 100 mg
Code Added

S0091 Granisetron hydrochloride, 1 mg (for circumstances falling under the medicare statute, use Q0166)
Code Added

S0092 Injection, hydromorphone hydrochloride, 250 mg (loading dose for infusion pump)
Code Added

S0093 Injection, morphine sulfate, 500 mg (loading dose for infusion pump)
Code Added

S0096 Injection, itraconazole, 200 mg
Code Deleted

S0155   Sterile dilutant for epoprostenol, 50 ml
Code Added

S0170   Anastrozole, oral, 1 mg
Code Added

S0171   Injection, bumetanide, 0.5 mg
Code Added

S0172   Chlorambucil, oral, 2 mg
Code Added

S0173   Dexamethasone, oral, 4 mg
Code Added

S0174   Dolasetron mesylate, oral 50 mg (for circumstances
falling under the medicare statute, use Q0180)
Code Added

S0175   Flutamide, oral, 125 mg
Code Added

S0176   Hydroxyurea, oral, 500 mg
Code Added

S0177   Levamisole hydrochloride, oral, 50 mg
Code Added

S0178   Lomustine, oral, 10 mg
Code Added

S0179   Megestrol acetate, oral, 20 mg
Code Added

S0181   Ondansetron hydrochloride, oral, 4 mg (for circumstances
falling under the medicare statute, use Q0179)
Code Added

S0182   Procarbazine hydrochloride, oral, 50 mg
Code Added

S0183   Prochlorperazine maleate, oral, 5 mg (for circumstances
falling under the medicare statute, use Q0164-Q0165)
Code Added

S0187   Tamoxifen citrate, oral, 10 mg
Code Added

S0189   Testosterone pellet, 75 mg
Code Added

S0190   Mifepristone, oral, 200 mg
Code Added

S0191   Misoprostol, oral, 200 mcg
Code Added

S0199   Medically induced abortion by oral ingestion of
medication including all associated services and supplies
(e.g., patient counseling, office visits, confirmation of
pregnancy by HCG, ultrasound to confirm duration of
pregnancy, ultrasound to confirm completion of abortion)
except drugs
Code Added

S0206   Procedure performed in surgery suite in physician's office
(list separately in addition to code for primary procedure
to denote use of facility and equipment)
Code Added

S0208   Paramedic intercept, hospital-based ALS service
(non-voluntary), non-transport
Code Added

S0209   Wheelchair van, mileage, per mile
Code Added

S0215   Non-emergency transportation; mileage
Code Added

S0250   Comprehensive geriatric assessment and treatment
planning performed by assessment team
Code Added

S0255   Hospice referral visit (advising patient and family of care
options) performed by nurse, social worker, or other
designated staff
Code Added

S0260   History and physical (outpatient or office) related to
surgical procedure (list separately in addition to code for
appropriate evaluation and management service)
Code Added

S0302   Completed early periodic screening diagnosis and
treatment (EPSDT) service (list in addition to code for
appropriate evaluation and management service)
Code Added

S0310   Hospitalist services (list separately in addition to code for appropriate evaluation and management service)
Code Added

S0340   Lifestyle modification program for management of coronary artery disease, including all supportive services; first quarter/stage
Code Added

S0341   Lifestyle modification program for management of coronary artery disease, including all supportive services; second or third quarter/stage
Code Added

S0342   Lifestyle modification program for management of coronary artery disease, including all supportive services; fourth quarter/stage
Code Added

S0395   Impression casting of a foot performed by a practitioner other than the manufacturer of the orthotic
Code Added

S0400   Global fee for extracorporeal shock wave lithotripsy treatment of kidney stone(s)
Code Added

S0500   Disposable contact lens, per lens
Code Added

S0504   Single vision prescription lens (safety, athletic or sunglass), per lens
Code Added

S0506   Bifocal vision prescription lens (safety, athletic or sunglass), per lens
Code Added

S0508   Trifocal vision prescription lens (safety, athletic or sunglass), per lens
Code Added

S0510   Non-prescription lens (safety, athletic or sunglass), per lens
Code Added

S0512   Daily wear specialty contact lens, per lens
Code Added

S0514   Color contact lens, per lens
Code Added

S0516   Safety eyeglass frames
Code Added

S0518   Sunglasses frames
Code Added

S0580   Polycarbonate lens (List this code in addition to the basic code for the lens)
Code Added

S0581   Nonstandard lens (List this code in addition to the basic code for the lens)
Code Added

S0590   Integral lens service, miscellaneous services reported separately
Code Added

S0592   Comprehensive contact lens evaluation
Code Added

S0622   Physical exam for college, new or established patient (list separately in addition to appropriate evaluation and management code)
Code Added

S0812   Phototherapeutic keratectomy (PTK)
Code Added

S1001   Deluxe item, patient aware (List in addition to code for basic item)
Code Added

S1002   Customized item (List in addition to code for basic item)
Code Added

S1025   Inhaled nitric oxide for the treatment of hypoxic respiratory failure in the neonate; per diem
Code Added

S1030   Continuous noninvasive glucose monitoring device, purchase (for physician interpretation of data, use CPT code)
Code Added

S1031   Continuous noninvasive glucose monitoring device, rental, including sensor, sensor replacement, and download to monitor (for physician interpretation of data, use CPT code)
Code Added

S2052   Transplantation of small intestine allograft (there are CPT codes available for intestinal allotransplantation - 44135 for graft from cadaver donor or 44136 for graft from living donor)
Code Deleted

S2065   Simultaneous pancreas kidney transplantation
Code Added

S2080   Laser-assisted uvulopalatoplasty (laup)
Code Added

S2112   Arthroscopy, knee, surgical for harvesting cartilage (chondrocyte cells)
Code Added

S2115   Osteotomy, periacetabular, with internal fixation
Code Added

S2150   Bone marrow or blood-derived peripheral stem cell harvesting and transplantation, allogenic or autologous, including pheresis, high-dose chemotherapy, and 28 days of post-transplant care (including drugs, hospitalization, medical, surgical, diagnostic and emergency services)
Code Added

S2210   Cryosurgical ablation (in situ destruction) of tumorous tissue, one or more lesions; liver
Code Deleted

S2220   Thrombectomy, coronary; by mechanical means (e.g. using rheolytic catheter)
Code Deleted

S2250   Uterine artery embolization for uterine fibroids
Code Added

S2260   Induced abortion, 17 to 24 weeks, any surgical method
Code Added

S2341   Chemodenervation of adductor muscle(s) of vocal cord
Code Added

S2342   Nasal endoscopy for post-operative debridement following functional endoscopic sinus surgery, nasal and/or sinus cavity(s), unilateral or bilateral
Code Added

S2360   Percutaneous vertebroplasty, one vertebral body, unilateral or bilateral injection; cervical
Code Added

S2361   Each additional cervical vertebral body (list separately in addition to code for primary procedure)
Code Added

S2400   Repair, congenital hernia in the fetus, procedure performed in utero
Code Added

S2401   Repair, urinary tract obstruction in the fetus, procedure performed in utero
Code Added

S2402   Repair, congenital cystic adenomatoid malformation in the fetus, procedure performed in utero
Code Added

S2403   Repair, extralobar pulmonary sequestration in the fetus, procedure performed in utero
Code Added

S2404   Repair, myelomeningocele in the fetus, procedure performed in utero
Code Added

S2409   Repair, congenital malformation of fetus, procedure performed in utero, not otherwise classified
Code Added

S2411   Fetoscopic laser therapy for treatment of twin-to-twin transfusion syndrome
Code Added

S3600   Stat laboratory request (situations other than S3601)
Code Added

S3601   Emergency stat laboratory charge for patient who is homebound or residing in a nursing facility
Code Added

S3630   Eosinophil count, blood, direct
Code Added

S3700   Bladder tumor-associated antigen test
Code Deleted

S3701   Immunoassay for nuclear matrix protein 22 (NMP-22), quantitative
Code Added

S3818   Complete gene sequence analysis; BRCA1 gene
Code Added

S3819   Complete gene sequense analysis; BRCA2 gene
Code Added

S3830   Complete mlh1 and mlh2 gene sequence analysis for hereditary nonpolyposis colorectal cancer (HNPCC) genetic testing
Code Added

S3831   Single-mutation analysis (in individual with a known mlh1 and mlh2 mutation in the family) for hereditary nonpolyposis colorectal cancer (HNPCC) genetic testing
Code Added

S3835   Complete gene sequence analysis for cystic fibrosis genetic testing
Code Added

S3837   Complete gene sequence analysis for hemochromatosis genetic testing
Code Added

S3900   Surface electromyography (EMG)
Code Added

S3906   Transfusion, direct, blood or blood components
Code Deleted

S4011   In vitro fertilization; including but not limited to identification and incubation of mature oocytes, fertilization with sperm, incubation of embryo(s), and subsequent visualization for determination of development
Code Added

S4015   Complete in vitro fertilization cycle, case rate
Code Added

S4016   Frozen in vitro fertilization cycle, case rate
Code Added

S4018 Frozen embryo transfer procedure canceled before transfer, case rate
Code Added

S4020 In vitro fertilization procedure canceled before aspiration, case rate
Code Added

S4021 In vitro fertilization procedure canceled after aspiration, case rate
Code Added

S4022 Assisted oocyte fertilization, case rate
Code Added

S4025 Donor services for in vitro fertilization (sperm or embryo), case rate
Code Added

S4026 Procurement of donor sperm from sperm bank
Code Added

S4027 Storage of previously frozen embryos
Code Added

S4028 Microsurgical epididymal sperm aspiration (mesa)
Code Added

S4030 Sperm procurement and cryopreservation services; initial visit
Code Added

S4031 Sperm procurement and cryopreservation services; subsequent visit
Code Added

S4980 Levonorgestrel - releasing intrauterine system, each
Code Deleted

S4981 Insertion of levonorgestrel-releasing intrauterine system
Code Added

S4989 Contraceptive intrauterine device (e.g., progestacert IUD), including implants and supplies
Code Added

S4990 Nicotine patches, legend
Code Added

S4991 Nicotine patches, non-legend
Code Added

S5002   Fat emulsion 10% in 250 ml, with administration set
Code Deleted

S5003   Fat emulsion 20% in 250 ml, with administration set
Code Deleted

S5016   Antibiotic administration supplies (with pump), per day
Code Deleted

S5017   Antibiotic administration supplies (without pump), per day
Code Deleted

S5018   Pain therapy administration supplies (pca or continuous), per day
Code Deleted

S5019   Chemotherapy administration supplies (with pump), per diem
Code Deleted

S5020   Chemotherapy administration supplies (without pump), per diem
Code Deleted

S5021   Hydration therapy administration supplies, per diem
Code Deleted

S5022   Growth hormone therapy (e.g., Protropin, humatrope)
Code Deleted

S5025   Infusion pump rental, per diem
Code Deleted

S5035   Home infusion therapy, routine service of infusion device (e.g., pump maintenance)
Code Added

S5036   Home infusion therapy, repair of infusion device (e.g., pump repair)
Code Added

S5497   Home infusion therapy, catheter care/maintenance, not otherwise classified; includes administrative services, professional pharmacy services, care coordination, and all necessary supplies and equipment (drugs and nursing visits coded separately), per diem
Code Added

S5498   Home infusion therapy, catheter care/maintenance, simple (single lumen), includes administrative services, professional pharmacy services, care coordination and all necessary supplies and equipment, (drugs and nursing visits coded separately), per diem
Code Added

S5501   Home infusion therapy, catheter care/maintenance, complex (more than one lumen), includes administrative services, professional pharmacy services, care coordination, and all necessary supplies and equipment (drugs and nursing visits coded separately), per diem
Code Added

S5502   Home infusion therapy, catheter care/maintenance, implanted access device, includes administrative services, professional pharmacy services, care coordination and all necessary supplies and equipment, (drugs and nursing visits coded separately), per diem (use this code for interim maintenance of vascular access not currently in use)
Code Added

S5503   Maintenance of implanted vascular access device, including supplies; per diem
Code Deleted

S5517   Home infusion therapy, all supplies necessary for restoration of catheter patency or declotting
Code Added

S5518   Home infusion therapy, all supplies necessary for catheter repair
Code Added

S5520   Home infusion therapy, all supplies (including catheter) necessary for a peripherally inserted central venous catheter (PICC) line insertion
Code Added

S5521   Home infusion therapy, all supplies (including catheter) necessary for a midline catheter insertion
Code Added

S5522   Home infusion therapy, insertion of peripherally inserted central venous catheter (PICC), nursing services only (no supplies or catheter included)
Code Added

S5523 Home infusion therapy, insertion of midline central venous catheter, nursing services only (no supplies or catheter included)
Code Added

S8001 Radiofrequency stimulation of the thalamus for tremor accomplished by stereotactic method, including burr holes, localizing and recording techniques and placement of the electrode(s)
Code Deleted

S8030 Scleral application of tantalum ring(s) for localization of lesions for proton beam therapy
Code Added

S8037 Magnetic resonance cholangiopancreatography (MRCP)
Code Added

S8055 Ultrasound guidance for multifetal pregnancy reduction(s), technical component (only to be used when the physician doing the reduction procedure does not perform the ultrasound, guidance is included in the CPT code for multifetal pregnancy reduction - 59866)
Code Added

S8095 Wig (for medically-induced or congenital hair loss)
Description Changed

S8097 Asthma kit (including but not limited to portable peak expiratory flow meter, instructional video, brochure, and/or spacer)
Code Added

S8100 Holding chamber or spacer for use with an inhaler or nebulizer; without mask
Code Added

S8101 Holding chamber or spacer for use with an inhaler or nebulizer; with mask
Code Added

S8180 Tracheostomy shower protector
Code Added

S8181 Tracheostomy tube holder
Code Added

S8182 Humidifier, heated, used with ventilator, non-servo-controlled
Code Added

S8183 Humidifier, heated, used with ventilator, dual servo-controlled with temperature monitoring
Code Added

S8185 Flutter device
Code Added

S8186 Swivel adaptor
Code Added

S8189 Tracheostomy supply, not otherwise classified
Code Added

S8190 Electronic spirometer (or microspirometer)
Code Added

S8400 Incontinence pants, each
Code Deleted

S8401 Child-size incontinence garment, diaper, each
Code Added

S8402 Diapers, each
Code Deleted

S8403 Adult-sized incontinence garment, disposable, pull-up brief, each
Code Added

S8404 Child-size incontinence garment, disposable, pull-up brief, each
Code Added

S8405 Disposable liner/shield for incontinence, each
Description Changed

S8415 Supplies for home delivery of infant
Code Added

S8420 Gradient pressure aid (sleeve and glove combination), custom made
Code Added

S8421 Gradient pressure aid (sleeve and glove combination), ready made
Code Added

S8422 Gradient pressure aid (sleeve), custom made, medium weight
Code Added

S8423 Gradient pressure aid (sleeve), custom made, heavy weight
Code Added

S8424 Gradient pressure aid (sleeve), ready made
Code Added

S8425 Gradient pressure aid (glove), custom made, medium weight
Code Added

S8426 Gradient pressure aid (glove), custom made, heavy weight
Code Added

S8427 Gradient pressure aid (glove), ready made
Code Added

S8428 Gradient pressure aid (gauntlet), ready made
Code Added

S8429 Gradient pressure exterior wrap
Code Added

S8430 Padding for compression bandage, roll
Code Added

S8431 Compression bandage, roll
Code Added

S8450 Splint, prefabricated, digit (specify digit by use of modifier)
Code Added

S8451 Splint, prefabricated, wrist or ankle
Code Added

S8452 Splint, prefabricated, elbow
Code Added

S8490 Insulin syringes (100 syringes, any size)
Code Added

S9023 Xenon regional cerebral blood flow studies
Code Deleted

S9035 Medical equipment or supplies distributed by home care provider without professional nursing intervention, per day
Code Deleted

S9061 Home administration of aerosolized drug therapy (e.g., pentamidine); administrative services, professional pharmacy services, care coordination, all necessary

supplies and equipment (drugs and nursing visits coded separately), per diem
Description Changed

S9083 Global fee urgent care centers
Code Added

S9085 Meniscal allograft transplantation
Code Deleted

S9088 Services provided in an urgent care center (list in addition to code for service)
Description Changed

S9098 Home visit, phototherapy services (e.g., Bili-lite), including equipment rental, nursing services, blood draw, supplies, and other services, per diem
Code Added

S9109 Congestive heart failure telemonitoring, equipment rental, including telescale, computer system and software, telephone connections, and maintenance, per month
Code Added

S9117 Back school, per visit
Code Added

S9131 Physical therapy; in the home, per diem
Code Added

S9200 Nursing services and all necessary supplies (including pca pump rental) for home administration of patient controlled analgesia (pca) per diem (drugs not included)
Code Deleted

S9208 Home management of pre-term labor, including administrative services, professional pharmacy services, care coordination, and all necessary supplies or equipment (drugs and nursing visits coded separately), per diem (do not use this code with any home infusion per diem code)
Code Added

S9209 Home management of pre-term premature rupture of membranes (PPROM), including administrative services, professional pharmacy services, care coordination, and all necessary supplies or equipment (drugs and nursing visits coded separately), per diem (do not use this code with any home infusion per diem code)
Code Added

S9210 Nursing services and all necessary equipment and supplies for continuous, uninterrupted infusion of epoprostenol (includes venous access device, infusion pump, back up pump, ice packs for cassettes, batteries, all related supplies, and all nursing services including follow-up visits, telephone monitoring, 24 hour/7 day a week availability, and all education to patient and care givers); per diem
Code Deleted

S9211 Home management of gestational hypertension, includes administrative services, professional pharmacy services, care coordination and all necessary supplies and equipment (drugs and nursing visits coded separately); per diem (do not use this code with any home infusion per diem code)
Code Added

S9212 Home management of postpartum hypertension, includes administrative services, professional pharmacy services, care coordination, and all necessary supplies and equipment (drugs and nursing visits coded separately), per diem (do not use this code with any home infusion per diem code)
Code Added

S9213 Home management of preeclampsia, includes administrative services, professional pharmacy services, care coordination, and all necessary supplies and equipment (drugs and nursing services coded separately); per diem (do not use this code with any home infusion per diem code)
Code Added

S9214 Home management of gestational diabetes, includes administrative services, professional pharmacy services, care coordination, and all necessary supplies and equipment (drugs and nursing visits coded separately); per diem (do not use this code with any home infusion per diem code)
Code Added

S9216 Nursing services and all necessary equipment and supplies for gestational hypertension program (includes maternal assessment as needed, telephonic collection of blood pressure, urine protein, weight and fetal movement counting via a home data collection system, patient status reports, 24 hour/7 day a week nursing support, and all education to the patient and care giver); per diem
Code Added

S9217   Nursing services and all necessary equipment and supplies for postpartum hypertension program (includes maternal assessment as needed, telephonic collection of blood pressure, urine protein, weight, compliance management support, patient status reports, 24 hour/7 day a week nursing support, and all education to the patient and care giver); per diem
Code Added

S9218   Nursing services and all necessary equipment and supplies for preeclampsia program (includes maternal assessment as needed, telephonic collection of blood pressure, urine protein, weight and daily fetal movement counts via a home data collection system, compliance management support, patient status reports, 24 hour/7 day a week nursing support, and all education to the patient and care giver); per diem
Code Added

S9220   Nursing services and all necessary equipment and supplies for home administration of controlled rate intravenous infusion (e.g. Dobutamine) requiring prolonged attendance by the nurse, per diem (drugs not included)
Code Deleted

S9225   Nursing services and all necessary equipment and supplies for home administration of intravenous tocolytic therapy, per diem - use new CPT code
Code Deleted

S9230   Nursing services and all necessary equipment and supplies for home administration of heparin, per diem
Code Deleted

S9300   Nursing services and all necessary supplies for home enteral feeding by gravity, per diem (enteral formula not included)
Code Deleted

S9308   Nursing services and all necessary supplies for home enteral feeding by pump, including pump rental, per diem (enteral formula not included)
Code Deleted

S9310   Nursing services and all necessary supplies for home parenteral nutrition without lipids, including pump rental, per diem (parenteral solutions not included)
Code Deleted

S9325 Home infusion therapy, pain management infusion; administrative services, professional pharmacy services, care coordination, and all necessary supplies and equipment, (drugs and nursing visits coded separately), per diem (do not use this code with S9326, S9327 or S9328)
Code Added

S9326 Home infusion therapy, continuous pain management infusion; administrative services, professional pharmacy services, care coordination and all necessary supplies and equipment (drugs and nursing visits coded separately), per diem
Code Added

S9327 Home infusion therapy, intermittent pain management infusion; administrative services, professional pharmacy services, care coordination, and all necessary supplies and equipment (drugs and nursing visits coded separately), per diem
Code Added

S9328 Home infusion therapy, implanted pump pain management infusion; administrative services, professional pharmacy services, care coordination, and all necessary supplies and equipment (drugs and nursing visits coded separately), per diem
Code Added

S9329 Home infusion therapy, chemotherapy infusion; administrative services, professional pharmacy services, care coordination, and all necessary supplies and equipment (drugs and nursing visits coded separately), per diem (do not use this code with S9330 or S9331)
Code Added

S9330 Home infusion therapy, continuous chemotherapy infusion; administrative services, professional pharmacy services, care coordination, and all necessary supplies and equipment (drugs and nursing visits coded separately), per diem
Code Added

S9331 Home infusion therapy, intermittent chemotherapy infusion; administrative services, professional pharmacy services, care coordination, and all necessary supplies and equipment (drugs and nursing visits coded separately), per diem
Code Added

S9336   Home infusion therapy, continuous anticoagulant infusion therapy (e.g., Heparin), administrative services, professional pharmacy services, care coordination and all necessary supplies and equipment (drugs and nursing visits coded separately), per diem
Code Added

S9338   Home infusion therapy, immunotherapy therapy; administrative services, professional pharmacy services, care coordination, and all necessary supplies and equipment (drug and nursing visits coded separately), per diem
Code Added

S9339   Home therapy; peritoneal dialysis, administrative services, professional pharmacy services, care coordination and all necessary supplies and equipment (drugs and nursing visits coded separately), per diem
Code Added

S9340   Home therapy; enteral nutrition; administrative services, professional pharmacy services, care coordination, and all necessary supplies and equipment (enteral formula and nursing visits coded separately), per diem
Code Added

S9341   Home therapy; enteral nutrition via gravity; administrative services, professional pharmacy services, care coordination, and all necessary supplies and equipment (enteral formula and nursing visits coded separately), per diem
Code Added

S9342   Home therapy; enteral nutrition via pump; administrative services, professional pharmacy services, care coordination, and all necessary supplies and equipment (enteral formula and nursing visits coded separately), per diem
Code Added

S9343   Home therapy; enteral nutrition via bolus; administrative services, professional pharmacy services, care coordination, and all necessary supplies and equipment (enteral formula and nursing visits coded separately), per diem
Code Added

S9345 Home infusion therapy, anti-hemophilic agent infusion therapy (e.g., Factor VIII); administrative services, professional pharmacy services, care coordination, and all necessary supplies and equipment (drugs and nursing visits coded separately), per diem
Code Added

S9346 Home infusion therapy, alpha-1-proteinase inhibitor (e.g., Prolastin); administrative services, professional pharmacy services, care coordination, and all necessary supplies and equipment (drugs and nursing visits coded separately), per diem
Code Added

S9347 Home infusion therapy, uninterrupted, long-term, controlled rate intravenous infusion therapy (e.g., Epoprostenol); administrative services, professional pharmacy services, care coordination, all necessary supplies and equipment (drugs and nursing visits coded separately), per diem
Code Added

S9348 Home infusion therapy, sympathomimetic/inotropic agent infusion therapy (e.g., Dobutamine); administrative services, professional pharmacy services, care coordination, all necessary supplies and equipment (drugs and nursing visits coded separately), per diem
Code Added

S9349 Home infusion therapy, tocolytic infusion therapy; administrative services, professional pharmacy services, care coordination, and all necessary supplies and equipment (drugs and nursing visits coded separately), per diem
Code Added

S9351 Home infusion therapy, continuous anti-emetic infusion therapy; administrative services, professional pharmacy services, care coordination, all necessary supplies and equipment (drugs and nursing visits coded separately), per diem
Code Added

S9353 Home infusion therapy, continuous insulin infusion therapy; administrative services, professional pharmacy services, care coordination, and all necessary supplies and equipment (drugs and nursing visits coded separately), per diem
Code Added

S9355   Home infusion therapy, chelation therapy; administrative services, professional pharmacy services, care coordination, and all necessary supplies and equipment (drugs and nursing visits coded separately), per diem
Code Added

S9357   Home infusion therapy, enzyme replacement intravenous therapy; (e.g., Imiglucerase); administrative services, professional pharmacy services, care coordination, and all necessary supplies and equipment (drugs and nursing visits coded separately), per diem
Code Added

S9359   Home infusion therapy, anti-tumor necrosis factor intravenous therapy; (e.g., Infliximab); administrative services, professional pharmacy services, care coordination, and all necessary supplies and equipment (drugs and nursing visits coded separately), per diem
Code Added

S9361   Home infusion therapy, diuretic intravenous therapy; administrative services, professional pharmacy services, care coordination, and all necessary supplies and equipment (drugs and nursing visits coded separately), per diem
Code Added

S9363   Home infusion therapy, anti-spasmotic intravenous therapy; administrative services, professional pharmacy services, care coordination, and all necessary supplies and equipment (drugs and nursing visits coded separately), per diem
Code Added

S9364   Home infusion therapy, total parenteral nutrition (TPN); administrative services, professional pharmacy services, care coordination, and all necessary supplies and equipment (includes standard TPN formula, lipids, specialty amino acid formulas, drugs, and nursing visits coded separately), per diem (do not use with home infusion codes S9365-S9368 using daily volume scales)
Code Added

S9365   Home infusion therapy, total parenteral nutrition (TPN); one liter per day, administrative services, professional pharmacy services, care coordination, and all necessary supplies and equipment (includes standard TPN formula, lipids, specialty amino acid formulas, drugs, and nursing visits coded separately), per diem
Code Added

S9366 Home infusion therapy, total parenteral nutrition (TPN); more than one liter but no more than two liters per day, administrative services, professional pharmacy services, care coordination, and all necessary supplies and equipment (includes standard TPN formula, lipids, specialty amino acid formulas, drugs, and nursing visits coded separately), per diem
Code Added

S9367 Home infusion therapy, total parenteral nutrition (TPN); more than two liters but no more than three liters per day, administrative services, professional pharmacy services, care coordination, and all necessary supplies and equipment (includes standard TPN formula; lipids, specialty amino acids, drugs, and nursing visits coded separately), per diem
Code Added

S9368 Home infusion therapy, total parenteral nutrition (TPN); more than three liters per day, administrative services, professional pharmacy services, care coordination, and all necessary supplies and equipment (includes standard TPN formula; lipids, specialty amino acid formulas, drugs, and nursing visits coded separately), per diem
Code Added

S9370 Home therapy, intermittent anti-emetic injection therapy; administrative services, professional pharmacy services, care coordination, and all necessary supplies and equipment (drugs and nursing visits coded separately), per diem
Code Added

S9372 Home therapy; intermittent anticoagulant injection therapy (e.g., heparin); administrative services, professional pharmacy services, care coordination, and all necessary supplies and equipment (drugs and nursing visits coded separately), per diem (do not use this code for flushing of infusion devices with heparin to maintain patency)
Code Added

S9373 Home infusion therapy, hydration therapy; administrative services, professional pharmacy services, care coordination, and all necessary supplies and equipment (drugs and nursing visits coded separately), per diem (do not use with hydration therapy codes S9374-S9377 using daily volume scales)
Code Added

S9374 Home infusion therapy, hydration therapy; one liter per day, administrative services, professional pharmacy services, care coordination, and all necessary supplies and equipment (drugs and nursing visits coded separately), per diem
Code Added

S9375 Home infusion therapy, hydration therapy; more than one liter but no more than two liters per day, administrative services, professional pharmacy services, care coordination, and all necessary supplies and equipment (drugs and nursing visits coded separately), per diem
Code Added

S9376 Home infusion therapy, hydration therapy; more than two liters but no more than three liters per day, administrative services, professional pharmacy services, care coordination, and all necessary supplies and equipment (drugs and nursing visits coded separately), per diem
Code Added

S9377 Home infusion therapy, hydration therapy; more than three liters per day, administrative services, professional pharmacy services, care coordination, and all necessary supplies (drugs and nursing visits coded separately), per diem
Code Added

S9379 Home infusion therapy, infusion therapy, not otherwise classified; administrative services, professional pharmacy services, care coordination, and all necessary supplies and equipment (drugs and nursing visits coded separately), per diem
Code Added

S9381 Delivery or service to high risk areas requiring escort or extra protection, per visit
Code Added

S9395 Nursing services and all necessary supplies and additives for home iv hydration (via gravity or pump), per diem (hydration solution and drugs not included)
Code Deleted

S9420 Nursing services and all necessary supplies for interim home maintenance of implanted vascular access port/catheter/reservoir, per diem
Code Deleted

S9423   Nursing services, patient assessment and education, follow-up visits, electronic programmer and equipment (use of computer), programming of the pump, all necessary supplies, products or services for intrathecal drug infusion, per diem
Code Deleted

S9425   Nursing services and all necessary supplies and additives for home iv chemotherapy (via iv push, gravity drip, stationary pump, ambulatory belt pump), per diem (hydration solution and drugs not included)
Code Deleted

S9441   Asthma education, non-physician provider, per session
Code Added

S9442   Birthing classes, non-physician provider, per session
Code Added

S9443   Lactation classes, non-physician provider, per session
Code Added

S9445   Patient education, not otherwise classified, non-physician provider, individual, per session
Code Added

S9446   Patient education, not otherwise classified, non-physician provider, group, per session
Code Added

S9494   Home infusion therapy, antibiotic, antiviral, or antifungal therapy; administrative services, professional pharmacy services, care coordination, and all necessary supplies and equipment (drug and nursing visits coded separately), per diem (do not use with home infusion codes for hourly dosing schedules S9497-S9504)
Code Added

S9497   Home infusion therapy, antibiotic, antiviral, or antifungal therapy; once every 3 hours; administrative services, professional pharmacy services, care coordination, and all necessary supplies and equipment (drugs and nursing visits coded separately), per diem
Code Added

S9500   Home infusion therapy, antibiotic, antiviral, or antifungal therapy; once every 24 hours; administrative services, professional pharmacy services, care coordination, and all

necessary supplies and equipment (drugs and nursing visits coded separately), per diem
Code Added

S9501   Home infusion therapy, antibiotic, antiviral, or antifungal therapy; once every 12 hours; administrative services, professional pharmacy services, care coordination, and all necessary supplies and equipment (drugs and nursing visits coded separately), per diem
Code Added

S9502   Home infusion therapy, antibiotic, antiviral, or antifungal therapy; once every 8 hours, administrative services, professional pharmacy services, care coordination, and all necessary supplies and equipment (drugs and nursing visits coded separately), per diem
Code Added

S9503   Home infusion therapy, antibiotic, antiviral, or antifungal; once every 6 hours; administrative services, professional pharmacy services, care coordination, and all necessary supplies and equipment (drugs and nursing visits coded separately), per diem
Code Added

S9504   Home infusion therapy, antibiotic, antiviral, or antifungal; once every 4 hours; administrative services, professional pharmacy services, care coordination, and all necessary supplies and equipment (drugs and nursing visits coded separately), per diem
Code Added

S9526   Skilled nursing visits for blood product administration, including pump and all related supplies; per service
Code Deleted

S9527   Insertion of a peripherally inserted central venous catheter (picc), including nursing services and all supplies
Code Deleted

S9528   Insertion of midline central venous catheter, including nursing services and all supplies
Code Deleted

S9529   Routine venipuncture for collection of specimen(s), single home bound, nursing home, or skilled nursing facility patient
Code Added

S9533   Pain management, intravenous, epidural or subcutaneous, including solution, equipment rental, nursing care, and supplies; daily (drugs not included)
Code Deleted

S9535   Administration of hematopoietic hormones (e.g. Erythropoietin, g-csf, gm-csf) or platelets, intravenously, in the home setting, including all nursing care, equipment, and supplies; per diem
Code Deleted

S9537   Home therapy; hematopoietic hormone injection therapy (e.g., Crythropoietin, g-csf, gm-csf); administrative services, professional pharmacy services, care coordination, and all necessary supplies and equipment (drugs and nursing visits coded separately), per diem
Code Added

S9538   Home transfusion of blood product(s); administrative services, professional pharmacy services, care coordination and all necessary supplies and equipment (blood products, drugs, and nursing visits coded separately), per diem
Code Added

S9539   Administration of antibiotics, intravenously, in the home setting, including all nursing care, equipment, and supplies; per diem
Code Deleted

S9542   Home injectable therapy; not otherwise classified, including administrative services, professional pharmacy services, coordination of care, and all necessary supplies and equipment (drugs and nursing visits coded separately), per diem
Code Added

S9545   Administration of immune globulin, intravenously, in the home setting, including all nursing care, equipment, and supplies; per diem
Code Deleted

S9550   Home iv therapy, hydration fluids and electrolytes, including all nursing care, equipment, and supplies; per diem
Code Deleted

S9555 Additional home infusion therapy, including all nursing care, equipment, and supplies; each therapy, per diem (S9555 should be used in addition to the code for the primary therapy)
Code Deleted

S9558 Home injectable therapy; growth hormone, including administrative services, professional pharmacy services, coordination of care, and all necessary supplies and equipment (drugs and nursing visits coded separately), per diem
Code Added

S9559 Home injectable therapy; interferon, including administrative services, professional pharmacy services, coordination of care, and all necessary supplies and equipment (drugs and nursing visits coded separately), per diem
Code Added

S9560 Home injectable therapy; hormonal therapy (e.g., leuprolide, goserelin), including administrative services, professional pharmacy services, care coordination, and all necessary supplies and equipment (drugs and nursing visits coded separately), per diem
Code Added

S9800 Home therapy; provision of infusion, specialty drug administration, and/or associated nursing services and procedures, by highly technical RN, per hour (do not use this code with S9524)
Code Added

S9810 Home therapy; professional pharmacy services for provision of infusion, specialty drug administration, and/or disease state management, not otherwise classified, per hour (do not use this code with any per diem code)
Code Added

S9981 Medical records copying fee, administrative
Code Added

S9982 Medical records copying fee, per page
Code Added

S9986 Not medically necessary service (patient is aware that service not medically necessary)
Code Added

S9989   Services provided outside of the United States of America (list in addition to code(s) for services(s))
Code Added

T1000   Private duty/independent nursing service(s), licensed, up to 15 minutes
Code Added

T1001   Nursing assessment/evaluation
Code Added

T1002   RN services, up to 15 minutes
Code Added

T1003   LPN/LVN services, up to 15 minutes
Code Added

T1004   Services of a qualified nursing aide, up to 15 minutes
Code Added

T1005   Respite care services, up to 15 minutes
Code Added

T1006   Alcohol and/or substance abuse services, family/couple counseling
Code Added

T1007   Alcohol and/or substance abuse services, treatment plan development and/or modification
Code Added

T1008   Day treatment for individual alcohol and/or substance abuse services
Code Added

T1009   Child sitting services for children of the individual receiving alcohol and/or substance abuse services
Code Added

T1010   Meals for individuals receiving alcohol and/or substance abuse services (when meals are not included in the program)
Code Added

T1011   Alcohol and/or substance abuse services, not otherwise classified
Code Added

T1012   Alcohol and/or substance abuse services, skills
development
Code Added

T1013   Sign language or oral interpreter services
Code Added

T1014   Telehealth transmission, per minute, professional services
bill separately
Code Added

T1015   Clinic visit/encounter, all-inclusive
Code Added

V5241   Dispensing fee, monaural hearing aid, any type
Code Added

V5242   Hearing aid, analog, monaural, cic (completely in the ear
canal)
Code Added

V5243   Hearing aid, analog, monaural, itc (in the canal)
Code Added

V5244   Hearing aid, digitally programmable analog, monaural, cic
Code Added

V5245   Hearing aid, digitally programmable, analog, monaural, itc
Code Added

V5246   Hearing aid, digitally programmable analog, monaural, ite
(in the ear)
Code Added

V5247   Hearing aid, digitally programmable analog, monaural,
bte (behind the ear)
Code Added

V5248   Hearing aid, analog, binaural, cic
Code Added

V5249   Hearing aid, analog, binaural, itc
Code Added

V5250   Hearing aid, digitally programmable analog, binaural, cic
Code Added

V5251   Hearing aid, digitally programmable analog, binaural, itc
Code Added

V5252   Hearing aid, digitally programmable, binaural, ite
         Code Added

V5253   Hearing aid, digitally programmable, binaural, bte
         Code Added

V5254   Hearing aid, digital, monaural, cic
         Code Added

V5255   Hearing aid, digital, monaural, itc
         Code Added

V5256   Hearing aid, digital, monaural, ite
         Code Added

V5257   Hearing aid, digital, monaural, bte
         Code Added

V5258   Hearing aid, digital, binaural, cic
         Code Added

V5259   Hearing aid, digital, binaural, itc
         Code Added

V5260   Hearing aid, digital, binaural, ite
         Code Added

V5261   Hearing aid, digital, binaural, bte
         Code Added

V5262   Hearing aid, disposable, any type, monaural
         Code Added

V5263   Hearing aid, disposable, any type, binaural
         Code Added

V5264   Ear mold/insert, not disposable, any type
         Code Added

V5265   Ear mold/insert, disposable, any type
         Code Added

V5266   Battery for use in hearing device
         Code Added

V5267   Hearing aid supplies/accessories
         Code Added

V5268   Assistive listening device, telephone amplifier, any type
         Code Added

V5269   Assistive listening device, alerting, any type
Code Added

V5270   Assistive listening device, television amplifier, any type
Code Added

V5271   Assistive listening device, television caption decoder
Code Added

V5272   Assistive listening device, TDD
Code Added

V5273   Assistive listening device, for use with cochlear implant
Code Added

V5274   Assistive learning device, not otherwise specified
Code Added

V5275   Ear impression, each
Code Added

APPENDIX C

HCPCS TABLE OF DRUGS

Directions for the Use of the Table:

1. All drugs are listed in strict alphabetical order by generic drug name.

2. HCPCS code numbers for drugs are listed only under the generic drug name. Users should first look for entries under generic names of drugs. When a drug is known only by brand name, look for the brand name and you will be directed to the generic name of the drug (see "generic name").

3. Cancer chemotherapy drugs are preceded by an asterisk (*).

4. In all cases except those preceded by a pound sign (#), the amount stated includes the amount as well as any amount "up to" that which is stated in the column. When a pound sign appears, it designated that the amount of the drug is only the amount listed.

5. A hyphen (—) appearing in a column signifies that no information is given for that particular variable for the drug listed.

6. Information which is indented and appears beneath the first line for a drug is to be considered a continuation of the line preceding it. All drug entries should be checked for indented lines beneath it as a continuation of that entry.

7. When one drug has more than one entry as a result of different routes of administration or different amounts, the drug name is not repeated. All entries for the same drug are listed beneath that drug.

8. The following abbreviations are used in the "routes of administration" column:

amp   = ampule

DME = durable medical equipment

EPI   = epidural

g   = gram

IA   = intra-arterial administration

IM   = intramuscular administration

INF   = infusion

INH   = administration by inhaled solution

INJ   = injection

IO   = intraocular

IT   = intrathecal

IU   = international unit

IV   = intravenous administration

mcg   = microgram

mg   = milligram

ml   = milliliter

ORAL= administered orally

OTH   = other routes of administration

PAR   = parenteral

SC   = subcutaneous administration

TABS = tablets

U   = units

VAR   = various routes of administration

A

Abbokinase (see Urokinase)			
Abbokinase, Open Cath (see Urokinase)			
Abciximab	10 mg	IV	J0130
Abelcet (see Amphotericin B Lipid Complex)			
ABLC (see Amphotericin B)			
Acetazolamide sodium	up to 500 mg	IM/IV	J1120
Acetylcysteine, unit dose form	per gram	INH	J7608
Achromycin (see Tetracycline)			
ACTH (see Corticotropin)			
Acthar (see Corticotropin)			
Actimmune (see Interferon gamma 1-B)			
Activase (see Alteplase recombinant)			
Adenocard (see Adenosine)			
Adenoscan (see Adenosine)			
Adenosine	6 mg	IV	J0150
	90 mg	IV	J0151
Adrenalin Chloride (see Adrenalin, epinephrine)			
Adrenalin, epinephrine	up to 1 ml amp	SC/IM	J0170
Adriamycin PFS or RDF (see Doxorubicin HCl)			
Adrucil (see Fluorouracil)			
Aggrastat (see Tirofiban hydrochloride)			

A-hydroCort (see Hydrocortisone sodium phosphate)			
Akineton (see Biperiden)			
Alatrofloxacin mesylate, injection	100 mg	IV	J0200
Albuterol, concentrated form	per mg	INH	J7618
Albuterol, unit dose form	per mg	INH	J7619
Aldesleukin	per single use vial	IM/IV	J9015
Aldomet (see Methyldopate HCl)			
Alferon N (see Interferon alfa-n3)			
Alglucerase	per 10 U	IV	J0205
Alkaban-AQ (see Vinblastine sulfate)			
Alkeran (see Melphalan, oral)			
Alpha 1 - proteinase inhibitor, human	10 mg	IV	J0256
Alprostadil, injection	1.25 mcg	OTH/ injection	J0270
Alprostadil, urethral suppository	—	OTH	J0275
Alteplase recombinant	1 mg	IV	J2997
Alupent (see Metaproterenol sulfate or Metaproterenol, compounded)			
Amcort (see Triamcinolone diacetate)			
A-methaPred (see Methylprednisolone sodium succinate)			
Amgen (see Interferon alphacon-1)			

Amifostine	500 mg	IV	J0207
Aminolevalinic acid HCl	unit dose (354 mg)	OTH	J7308
Aminophylline/Aminophylli	up to 250 mg	IV	J0280
Amiodarone HCl	30 mg	IV	J0282
Amitriptyline HCl	up to 20 mg	IM	J1320
Amobarbital	up to 125 mg	IM/IV	J0300
Amphocin (see Amphotericin B)			
Amphotericin B	50 mg	IV	J0285
Amphotericin B, lipid complex	50 mg	IV	J0286
Ampicillin sodium	up to 500 mg	IM/IV	J0290
Ampicillin sodium/ sulbactam sodium	per 1.5 g	IM/IV	J0295
Amygdalin (see Laetrile, Amygdalin, vitamin B-17)			
Amytal (see Amobarbital)			
Anabolin LA 100 (see Nandrolone decanoate)			
Ancef (see Cefazolin sodium)			
Andrest 90-4 (see Testosterone enanthate and estradiol valerate)			
Andro-Cyp (see Testosterone cypionate)			
Andro-Cyp 200 (see Testosterone cypionate)			
Andro LA 200 (see Testosterone enanthate)			
Andro-Estro 90-4 (see Testosterone enanthate and estradiol valerate)			

Andro/Fem (see
  Testosterone cypionate
  and estradiol cypionate)

Androgyn LA (see
  Testosterone enanthate
  and estradiol valerate)

Androlone-50 (see
  Nandrolone
  phenpropionate)

Androlone-D 100 (see
  Nandrolone decanoate)

Andronaq-50 (see
  Testosterone suspension)

Andronaq-LA (see
  Testosterone cypionate)

Andronate -100 or -200
  (see Testosterone
  cypionate)

Andropository 100 (see
  Testosterone enanthate)

Andryl 200 (see
  Testosterone enanthate)

Anectine (see
  Succinylcholine chloride)

Anergan 25 or 50 (see
  Promethazine HCl)

Anistreplase	per 30 U	IV	J0350
Anti-inhibitor	per IU	IV	J7198

Antispas (see Dicyclomine
  HCl)

Antithrombin III (human)	per IU	IV	J7197

Anzemet (see Dolasetron
  mesylate injection)

A.P.L. (see Chorionic
  gonadotropin)

Apresoline (see
  Hydralazine HCl)

Aprotinin	10,000 KIU	—	Q2003
AquaMEPHYTON (see Vitamin K)			
Aralen (see Chloroquine HCl)			
Aramine (see Metaraminol)			
Arbutamine HCl	1 mg	IV	J0395
Aredia (see Pamidronate disodium)			
Arfonad (see Trimethaphan camsylate)			
Aristocort Forte or Intralesional (see Triamcinolone diacetate)			
Aristospan Intra-Articular or Intralesional (see Triamcinolone hexacetonide)			
Arrestin (see Trimethobenzamide HCl)			
Arsenic trioxide	1 mg	IV	J9017
Asparaginase	10,000 U	IV/IM	J9020
Astramorph PF (see Morphine sulfate)			
Atgam (see Lymphocyte immune globulin)			
Ativan (see Lorazepam)			
Atropine, concentrated form	per mg	INH	J7635
Atropine, unit dose form	per mg	INH	J7636
Atropine sulfate	up to 0.3 mg	IV/IM/SC	J0460
Atrovent (see Ipratropium bromide)			
Aurothioglucose	up to 50 mg	IM	J2910
Autologous cultured chondrocytes, implant	—	—	J7330

Autoplex T (see Hemophilia clotting factors)			
Avonex (see Interferon beta-1a)			
Azathioprine	50 mg	ORAL	J7500
Azathioprine, parenteral	100 mg	IV	J7501
Azithromycin, injection	500 mg	IV	J0456

B

Baclofen	10 mg	IT	J0475
Baclofen for intrathecal trial	50 mcg	OTH	J0476
Bactocill (see Oxacillin sodium)			
BAL in oil (see Dimercaprol)			
Banflex (see Orphenadrine citrate)			
Basiliximab	20 mg	—	Q2019
BCG (Bacillus Calmette & Guerin) live instillation	per instillation	IV	J9031
Beclomethasone inhalation solution, unit dose form	per mg	INH	J7622
Bena-D 10 or 50 (see Diphenhydramine HCl)			
Benadryl (see Diphenhydramine HCl)			
Benahist 10 or 50 (see Diphenhydramine HCl)			
Ben-Allergin-50 (see Diphenhydramine HCl)			
Benefix (see Factor IX, recombinant)			

Benoject-10 or -50 (see Diphenhydramine HCl)			
Bentyl (see Dicyclomine)			
Benztropine mesylate	per 1 mg	IM/IV	J0515
Berubigen (see Vitamin B-12 cyanocobalamin)			
Betalin 12 (see Vitamin B-12 cyanocobalamin)			
Betameth (see Betamethasone sodium phosphate)			
Betamethasone acetate & Betamethasone sodium phosphate	per 3 mg	IM	J0702
Betamethasone inhalation solution, unit dose form	per mg	INH	J7624
Betamethasone sodium phosphate	per 4 mg	IM/IV	J0704
Betaseron (see Interferon beta-1b)			
Bethanechol chloride	up to 5 mg	SC	J0520
Bicillin C-R, and Bicillin C-R 900/300 (Penicillin G procaine & Penicillin G benzathine)			
Bicillin L-A (see Penicillin G benzathine)			
BiCNU (see Carmustine)			
Biperiden lactate	per 5 mg	IM/IV	J0190
Bitolterol mesylate, concentrated form	per mg	INH	J7628
Bitolterol mesylate, unit dose form	per mg	INH	J7629
Blenoxane (see Bleomycin sulfate)			
Bleomycin sulfate	15 U	IM/IV/SC	J9040
Botulinum toxin type A	per unit	IM	J0585

Botulinum toxin type B	per 100 U	IM	J0587
Brethine (see Terbutaline sulfate or Terbutaline, compounded)			
Bricanyl subcutaneous (see Terbutaline sulfate)			
Brompheniramine maleate	per 10 mg	IM/SC/IV	J0945
Bronkephrine (see Ethylnorepinephrine HCl)			
Bronkosol (see Isoetharine HCl)			
Budesonide inhalation solution, unit dose form	0.25 mg	INH	J7626
Busulfan	2 mg	ORAL	J8510

C

Cabergoline	0.5 mg	ORAL	Q2001
Cafcit (see Caffeine citrate)			
Caffeine citrate	5 mg	IV	J0706
Caine-1 or -2 (see Lidocaine HCl)			
Calcijex (see Calcitriol)			
Calcimar (see Calcitonin-salmon)			
Calcitonin-salmon	up to 400 U	SC/IM	J0630
Calcitriol	1 mcg amp	IM	J0635
Calcium disodium versenate (see Edetate calcium disodium)			
Calcium gluconate	per 10 ml	IV	J0610
Calcium glycerophosphate and calcium lactate	per 10 ml	IM/SC	J0620

Calphosan (see Calcium
  glycerophosphate and
  calcium lactate)

Camptosar (see Irinotecan)

| Capecitabine | 150 mg | ORAL | J8520 |
| | 500 mg | ORAL | J8521 |

Carbocaine (see
  Mepivacaine)

Carbocaine with
  Neo-Cobefrin (see
  Mepivacaine)

| Carboplatin | 50 mg | IV | J9045 |
| Carmustine | 100 mg | IV | J9050 |

Carnitor (see
  Levocarnitine)

Carticel (see Autologous
  cultured chondrocytes)

Cefadyl (see Cephapirin
  sodium)

| Cefazolin sodium | up to 500 mg | IV/IM | J0690 |
| Cefepime hydrochloride | 500 mg | IV | J0692 |

Cefizox (see Ceftizoxime
  sodium)

Cefotaxime sodium	per gram	IV/IM	J0698
Cefoxitin sodium	1 g	IV/IM	J0694
Ceftazidime	per 500 mg	IV/IM	J0713
Ceftizoxime sodium	per 500 mg	IV/IM	J0715
Ceftriaxone sodium	per 250 mg	IV/IM	J0696
Cefuroxime sodium, sterile	per 750 mg	IM/IV	J0697

Celestone phosphate (see
  Betamethasone sodium
  phosphate)

Celestone soluspan (see
  Betamethasone acetate
  and betamethasone
  sodium phosphate)

CellCept (see Mycophenolate mofetil)			
Cel-U-Jec (see Betamethasone sodium phosphate)			
Cenacort Forte (see Triamcinolone diacetate)			
Cenacort A-40 (see Triamcinolone acetonide)			
Cephalothin sodium	up to 1 g	IM/IV	J1890
Cephapirin sodium	up to 1 g	IV/IM	J0710
Ceredase (see Alglucerase)			
Cerezyme (see Imiglucerase)			
Cerubidine (see Daunorubicin HCl)			
Chealamide (see Endrate ethylenediamine-tetra-acetic acid)			
Chloramphenicol sodium succinate	up to 1 g	IV	J0720
Chlordiazepoxide HCl	up to 100 mg	IM/IV	J1990
Chloromycetin sodium succinate (see Chloramphenicol sodium succinate)			
Chloroprocaine HCl	per 30 ml	VAR	J2400
Chloroquine HCl	up to 250 mg	IM	J0390
Chlorothiazide sodium	per 500 mg	IV	J1205
Chlorpromazine HCl	up to 50 mg	IM/IV	J3230
Chlorpromazine HCl, oral	10 mg	ORAL	Q0171
	25 mg	ORAL	Q0172
Chlorprothixene	up to 50 mg	IM	J3080
Chorex-5 or -10 (see Chorionic gonadotropin)			

Chorignon (see Chorionic gonadotropin)			
Chorionic gonadotropin	per 1,000 USP U	IM	J0725
Choron 10 (see Chorionic gonadotropin)			
Cidofovir	375 mg	IV	J0740
Cilastatin sodium/ imipenem	per 250 mg	IV/IM	J0743
Cipro IV (see Ciprofloxacin)			
Ciprofloxacin	200 mg	IV	J0706
Cisplatin, powder or soln.	per 10 mg	IV	J9060
Cisplatin	50 mg	IV	J9062
Cladribine	per 1 mg	IV	J9065
Claforan (see Cefotaxime sodium)			
Clonidine hydrochloride	1 mg	EPI	J0735
Cobex (see Vitamin B-12 cyanocobalamin)			
Codeine phosphate	per 30 mg	IM/IV/SC	J0745
Codimal-A (see Brompheniramine maleate)			
Cogentin (see Benztropine mesylate)			
Colchicine	per 1 mg	IV	J0760
Colistimethate sodium	up to 150 mg	IM/IV	J0770
Coly-Mycin M (see Colistimethate sodium)			
Compa-Z (see Prochlorperazine)			
Compazine (see Prochlorperazine)			
Cophene-B (see Brompheniramine maleate)			

Copper contraceptive, intrauterine	—	OTH	J7300
Cordarone (see Amiodarone HCl)			
Corgonject-5 (see Chorionic gonadotropin)			
Corticorelin ovine triflutate	per dose	—	Q2005
Corticotropin	up to 40 U	IV/IM/SC	J0800
Cortisone acetate (see Cortisone)			
Cortisone	up to 50 mg	IM	J0810
Cortrosyn (see Cosyntropin)			
Cosmegen (see Dactinomycin)			
Cosyntropin	per 0.25 mg	IM/IV	J0835
Cotranzine (see Prochlorperazine)			
Cromolyn sodium, unit dose form	per 10 mg	INH	J7631
Crysticillin 300 A.S. or 600 A.S. (see Penicillin G procaine)			
Cyclophosphamide	100 mg	IV	J9070
	200 mg	IV	J9080
	500 mg	IV	J9090
	1.0 g	IV	J9091
	2.0 g	IV	J9092
Cyclophosphamide, lyophilized	100 mg	IV	J9093
	200 mg	IV	J9094
	500 mg	IV	J9095
	1.0 g	IV	J9096
	2.0 g	IV	J9097
Cyclophosphamide, oral	25 mg	ORAL	J8530

Cyclosporine, oral	25 mg	ORAL	J7515
	100 mg	ORAL	J7502
Cyclosporine, parenteral	250 mg	IV	J7516
Cytarabine	100 mg	SC/IV	J9100
	500 mg	SC/IV	J9110
Cytomegalovirus immune globulin intravenous (human)	per vial	IV	J0850
Cytostar-U (see Cytarabine)			
Cytovene (see Ganciclovir sodium)			
Cytoxan (see Cyclophosphamide; cyclophosphamide, lyophilized; and cyclophosphamide, oral)			

D

D-5-W, infusion	1,000 cc	IV	J7070
Dacarbazine	100 mg	IV	J9130
	200 mg	IV	J9140
Daclizumab, parenteral	25 mg	IV	J7513
Dactinomycin	0.5 mg	IV	J9120
Dalalone (see Dexamethasone sodium phosphate)			
Dalalone-LA (see Dexamethasone acetate)			
Dalteparin sodium	per 2,500 IU	SC	J1645
Daunorubicin citrate, liposomal formulation	10 mg	IV	J9151
Daunorubicin	10 mg	IV	J9150
Daunoxome (see Daunorubicin citrate)			

DDAVP (see
  Desmopressin acetate)

Decadron (see
  Dexamethasone sodium
  phosphate)

Decadron-LA (see
  Dexamethasone acetate)

Decadron Phosphate (see
  Dexamethasone sodium
  phosphate)

Deca-Durabolin (see
  Nandrolone decanoate)

Decaject (see
  Dexamethasone sodium
  phosphate)

Decaject-LA (see
  Dexamethasone acetate)

Decolone-50 or -100 (see
  Nandrolone decanoate)

De-Comberol (see
  Testosterone cypionate
  and estradiol cypionate)

Deferoxamine mesylate   500 mg   IM/SC/IV   J0895

Dehist (see
  Brompheniramine
  maleate)

Deladumone or
  Deladumone OB (see
  Testosterone enanthate
  and estradiol valerate)

Delatest (see Testosterone
  enanthate)

Delatestadiol (see
  Testosterone enanthate
  and estradiol valerate)

Delatestryl (see
  Testosterone enanthate)

Delestrogen (see Estradiol valerate)

Delta-Cortef (see Prednisolone, oral)

Demadex (see Torsemide)

Demerol HCl (see Meperidine HCl)

| Denileukin diftitox | 300 mcg | — | J9160 |

DepAndro 100 or 200 (see Testosterone cypionate)

DepAndrogyn (see Testosterone cypionate and estradiol cypionate)

DepGynogen (see Depo-estradiol cypionate)

DepMedalone 40 or 80 (see Methylprednisolone acetate)

| Depo-estradiol cypionate | up to 5 mg | IM | J1000 |

Depogen (see Depo-estradiol cypionate)

Depoject (see Methylprednisolone acetate)

Depo-Medrol (see Methylprednisolone acetate)

Depopred 40 or 80 (see Methylprednisolone acetate)

Depo-Provera (see Medroxyprogesterone acetate)

Depotest (see Testosterone cypionate)

Depo-Testadiol (see
  Testosterone cypionate
  and estradiol cypionate)

Depotestogen (see
  Testosterone cypionate
  and estradiol cypionate)

Depo-Testosterone (see
  Testosterone cypionate)

Desferal Mesylate (see
  Deferoxamine mesylate)

Desmopressin acetate	per 1 mcg	IV/SC	J2597

Dexacen-4 (see
  Dexamethasone sodium
  phosphate)

Dexacen LA-8 (see
  Dexamethasone acetate)

Dexamethasone, concentrated form	per mg	INH	J7637
Dexamethasone, unit form	per mg	INH	J7638
Dexamethasone acetate	per 8 mg	IM	J1095
Dexamethosone sodium phosphate	1 mg	IM/IV/OTH	J1100

Dexasone (see
  Dexamethasone sodium
  phosphate)

Dexasone LA (see
  Dexamethasone acetate)

Dexferrum (see Iron
  dextran)

Dexone (see
  Dexamethasone sodium
  phosphate)

Dexone LA (see
  Dexamethasone acetate)

Dexrazoxane hydrochloride	per 250 mg	IV	J1190
Dextran 40, infusion	500 ml	IV	J7100
Dextran 75, infusion	500 ml	IV	J7110

Dextrose 5%/normal saline	500 ml = 1 U	IV	J7042
Dextrose/water (5%)	500 ml = 1 U	IV	J7060
D.H.E. 45 (see Dihydroergotamine)			
Diamox (see Acetazolamide sodium)			
Diazepam	up to 5 mg	IM/IV	J3360
Diazoxide	up to 300 mg	IV	J1730
Dibent (see Dicyclomine HCl)			
Dicylomine HCl	up to 20 mg	IM	J0500
Didronel (see Etidronate disodium)			
Diethylstilbestrol diphosphate	250 mg	IV	J9165
Diflucan (see Fluconazole)			
Digoxin	up to 0.5 mg	IM/IV	J1160
Digoxin immune fab (ovine)	per vial	—	Q2006
Dihydrex (see Diphenhydramine HCl)			
Dihydroergotamine mesylate	per 1 mg	IM/IV	J1110
Dilantin (see Phenytoin sodium)			
Dilaudid (see Hydromorphone HCl)			
Dilocaine (see Lidocaine HCl)			
Dilomine (see Dicyclomine HCl)			
Dilor (see Dyphylline)			
Dimenhydrinate	up to 50 mg	IM/IV	J1240
Dimercaprol	per 100 mg	IM	J0470

Dimethyl sulfoxide (see
DMSO, Dimethyl-
sulfoxide)

Dinate (see
Dimenhydrinate)

Dioval or Dioval 40 or
Dioval XX (see
Estradiol valerate)

Diphenacen-50 (see
Diphenhydramine HCl)

Diphenhydramine HCl, injection	up to 50 mg	IV/IM	J1200
Diphenhydramine HCl, oral	50 mg	ORAL	Q0163
Dipyridamole	per 10 mg	IV	J1245

Disotate (see Endrate
ethylenediamine-tetra-
acetic acid)

Di-Spaz (see Dicyclomine
HCl)

Ditate-DS (see
Testosterone enanthate
and estradiol valerate)

Diural sodium (see
Chlorothiazide sodium)

D-Med 80 (see
Methylprednisolone
acetate)

DMSO, Dimethyl sulfoxide	50%, 50 ml	OTH	J1212
Dobutamine HCl	per 250 mg	IV	J1250

Dobutrex (see Dobutamine
HCl)

Docetaxel	20 mg	IV	J9170
Dolasetron mesylate, injection	10 mg	IV	J1260
Dolasetron mesylate, tablets	100 mg	ORAL	Q0180

Dolophine HCl (see Methadone HCl)			
Dommanate (see Dimenhydrinate)			
Dornase alpha, inhalation solution, unit dose form	per mg	INH	J7639
Doxercalciferol	1 mcg	IV	J1270
Doxil (see Doxorubicin HCl, lipid)			
Doxorubicin HCl	10 mg	IV	J9000
Doxorubicin HCl, all lipid	10 mg	IV	J9001
Dramamine (see Dimenhydrinate)			
Dramanate (see Dimenhydrinate)			
Dramilin (see Dimenhydrinate)			
Dramocen (see Dimenhydrinate)			
Dramoject (see Dimenhydrinate)			
Dronabinol, oral	2.5 mg	ORAL	Q0167
	5 mg	ORAL	Q0168
Droperidol	up to 5 mg	IM/IV	J1790
Droperidol and fentanyl citrate	up to 2 ml amp	IM/IV	J1810
Drug(s) administered through metered dose inhaler	—	INH	J3535
DTIC-Dome (see Dacarbazine)			
Dua-Gen LA (see Testosterone enanthate and estradiol valerate cypionate)			

Duoval PA (see
  Testosterone enanthate
  and estradiol valerate)

Durabolin (see Nandrolone
  phenpropionate)

Duraclon (see Clonidine
  HCl)

Dura-Estrin (see
  Depo-estradiol
  cypionate)

Duracillin A.S. (see
  Penicillin G procaine)

Duragen-10, -20, or -40
  (see Estradiol valerate)

Duralone-40 or -80 (see
  Methylprednisolone
  acetate)

Duralutin (see
  Hydroxyprogesterone
  caproate)

Duramorph (see Morphine
  sulfate)

Duratest-100 or -200 (see
  Testosterone cypionate)

Duratestrin (see
  Testosterone cypionate
  and estradiol cypionate)

Durathate 200 (see
  Testosterone enanthate)

Dymenate (see
  Dimenhydrinate)

Dyphylline	up to 500 mg	IM	J1180

E

Edetate calcium disodium	up to 1,000 mg	IV/SC/IM	J0600
Edetate disodium	per 150 mg	IV	J3520

Elavil (see Amitriptyline HCl)			
Ellence (see Epirubicin HCl)			
Elliots b solution	per ml	OTH	Q2002
Elspar (see Asparaginase)			
Emete-Con (see Benzquinamide)			
Eminase (see Anisteplase)			
Enbrel (see Etanercept)			
Endrate ethylenediamine-tetra-acetic acid (see Edetate disodium)			
Enovil (see Amitriptyline HCl)			
Enoxaparin sodium	10 mg	SC	J1650
Epinephrine, adrenalin	up to 1 ml amp	SC/IM	J0170
Epirubicin hydrochloride	50 mg	—	J9180
Epoprostenol	0.5 mg	IV	J1325
Eptifibatide, injection	5 mg	IM/IV	J1327
Ergonovine maleate	up to 0.2 mg	IM/IV	J1330
Erythromycin lactobionate	500 mg	IV	J1364
Estra-D (see Depo-estradiol cypionate)			
Estra-L 20 or 40 (see Estradiol valerate)			
Estra-Testrin (see Testosterone enanthate and estradiol valerate)			
Estradiol cypionate (see Depo-estradiol cypionate)			

Estradiol LA, or Estradiol LA-20, or Estradiol LA-40 (see Estradiol valerate)			
Estradiol valerate	up to 10 mg	IM	J1380
	up to 20 mg	IM	J1390
	up to 40 mg	IM	J0970
Estro-Cyp (see Depo-estradiol cypionate)			
Estrogen, conjugated	per 25 mg	IV/IM	J1410
Estroject LA (see Depo-estradiol cypionate)			
Estrone	per 1 mg	IM	J1435
Estrone 5 (see Estrone)			
Estrone aqueous (see Estrone)			
Estronol (see Estrone)			
Estronol-LA (see Depo-estradiol cypionate)			
Etanercept, injection	25 ml	IM/IV	J1438
Ethanolamine	100 mg	—	Q2007
Ethyol (see Amifostine)			
Etidronate disodium	per 300 mg	IV	J1436
Etopophos (see Etoposide)			
Etoposide	10 mg	IV	J9181
	100 mg	IV	J9182
Etoposide, oral	50 mg	ORAL	J8560
Everone (see Testosterone enanthate)			

F

Factor VIIa (coagulation factor, recombinant)	per mg	IV	Q0187
Factor VIII (anti-hemophilic factor, human)	per IU	IV	J7190
Factor VIII (anti-hemophilic factor, porcine)	per IU	IV	J7191
Factor VIII (anti-hemophilic factor, recombinant)	per IU	IV	J7192
Factor IX (anti-hemophilic factor, purified, non-recombinant)	per IU	IV	Q0160
Factor IX (anti-hemophilic factor, recombinant)	per IU	IV	Q0161
Factor IX, complex	per IU	IV	J7194
Factors, other hemophilia clotting	per IU	IV	J7196
Factrel (see Gonadorelin HCl)			
Feiba VH Immuno (see Factors, other hemophilia clotting)			
Fentanyl citrate	0.1 mg	IM/IV	J3010
Ferrlecit (see Sodium ferricgluconate complex in sucrose injection)			
Filgrastim (G-CSF)	300 mcg	SC/IV	J1440
	480 mcg	SC/IV	J1441
Flexoject (see Orphenadrine citrate)			
Flexon (see Orphenadrine citrate)			
Flolan (see Epoprostenol)			

Floxuridine	500 mg	IV	J9200
Fluconazole	200 mg	IV	J1450
Fludara (see Fludarabine phosphate)			
Fludarabine phosphate	50 mg	IV	J9185
Flunisolide inhalation solution, unit dose form	per mg	INH	J7641
Fluorouracil	500 mg	IV	J9190
Folex, or Folex PFS (see Methotrexate sodium)			
Follutein (see Chorionic gonadotropin)			
Fomepizole	1.5 mg	—	Q2008
Fomivirsen	1.65 mg	IO	J1452
Fortaz (see Ceftazidime)			
Foscarnet sodium	per 1,000 mg	IV	J1455
Foscavir (see Foscarnet sodium)			
Fosphenytoin	50 mg	—	Q2009
FUDR (see Floxuridine)			
Fungizone intravenous (see Amphotericin B)			
Furomide M.D. (see Furosemide)			
Furosemide	up to 20 mg	IM/IV	J1940

G

Gamastan (see Gamma globulin and immune globulin)

Gamma globulin	1cc	IM	J1460
	2cc	IM	J1470
	3cc	IM	J1480
	4cc	IM	J1490
	5cc	IM	J1500
	6cc	IM	J1510
	7cc	IM	J1520
	8cc	IM	J1530
	9cc	IM	J1540
	10cc	IM	J1550
	over 10cc	IM	J1560
Gammar (see Gamma globulin and immune globulin)			
Gammar-IV (see Immune globulin intravenous (human))			
Gamulin RH (see Rho(D) immune globulin)			
Ganciclovir, implant	4.5 mg	OTH	J7310
Ganciclovir sodium	500 mg	IV	J1570
Garamycin, gentamicin	up to 80 mg	IM/IV	J1580
Gatifloxacin	10 mg	IV	J1590
Gemcitabine HCl	200 mg	IV	J9201
Gemsar (see Gemcitabine HCl)			
Gemtuzumab ozogamicin	5 mg	IV	J9300
Gentamicin sulfate (see Garamycin, gentamicin)			
Gentran (see Dextran 40)			
Gentran 75 (see Dextran 75)			
Gesterol 50 (see Progesterone)			
Glatiramer acetate	per dose	—	Q2010
Glucagon HCl	per 1 mg	SC/IM/IV	J1610

Glukor (see Chorionic gonadotropin)			
Glycopyrrolate, concentrated form	per 1 mg	INH	J7642
Glycopyrrolate, unit dose form	per 1 mg	INH	J7643
Gold sodium thiomalate	up to 50 mg	IM	J1600
Gonadorelin HCl	per 100 mcg	SC/IV	J1620
Gonic (see Chorionic gonadotropin)			
Goserelin acetate implant	per 3.6 mg	SC	J9202
Granisetron HCl, injection	100 mcg	IV	J1626
Granisetron HCl, oral	1 mg	ORAL	Q0166
Gynogen LA-10, -20, or -40 (see Estradiol valerate)			

H

Haldol (see Haloperidol)			
Haloperidol	up to 5 mg	IM/IV	J1630
Haloperidol decanoate	per 50 mg	IM	J1631
Hectoral (see Doxercalciferol)			
Hemin	per 1 mg	—	Q2011
Hemofil M (see Factor VIII)			
Hemophilia clotting factors (e.g., anti-inhibitors)	per IU	IV	J7198
Hemophilia clotting factors, NOC	per IU	IV	J7199
Hepatitis B vaccine	5 mcg	IM	Q3018

Hep-Lock or Hep-Lock U/P (see Heparin sodium (heparin lock flush))			
Heparin sodium	1,000 U	IV/SC	J1644
Heparin sodium (heparin lock flush)	per 10 U	IV	J1642
Herceptin (see Trastuzumab)			
Hexadrol Phosphate (see Dexamethasone sodium phosphate)			
Histaject (see Brompheniramine maleate)			
Histerone 50 or 100 (see Testosterone suspension)			
Histrelin acetate	10 mg	—	Q2020
Hyalgan (see Sodium hyaluronate)			
Hyaluronidase	up to 150 U	SC/IV	J3470
Hyate:C (see Factor VIII (anti-hemophilic factor (porcine)))			
Hybolin improved (see Nandrolone phenpropionate)			
Hybolin decanoate (see Nandrolone decanoate)			
Hycamtin (see Topotecan)			
Hydralazine HCl	up to 20 mg	IV/IM	J0360
Hydrate (see Dimenhydrinate)			
Hydrocortisone acetate	up to 25 mg	IV/IM/SC	J1700
Hydrocortisone sodium phosphate	up to 50 mg	IV/IM/SC	J1710

Hydrocortisone succinate sodium	up to 100 mg	IV/IM/SC	J1720
Hydrocortone acetate (see Hyrocortisone acetate)			
Hydrocortone Phosphate (see Hydrocortisone sodium phosphate)			
Hydromorphone	up to 4 mg	SC/IM/IV	J1170
Hydroxyzine HCl	up to 25 mg	IM	J3410
Hydroxyzine pamoate	25 mg	ORAL	Q0177
	50 mg	ORAL	Q0178
Hylan G-F 20	16 mg	OTH	J7320
Hyoscyamine sulfate	up to 0.25 mg	SC/IM/IV	J1980
Hyperstat IV (see Diazoxide)			
Hyper-Tet (see Tetanus immune globulin, human)			
HypRho-D (see Rho(D) immune globulin)			
Hyrexin-50 (see Diphenhydramine HCl)			
Hyzine-50 (see Hydroxyzine HCl)			

I

Ibutilide fumarate	1 mg	IV	J1742
Idamycin (see Idarubicin HCl)			
Idarubicin HCl	5 mg	IV	J9211
Ifex (see Ifosfamide)			
Ifosfamide	1 g	IV	J9208
Ilotycin (see Erythromycin gluceptate)			
Imferon (see Iron dextran)			

Imiglucerase	per U	IV	J1785
Imipramine HCl	up to 25 mg	IM	J3270
Imitrex (see Sumatriptan succinate)			
Immune globulin	500 mg	IV	J1561
Immune globulin, anti-thymocyte globulin	250 mg	IV	J7504
Immune globulin, intravenous	1 g	IV	J1563
Immunosuppressive drug, not otherwise classified	—	—	J7599
Imuran (see Azathioprine)			
Inapsine (see Droperidol)			
Inderal (see Propranolol HCl)			
Infed (see Iron dextran)			
Infergen (see Interferon alfa-1)			
Infliximab, injection	10 mg	IM/IV	J1745
Innohep (see Tinzarparin)			
Innovar (see Droperidol with fentanyl citrate)			
Insulin	up to 100 U	SC	J1820
Insulin lispro	up to 50 U	SC	K0548
Intal (see Cromolyn sodium or Cromolyn sodium, compounded)			
Integrilin, injection (see Eptifibatide)			
Interferon			
alphacon-1, recombinant	1 mcg	SC	J9212
alfa-2A, recombinant	3 million U	SC/IM	J9213
alfa-2B, recombinant	1 million U	SC/IM	J9214
alfa-N3, (human leukocyte derived)	250,000 IU	IM	J9215

beta-1A	33 mcg	IM	J1825
beta-1B	0.25 mg	SC	J1830
gamma-1B	3 million U	SC	J9216
Intrauterine copper contraceptive (see Copper contraceptive, intrauterine)			
Ipratropium bromide, unit dose form	per mg	INH	J7644
Irinotecan	20 mg	IV	J9206
Iron dextran	50 mg	IV/IM	J1750
Iron sucrose	20 mg	IV	J1755
Irrigation solution for Tx of bladder calculi	per 50 ml	OTH	Q2004
Isocaine HCl (see Mepivacaine)			
Isoetharine HCl, concentrated form	per mg	INH	J7648
Isoetharine HCl, unit dose form	per mg	INH	J7649
Isoproterenol HCl, concentrated form	per mg	INH	J7658
Isoproterenol HCl, unit dose form	per mg	INH	J7659
Isuprel (see Isoproterenol HCl)			
Itraconazole	50 mg	IV	J1835

J

Jenamicin (see Garamycin, gentamicin)

K

Kabikinase (see Streptokinase)			
Kaleinate (see Calcium gluconate)			
Kanamycin sulfate	up to 75 mg	IM/IV	J1850
	up to 500 mg	IM/IV	J1840
Kantrex (see Kanamycin sulfate)			
Keflin (see Cephalothin sodium)			
Kefurox (see Cefuroxime sodium)			
Kefzol (see Cefazolin sodium)			
Kenaject-40 (see Triamcinolone acetonide)			
Kenalog-10 or -40 (see Triamcinolone acetonide)			
Kestrone 5 (see Estrone)			
Ketorolac tromethamine	per 15 mg	IM/IV	J1885
Key-Pred 25 or 50 (see Prednisolone acetate)			
Key-Pred-SP (see Prednisolone sodium phosphate)			
K-Flex (see Orphenadrine citrate)			
Klebcil (see Kanamycin sulfate)			
Koate-HP (see Factor VIII)			
Kogenate (see Factor VIII)			
Konakion (see Vitamin K, phytonadione, etc.)			

Konyne-80 (see Factor IX, complex)

Kutapressin	up to 2 ml	SC/IM	J1910

Kytril (see Granisetron HCl)

L

L.A.E. 20 (see Estradiol valerate)

Laetrile, amygdalin, vitamin B-17	—	—	J3570

Lanoxin (see Digoxin)

Largon (see Propiomazine HCl)

Lasix (see Furosemide)

L-Caine (see Lidocaine HCl)

Lepirudin	50 mg	—	Q2021
Leucovorin calcium	per 50 mg	IM/IV	J0640

Leukine (see Sargramostim (GM-CSF))

Leuprolide acetate	per 1 mg	IM	J9218
Leuprolide acetate, implant	65 mg	—	J9219
Leuprolide acetate (for depot suspension)	3.75 mg	IM	J1950
	7.5 mg	IM	J9217

Leustatin (see Cladribine)

Levabuterol HCl, concentrated form	0.5 mg	INH	J7618
Levabuterol HCl, unit dose form	0.5 mg	INH	J7619

Levaquin I.U. (see Levofloxacin)

Levocarnitine	per 1 g	IV	J1955

Levo-Dromoran (see Levorphanol tartrate)			
Levofloxacin	250 mg	IV	J1956
Levonorgestrel releasing intrauterine contraceptive	52 mg	OTH	J7302
Levorphanol tartrate	up to 2 mg	SC/IV	J1960
Levsin (see Hyoscyamine sulfate)			
Levulan Kerastick (see Aminolevulinic acid HCl)			
Librium (see Chlordiazepoxide HCl)			
Lidocaine HCl	50cc	VAR	J2000
Lidoject-1 or -2 (see Lidocaine HCl)			
Lincocin (see Lincomycin HCl)			
Lincomycin HCl	up to 300 mg	IV	J2010
Linezolid	200 mg	IV	J2020
Liquaemin sodium (see Heparin sodium)			
Lioresal (see Baclofen)			
LMD (10%) (see Dextran 40)			
Lorazepam	2 mg	IM/IV	J2060
Lovenox (see Enoxaparin sodium)			
Lufyllin (see Dyphylline)			
Luminal sodium (see Phenobarbital sodium)			
Lunelle (see Medroxyprogesterone acetate/estradiol cypionate)			

Lupron (see Leuprolide acetate)			
Lymphocyte immune globulin, anti-thymocyte globulin, equine	250 mg	IV	J7504
Lymphocyte immune globulin, anti-thymocyte globulin, rabbit	25 mg	IV	J7511
Lyophilized (see Cyclophosphamide, lyophilized)			

M

Magnesium sulfate	per 500 mg	—	J3475
Mannitol	25% in 50 ml	IV	J2150
Marmine (see Dimenhydrinate)			
Maxipime (see Cefepime hydrochloride)			
Mechlorethamine HCl (nitrogen mustard), HN2	10 mg	IV	J9230
Medralone 40 or 80 (see Methylprednisolone acetate)			
Medrol (see Methylprednisolone)			
Medroxyprogesterone acetate	100 mg	IM	J1050
	150 mg	IM	J1055
Medroxyprogesterone acetate/estradiol cypionate	5 mg/25mg	IM	J1056
Mefoxin (see Cefoxitin sodium)			
Melphalan HCl	50 mg	IV	J9245

Melphalan, oral	2 mg	ORAL	J8600
Menoject LA (see Testosterone cypionate and estradiol cypionate)			
Mepergan injection (see Meperidine and promethazine HCl)			
Meperidine HCl	per 100 mg	IM/IV/SC	J2175
Meperidine and promethazine HCl	up to 50 mg	IM/IV	J2180
Mephentermine sulfate	up to 30 mg	IM/IV	J3450
Mepivacaine HCl	per 10 ml	VAR	J0670
Mesna	200 mg	IV	J9209
Mesnex (see Mesna)			
Metaprel (see Metaproterenol sulfate)			
Metaproterenol sulfate, concentrated form	per 10 mg	INH	J7668
Metaproterenol sulfate, unit dose form	per 10 mg	INH	J7669
Metaraminol bitartrate	per 10 mg	IV/IM/SC	J0380
Metastron (see Strontium-89 chloride)			
Methadone HCl	up to 10 mg	IM/SC	J1230
Methergine (see Methylergonovine maleate)			
Methicillin sodium	up to 1 g	IM/IV	J2970
Methocarbamol	up to 10 ml	IV/IM	J2800
Methotrexate, oral	2.5 mg	ORAL	J8610
Methotrexate sodium	5 mg	IV/IM/IT/IA	J9250
	50 mg	IV/IM/IT/IA	J9260
Methotrexate LPF (see Methotrexate sodium)			
Methyldopa HCl	up to 250 mg	IV	J0210

Methylergonovine maleate	up to 0.2 mg	IM/IV	J2210
Methylprednisolone, oral	per 4 mg	ORAL	J7509
Methylprednisolone acetate	20 mg	IM	J1020
	40 mg	IM	J1030
	80 mg	IM	J1040
Methylprednisone sodium succinate	up to 40 mg	IM/IV	J2920
	up to 125 mg	IM/IV	J2930
Metoclopramide HCl	up to 10 mg	IV	J2765
Miacalcin (see Calcitonin-salmon)			
Midazolam HCl	per 1 mg	IM/IV	J2250
Milrinone lactate	5 ml	IV	J2260
Mirena (see Levonorgestrel releasing intrauterine contraceptive)			
Mithracin (see Plicamycin)			
Mitomycin	5 mg	IV	J9280
	20 mg	IV	J9290
	40 mg	IV	J9291
Mitoxantrone HCl	per 5 mg	IV	J9293
Monocid (see Cefonicid sodium)			
Monoclate-P (see Factor VIII)			
Monoclonal antibodies, parenteral	5 mg	IV	J7505
Mononine (see Factor IX, purified, non-recombinant)			
Morphine sulfate	up to 10 mg	IM/IV/SC	J2270
	100 mg	IM/IV/SC	J2271
Morphine sulfate, preservative free, sterile solution	per 10 mg	SC/IM/IV	J2275

M-Prednisol-40 or -80
(see Methylprednisolone
acetate)

Mucomyst (see
Acetylcysteine or
Acetylcysteine,
compounded)

Mucosol (see
Acetylcysteine)

Muromonab-CD3	5 mg	IV	J7505

Muse (see Alprostadil)

Mustargen (see
Mechlorethamine HCl)

Mutamycin (see
Mitomycin)

Mycophenolate mofetil	250 mg	ORAL	J7517

Myleran (see Busulfan)

Mylotarg (see
Gemtuzumab
ozogamicin)

Myobloc (see Botulinum
toxin type B)

Myochrysine (see Gold
sodium thiomalate)

Myolin (see Orphenadrine
citrate)

N

Nalbuphine HCl	per 10 mg	IM/IV/SC	J2300
Naloxone HCl	per 1 mg	IM/IV/SC	J2310
Nandrobolic LA (see Nandrolone decanoate)			
Nandrolone decanoate	up to 50 mg	IM	J2320
	up to 100 mg	IM	J2321
	up to 200 mg	IM	J2322

Narcan (see Naloxone HCl)

Naropin (see Ropivacaine
   HCl)

Nasahist B (see
   Brompheniramine
   maleate)

Nasal vaccine inhalation	—	INH	J3530

Navane (see Thiothixene)

Navelbine (see Vinorelbine
   tartrate)

ND Stat (see
   Brompheniramine
   maleate)

Nebcin (see Tobramycin
   sulfate)

NebuPent (see
   Pentamidine isethionate)

Nembutal sodium solution
   (see Pentobarbital
   sodium)

Neocyten (see
   Orphenadrine citrate)

Neo-Durabolic (see
   Nandrolone decanoate)

Neoquess (see
   Dicyclomine HCl)

Neosar (see
   Cyclophosphamide)

Neostigmine methylsulfate	up to 0.5 mg	IM/IV/SC	J2710

Neo-Synephrine (see
   Phenylephrine HCl)

Nervocaine 1% or 2%
   (see Lidocaine HCl)

Nesacaine or
   Nesacaine-MPF (see
   Chloroprocaine HCl)

Neumega (see Oprelvekin)

Neupogen (see Filgrastim (G-CSF))

Neutrexin (see Trimetrexate glucuronate)

Nipent (see Pentostatin)

Nordryl (see Diphenhydramine HCl)

Norflex (see Orphenadrine citrate)

Norzine (see Thiethylperazine maleate)

Not otherwise classified drugs	—	—	J3490
Not otherwise classified drugs, other than INH administered through DME	—	—	J7799
Not otherwise classified drugs	—	INH admin thru DME	J7699
Not otherwise classified drugs, anti-neoplastic	—	—	J9999
Not otherwise classified drugs, chemothera-peutic	—	ORAL	J8999
Not otherwise classified drugs, immunosup-pressive	—	—	J7599
Not otherwise classified drugs, non-chemothera-peutic	—	ORAL	J8499

Novantrone (see Mitoxantrone HCl)

Novo Seven (see Factor VIIa)

NPH (see Insulin)

Nubain (see Nalbuphine
HCl)

Nulicaine (see Lidocaine
HCl)

Numorphan or Numorphan
H.P. (see Oxymorphone
HCl)

O

Octreotide acetate, injection	1 mg	IM/IV	J2352
Oculinum (see Botulinum toxin type A)			
O-Flex (see Orphenadrine citrate)			
Omnipen-N (see Ampicillin)			
Oncaspar (see Pegaspargase)			
Oncovin (see Vincristine sulfate)			
Ondansetron HCl	1 mg	IV	J2405
Ondansetron HCl, oral	8 mg	ORAL	Q0179
Oprelvekin	5 mg	SC	J2355
Oraminic II (see Brompheniramine maleate)			
Ormazine (see Chlorpromazine HCl)			
Orphenadrine citrate	up to 60 mg	IV/IM	J2360
Orphenate (see Orphenadrine citrate)			
Or-Tyl (see Dicyclomine)			
Oxacillin sodium	up to 250 mg	IM/IV	J2700

Oxymorphone HCl	up to 1 mg	IV/SC/IM	J2410
Oxytetracycline HCl	up to 50 mg	IM	J2460
Oxytocin	up to 10 U	IV/IM	J2590

P

Paclitaxel	30 mg	IV	J9265
Pamidronate disodium	per 30 mg	IV	J2430
Papaverine HCl	up to 60 mg	IV/IM	J2440
Paragard T 380 A (see Copper contraceptive, intrauterine)			
Paraplatin (see Carboplatin)			
Paricalcitol, injection	5 mcg	IV/IM	J2500
Pegademase bovine	25 IU	—	Q2012
Pegaspargase	single dose vial	IM/IV	J9266
Penicillin G benzathine	up to 600,000U	IM	J0560
	up to 1,200,000U	IM	J0570
	up to 2,400,000U	IM	J0580
Penicillin G benzathine & penicillin G procaine	up to 600,000U	IM	J0530
	up to 1,200,000U	IM	J0540
	up to 2,400,000U	IM	J0550
Penicillin G potassium	up to 600,000U	IM/IV	J2540
Penicillin G procaine, aqueous	up to 600,000U	IM/IV	J2510
Pentamidine isethionate	per 300 mg	INH	J2545
Pentastarch, 10%	per 100 ml	—	Q2013
Pentazocine HCl	up to 30 mg	IM/SC/IV	J3070
Pentobarbital sodium	per 50 mg	IM/IV/OTH	J2515
Pentostatin	per 10 mg	IV	J9268
Permapen (see Penicillin G benzathine)			
Perphenazine, injection	up to 5 mg	IM/IV	J3310

Perphenazine, tablets	4 mg	ORAL	Q0175
	8 mg	ORAL	Q0176
Persantine IV (see Dipyridamole)			
Pfizerpen (see Penicillin G potassium)			
Pfizerpen AS (see Penicillin G procaine)			
Phenazine 25 or 50 (see Promethazine HCl)			
Phenergan (see Promethazine HCl)			
Phenobarbital sodium	up to 120 mg	IM/IV	J2560
Phentolamine mesylate	up to 5 mg	IM/IV	J2760
Phenylephrine HCl	up to 1 ml	SC/IM/IV	J2370
Phenytoin sodium	per 50 mg	IM/IV	J1165
Photofrin (see Porfimer sodium)			
Phytonadione (Vitamin K)	per 1 mg	IM/SC/IV	J3430
Piperacillin sodium/Tazobactam sodium, injection	1.125 g	IV	J2543
Pitocin (see Oxytocin)			
Plas + SD (see Plasma, pooled multiple donor)			
Plasma, cryoprecipitate reduced	each U	—	P9044
Plasma, pooled multiple donor, frozen	each U	IV	P9023
Platinol or Platinol AQ (see Cisplatin)			
Plicamycin	2,500 mcg	IV	J9270
Polocaine (see Mepivacaine)			
Polycillin-N (see Ampicillin)			

Porfimer sodium	75 mg	IV	J9600
Potassium chloride	per 2 mEq	IV	J3480
Pralidoxime chloride	up to 1 g	IV/IM/SC	J2730
Predalone-50 (see Prednisolone acetate)			
Predcor-25 or -50 (see Prednisolone acetate)			
Predicort-50 (see Prednisolone acetate)			
Prednisone	per 5 mg	ORAL	J7506
Prednisolone, oral	per 5 mg	ORAL	J7510
Prednisolone acetate	up to 1 ml	IM	J2650
Predoject-50 (see Prednisolone acetate)			
Pregnyl (see Chorionic gonadotropin)			
Premarin Intravenous (see Estrogen, conjugated)			
Prescription, chemotherapeutic, NOS	—	ORAL	J8999
Prescription, nonchemotherapeutic, NOS	—	ORAL	J8499
Primacor (see Milrinone lactate)			
Primaxin IM or IV (see Cilastatin sodium, imipenem)			
Priscoline HCl (see Tolazoline HCl)			
Pro-Depo (see Hydroxyprogesterone caproate)			
Procainamide HCl	up to 1 g	IM/IV	J2690
Prochlorperazine	up to 10 mg	IM/IV	J0780

Prochlorperazine maleate, oral	5 mg	ORAL	Q0164
	10 mg	ORAL	Q0165
Profasi HP (see Chorionic gonadotropin)			
Profilnine Heat-Treated (see Factor IX)			
Progestaject (see Progesterone)			
Prograf (see Tacrolimus, oral or parenteral)			
Prokine (see Sargramostim (GM-CSF))			
Prolastin (see Alpha 1 -proteinase inhibitor, human)			
Proleukin (see Aldesleukin)			
Prolixin decanoate (see Fluphenazine decanoate)			
Promazine HCl	up to 25 mg	IM	J2950
Promethazine HCl, injection	up to 50 mg	IM/IV	J2550
Promethazine HCl, oral	12.5 mg	ORAL	Q0169
	25 mg	ORAL	Q0170
Pronestyl (see Procainamide HCl)			
Proplex T or SX-T (see Factor IX)			
Propranolol HCl	up to 1 mg	IV	J1800
Prorex-25 or -50 (see Promethazine HCl)			
Prostaphlin (see Procainamide HCl)			
Prostigmin (see Neostigmine methylsulfate)			
Protamine sulfate	per 10 mg	IV	J2720

Protirelin	per 250 mcg	IV	J2725
Prothazine (see Promethazine HCl)			
Protopam chloride (see Pralidoxime chloride)			
Proventil (see Albuterol sulfate, compounded)			
Prozine-50 (see Promazine HCl)			
Pulminicort respules (see Budesonide)			

Q

Quelicin (see Succinylcholine chloride)			
Quinupristin/dalfopristin	500 mg (150/350)	IV	J2770

R

Ranitidine HCl, injection	25 mg	IV/IM	J2780
Rapamune (see Sirolimus)			
Recombinant (see Factor VIII)			
Redisol (see Vitamin B-12 cyanocobalamin)			
Regitine (see Phentolamine mesylate)			
Reglan (see Metoclopramide HCl)			
Regular (see Insulin)			
Relefact TRH (see Protirelin)			
Remicade (see Infliximab, injection)			
Reo Pro (see Abciximab)			

Rep-Pred 40 or 80 (see Methylprednisolone acetate)			
RespiGam (see Respiratory syncytial virus)			
Respiratory syncytial virus immuneglobulin	50mg	IV	J1565
Retavase (see Reteplase)			
Reteplase	18.8 mg	IV	J2993
Retrovir (see Zidovudine)			
Rheomacrodex (see Dextran 40)			
Rhesonativ (see Rho(D) immune globulin, human)			
Rheumatrex Dose Pack (see Methotrexate, oral)			
Rho(D) immune globulin, human	1 dose pkg	IM	J2790
Rho(D) immune globulin, human, solvent detergent	100 IU	IV	J2792
RhoGAM (see Rho(D) immune globulin, human)			
Ringer's lactate infusion	up to 1,000 cc	IV	J7120
Rituxan (see Rituximab)			
Rituximab	100 mg	IU	J9310
Robaxin (see Methocarbamol)			
Rocephin (see Ceftriaxone sodium)			
Roferon-A (see Interferon alfa-2A, recombinant)			
Ropivacaine HCl	1 mg	—	J2795

Rubex (see Doxorubicin HCl)

Rubramin PC (see Vitamin B-12 cyanocobalamin)

S

Saline solution, 5% dextrose	500 ml	IV	J7042
Saline solution, normal infusion	250 cc	IV	J7050
	1,000 cc	IV	J7030
Saline solution, sterile	500 ml = 1 U	IV/OTH	J7040
Saline solution or water, sterile	up to 5 cc	IV/OTH	J7051
Sandimmune (see Cyclosporine)			
Sandoglobulin (see Immune globulin intravenous (human))			
Sandostatin Lar Depot (see Octreotide)			
Sargramostim (GM-CSF)	50 mcg	IV	J2820
Secobarbital sodium	up to 250 mg	IM/IV	J2860
Seconal (see Secobarbital sodium)			
Selestoject (see Betamethasone sodium phosphate)			
Sermorelin acetate	0.5 mg	—	Q2014
Sinusol-B (see Brompheniramine maleate)			
Sirolimus	1 mg	ORAL	J7520
Sodium chloride 0.9%	per 2 ml	IV	J2912

Sodium ferricgluconate in sucrose	62.5 mg	—	J2915
Sodium hyaluronate	5 mg	OTH	J7316
Solganal (see Aurothioglucose)			
Solu-Cortef (see Hydrocortisone sodium phosphate (J1710))			
Solu-Medrol (see Methylprednisolone sodium succinate)			
Solurex (see Dexamethasone sodium phosphate)			
Solurex LA (see Dexamethasone acetate)			
Somatrem	1 mg	—	J2940
Somatropin	1 mg	—	J2941
Sparine (see Promazine HCl)			
Spasmoject (see Dicyclomine HCl)			
Spectinomycin HCl	up to 2 g	IM	J3320
Sporanox (see Itraconazole)			
Staphcillin (see Methicillin sodium)			
Stilphostrol (see Diethylstilbestrol diphosphate)			
Streptase (see Streptokinase)			
Streptokinase	per 250,000 IU	IV	J2995
Streptomycin	up to 1 g	IM	J3000
Streptomycin sulfate (see Streptomycin)			
Streptozocin	1 g	IV	J9320

Strontium-89 chloride	per 10 ml	IV	J3005
Sublimaze (see Fentanyl citrate)			
Succinylcholine chloride	up to 20 mg	IV/IM	J0330
Sumatriptan succinate	6 mg	SC	J3030
Supartz (see Sodium hyaluronate)			
Surostrin (see Succinycholine chloride)			
Sus-Phrine (see Adrenalin, epinephrine)			
Synercid (see Quinupristan/dalfopristin)			
Synkavite (see Vitamin K, phytonadione, etc.)			
Syntocionon (see Oxytocin)			
Synvisc (see Hylan G-F 20)			
Sytobex (see Vitamin B-12 cyanocobalamin)			

T

Tacrolimus, oral	per 1 mg	ORAL	J7507
	per 5 mg	ORAL	J7508
Tacrolimus, parenteral	5mg	—	J7515
Talwin (see Pentazocine HCl)			
Taractan (see Chlorprothixene)			
Taxol (see Paclitaxel)			
Taxotere (see Docetaxel)			
Tazidime (see Ceftazidime)			
Technetium Tc sestamibi	per dose	—	A9500

TEEV (see Testosterone enanthate and Estradiol valerate)			
Temozolmide	5 mg	ORAL	J8700
Tenecteplase	50 mg	—	J3100
Teniposide	50 mg	—	Q2017
Tequin (see Gatifloxin)			
Terbutaline sulfate	up to 1 mg	SC/IV	J3105
Terbutaline sulfate, concentrated form	per 1 mg	INH	J7680
Terbutaline sulfate, unit dose form	per 1 mg	INH	J7681
Terramycin IM (see Oxytetracycline HCl)			
Testa-C (see Testosterone cypionate)			
Testadiate (see Testosterone enanthate and Estradiol valerate)			
Testadiate-Depo (see Testosterone cypionate)			
Testaject-LA (see Testosterone cypionate)			
Testaqua (see Testosterone suspension)			
Test-Estro Cypionates or Test-Estro-C (see Testosterone cypionate and Estradiol cypionate)			
Testex (see Testosterone propionate)			
Testoject-50 (see Testosterone suspension)			
Testoject-LA (see Testosterone cypionate)			

Testone LA 100 or 200 (see Testosterone enanthate)			
Testosterone aqueous (see Testosterone suspension)			
Testosterone cypionate	up to 100 mg	IM	J1070
	1 cc, 200 mg	IM	J1080
Testosterone cypionate & estradiol cypionate	up to 1 ml	IM	J1060
Testosterone enanthate	up to 100 mg	IM	J3120
	up to 200 mg	IM	J3130
Testosterone enanthate & estradiol valerate	up to 1 cc	IM	J0900
Testosterone propionate	up to 100 mg	IM	J3150
Testosterone suspension	up to 50 mg	IM	J3140
Testradiol 90/4 (see Testosterone enanthate and Estradiol valerate)			
Testrin PA (see Testosterone enanthate)			
Tetanus immune globulin, human	up to 250 U	IM	J1670
Tetracycline	up to 250 mg	IM/IV	J0120
Thallous chloride Tl 201	per mci	—	A9505
Theelin Aqueous (see Estrone)			
Theophylline	per 40 mg	IV	J2810
TheraCys (see BCG live)			
Thiethylperazine maleate, injection	up to 10 mg	IM	J3280
Thiethylperazine maleate, oral	10 mg	ORAL	Q0174
Thiotepa	15 mg	IV	J9340
Thorazine (see Chlorpromazine HCl)			

Thymoglobulin (see Immune globulin, anti-thymocyte)			
Thypinone (see Protirelin)			
Thyrogen (see Thyrotropin alfa)			
Thyrotropin alfa, injection	0.9 mg	IM/SC	J3240
Tice BCG (see BCG live)			
Ticon (see Trimethobenzamide HCl)			
Tigan (see Trimethobenzamide HCl)			
Tiject-20 (see Trimethobenzamide HCl)			
Tinzarparin	1,000 IU	SC	J1655
Tirofiban hydrochloride, injection	12.5 mg	IM/IV	J3245
TNKase (see Tenecteplase)			
Tobi (see Tobramycin, inhalation solution)			
Tobramycin, inhalation solution	300 mg	INH	J7682
Tobramycin sulfate	up to 80 mg	IM/IV	J3260
Tofranil (see Imipramine HCl)			
Tolazoline HCl	up to 25 mg	IV	J2670
Topotecan	4 mg	IV	J9350
Toradol (see Ketorolac tromethamine)			
Torecan (see Thiethylperazine maleate)			
Tornalate (see Bitolterol mesylate)			
Torsemide	10 mg/ml	IV	J3265

Totacillin-N (see Ampicillin)			
Trastuzumab	10 mg	IV	J9355
Tri-Kort (see Triamcinolone acetonide)			
Triam-A (see Triamcinolone acetonide)			
Triamcinolone, concentrated form	per 1 mg	INH	J7683
Triamcinolone, unit form	per 1 mg	INH	J7684
Triamcinolone acetonide	per 10 mg	IM	J3301
Triamcinolone diacetate	per 5 mg	IM	J3302
Triamcinolone hexacetonide	per 5 mg	VAR	J3303
Triflupromazine HCl	up to 20 mg	IM/IV	J3400
Trilafon (see Perphenazine)			
Trilog (see Triamcinolone acetonide)			
Trilone (see Triamcinolone diacetate)			
Trimethobenzamide HCl, injection	up to 200 mg	IM	J3250
Trimethobenzamide HCl, oral	250 mg	ORAL	Q0173
Trimetrexate glucoronate	per 25 mg	IV	J3305
Trisenox (see Arsenic trioxide)			
Trobicin (see Spectinomycin HCl)			
Trovan (see Alatrofloxacin mesylate)			

U

Ultrazine-10 (see Prochlorperazine)			

Unasyn (see Ampicillin sodium/sulbactam sodium)			
Unclassified drugs (see also Not elsewhere classified)	—	—	J3490
Unspecified oral antiemetic	—	—	Q0181
Urea	up to 40 g	IV	J3350
Ureaphil (see Urea)			
Urecholine (see Bethanechol chloride)			
Urofollitropin	75 IU	—	Q2018
Urokinase	5,000 IU vial	IV	J3364
	250,000 IU vial	IV	J3365

V

V-Gan 25 or 50 (see Promethazine HCl)			
Valergen 10, 20, or 40 (see Estradiol valerate)			
Valertest No. 1 or No. 2 (see Testosterone enanthate and Estradiol valerate)			
Valium (see Diazepam)			
Valrubicin, intravesical	200 mg	OTH	J9357
Valstar (see Valrubicin)			
Vancocin (see Vancomycin HCl)			
Vancoled (see Vancomycin HCl)			
Vancomycin HCl	up to 500 mg	IV/IM	J3370
Vasoxyl (see Methoxamine HCl)			

Velban (see Vinblastine
sulfate)

Velsar (see Vinblastine
sulfate)

Venofer (see Iron sucrose)

Ventolin (see Albuterol
sulfate)

VePesid (see Etoposide
and Etoposide, oral)

Versed (see Midazolam
HCl)

Verteporfin	15 mg	IV	J3395

Vesprin (see
Triflupromazine HCl)

Viadur (see Leuprolide
acetate implant)

Vinblastine sulfate	1 mg	IV	J9360

Vincasar PFS (see
Vincristine sulfate)

Vincristine sulfate	1 mg	IV	J9370
	2 mg	IV	J9375
	5 mg	IV	J9380
Vinorelbine tartrate	per 10 mg	IV	J9390

Vistaject-25 (see
Hydroxyzine HCl)

Vistaril (see Hydroxyzine
HCl)

Vistide (see Cidofovir)

Visudyne (see Verteporfin)

Vitamin B-12 cyanocobalamin	up to 1,000 mcg	IM/SC	J3420
Vitamin K, phytonadione	per 1 mg	IM/SC/IV	J3430
Von Willebrand factor complex, human	per IU	IV	Q2022

W

Wehamine (see
  Dimenhydrinate)

Wehdryl (see
  Diphenhydramine HCl)

Wellcovorin (see
  Leucovorin calcium)

Win Rho SD (see Rho(D)
  immuneglobulin,
  human, solvent
  detergent)

Wyamine sulfate (see
  Mephentermine sulfate)

Wycillin (see Penicillin G
  procaine)

Wydase (see
  Hyaluronidase)

X

Xeloda (see Capecitabine)

Xopenex (see Albuterol)

Xylocaine HCl (see
  Lidocaine HCl)

Z

Zanosar (see Streptozocin)

Zantac (see Ranitidine
  HCl)

Zemplar (see Paricalcitol)

Zenapax (see Daclizumab)

Zetran (see Diazepam)

Zidovudine	10 mg	IV	J3485

Zinacef (see Cefuroxime
  sodium)

Zithromax (see
  Azithromycin dihydrate)

Zithromax I.V. (see
  Azithromycin, injection)

Zofran (see Ondansetron
  HCl)

Zoladex (see Goserelin
  acetate implant)

Zolicef (see Cefazolin
  sodium)

Zosyn (see Piperacillin)

Zyvox (see Linezoid)

INDEX

A

INDEX

B

C

D

E

F

Filter—*continued*

G

H

L

M

N

O

P

Q

R

S

T

U

X

Z